Chemical
Carcinogenesis

NATO ADVANCED STUDY INSTITUTES SERIES

A series of edited volumes comprising multifaceted studies of contemporary scientific issues by some of the best scientific minds in the world, assembled in cooperation with NATO Scientific Affairs Division.

Series A: Life Sciences

Recent Volumes in this Series

Volume 43 — Advanced Topics on Radiosensitizers of Hypoxic Cells
edited by A. Breccia, C. Rimondi, and G. E. Adams

Volume 44 — Cell Regulation by Intracellular Signals
edited by Stéphane Swillens and Jacques E. Dumont

Volume 45 — Structural Molecular Biology: Methods and Applications
edited by David B. Davies, Wolfram Saenger, and Steven S. Danyluk

Volume 46 — Post-Harvest Physiology and Crop Preservation
edited by Morris Lieberman

Volume 47 — Targeting of Drugs
edited by Gregory Gregoriadis, Judith Senior, and André Trouet

Volume 48 — Neurotransmitter Interaction and Compartmentation
edited by H. F. Bradford

Volume 49 — Biological Effects and Dosimetry of Nonionizing Radiation
edited by Martino Grandolfo, Sol M. Michaelson, and Alessandro Rindi

Volume 50 — Somatic Cell Genetics
edited by C. Thomas Caskey and D. Christopher Robbins

Volume 51 — Factors in Formation and Regression of the Atherosclerotic Plaque
edited by Gustav R. V. Born, Alberico L. Catapano, and
Rodolfo Paoletti

Volume 52 — Chemical Carcinogenesis
edited by Claudio Nicolini

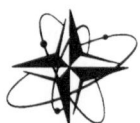

This series is published by an international board of publishers in conjunction with NATO Scientific Affairs Division

A Life Sciences	Plenum Publishing Corporation
B Physics	London and New York
C Mathematical and Physical Sciences	D. Reidel Publishing Company Dordrecht, The Netherlands and Hingham, Massachusetts, USA
D Behavioral and Social Sciences	Martinus Nijhoff Publishers The Hague, The Netherlands
E Applied Sciences	

Chemical Carcinogenesis

Edited by
Claudio Nicolini
Temple University Health Sciences Center
Philadelphia, Pennsylvania
and National Research Council
Genoa, Italy

PLENUM PRESS • NEW YORK AND LONDON
Published in cooperation with NATO Scientific Affairs Division

Library of Congress Cataloging in Publication Data

Main entry under title:

Chemical carcinogenesis.

(NATO advanced study institutes series. Series A, Life sciences; v. 52)
"Proceedings of a NATO Advanced Study Institute, which was the second course of
the International School of Pure and Applied Biostructure, held October 18-30, 1981, at
the Ettore Majorana Center for Scientific Culture, Erice, Italy" — Verso of t.p.
  Includes bibliographical references and indexes.
  1. Carcinogenesis — Congresses. 2. Carcinogen — Congresses. I. Nicolini, Claudio
A. II. Series. [DNLM: 1. Carcinogens — Congresses. 2. Neoplasms — Chemically induced
— Congresses. QZ 202 I59 1981c]
RC268.5.C48 1982   616.99'4071   82-13140
ISBN-13: 978-1-4684-4336-3   e-ISBN-13: 978-1-4684-4334-9
DOI: 10.1007/978-1-4684-4334-9

Dedicated to my Mother and Father

Proceedings of a NATO Advanced Study Institute, which was the
second course of the International School of Pure and Applied
Biostructure, held October 18-30, 1981, at the Ettore Majorana
Center for Scientific Culture, Erice, Italy

© 1982 Plenum Press, New York
Softcover reprint of the hardcover 1st edition   1982
A Division of Plenum Publishing Corporation
233 Spring Street, New York, N.Y. 10013

PREFACE

During October 18-30, 1981, the second course of the International
School of Pure and Applied Biostructure, a NATO Advanced Study
Institute, was held at the Ettore Majorana Center for Scientific
Culture in Erice, Italy, co-sponsored by the International Union
Against Cancer, the Italian League Against Cancer, the Italian
Ministry of Public Education, the Italian Ministry of Scientific
and Technological Research, the North Atlantic Treaty Organization,
the Italian National Research Council, the Sicilian Regional
Government and two pharmaceutical Companies (Zambeletti and
Farmitalia). The subject of the course was "Chemical Carcino-
genesis" with participants selected world-wide from 18 different
countries.

It is now eminently clear that the bulk of human cancers are
related to one of several types of environmental exposure. Of the
environmental hazards, chemicals are among the best characterized
carcinogens. However, how chemicals induce cancer is still poorly
understood. Because of the magnitude of the problem and the obvious need for a much more critical scientific analysis of the
process by which cancer is induced (carcinogenesis), it was highly
desirable to expose a greater number of scientists with varying
background to some of the latest thinking in chemical carcinogenesis. The course had this as its major objective and the resulting book does reflect it.

The participants were exposed to a critical evaluation of a current
knowledge about chemical and how this might induce cancer and to
some of the key problems that remain as stumbling blocks to our
eventual understanding of this important biological and medical
problem. Through the media of formal and informal lectures, work-
shops, symposia and informal discussions, a select group of interested young and senior scientists were acquainted with many of the
aspects of cancer development with chemicals.

The conduction of the course (a joint effort with Professor
E. Farber) was a little bit different than the conventional one
in that it made a sharp distinction between agents and processes.

We think this is terribly important since carcinogenesis is often erroneously equated with carcinogens. If we are ever to understand cancer induction, we must begin to understand the processes in terms far broader than in terms of the agents.

This book is the result of this Advanced Study Institute and is the third of a series, begun with "Chromatin Structure and Function" (1979, Vol. A21 & B) and continued with "Cell Growth" (1982, Vol. A38), edited by myself and published by Plenum within the NATO ASI Life Science Series. It aims to present a structured and interdisciplinary view of the current knowledge on chemical-macromolecules interaction, up to the possible molecular and cellular mechanisms leading to cancer initiation and promotion.

For completeness, I have included a chapter by T. Brinkley, who lectured at my previous course on "Cell Growth", on the emerging and critical role of the cytoskeleton in controlling neoplastic cell transformation, as induced by virus or chemicals. I wish to express my gratitude to Emanuel Farber for his active co-leadership in the conduction of the course at Erice, to Silvio Parodi for his invaluable and critical cooperation prior and during the Institute, and to Donatella Ugolini for her excellent organizational assistance. A final thanks to Julia Nicolini for her brilliant editorial assistance in the preparation of this volume.

                                        Claudio Nicolini

CONTENTS

SECTION I: CHEMICALS AS CARCINOGENS

SECTION II: DNA ADDUCTS

SECTION I

CHEMICALS AS CARCINOGENS

CHEMICAL CARCINOGENESIS BY POLYCYCLIC AROMATIC HYDROCARBONS

Franz Oesch

Department of Toxicology
Institute of Pharmacology and Toxicology
University of Mainz
D-6500 Mainz, FRG

INTRODUCTION

The realization that for a vast number of toxic effects, not the given compound itself was responsible but rather a metabolite that was produced from the compound, brought about an enormous step forward in chemical carcinogenesis and in toxicology in general (1-15). In chemical mutagenesis and in chemical carcinogenesis very often coumpounds, which by themselves are chemically inert, will produce mutagenic and carcinogenic effects. A prime example of this is the polycyclic aromatic hydrocarbons, which consisting of condensed aromatic rings are chemically inert, yet do produce mutagenic and carcinogenic effects. During the last 10 to 20 years researchers have started to realize that this is because they are metabolized to electrophilic metabolites which chemically react and combine with nucleophilic sites in the tissue (1-15). These nucleophilic sites include nitrogen atoms, sulphur atoms, and oxygen atoms in nucleic acids, in proteins and in carbohydrates, e.g. in carbohydrates which are parts of cellular membranes. This brings about two levels of control, the first determined by the chemical properties of the reactive metabolite, the second determined by the enzymic control of its concentration.

RELATIONSHIPS BETWEEN CHEMICAL PROPERTIES OF REACTIVE METABO-LITES AND TOXIC EFFECTS

Fig. 1 shows a study on the congeners of benzene oxide which is derived from the most simple aromatic compound, benzene. This

F. OESCH

Compound No.	Structure	TA 98 per µmole	TA 98 per dose [col/µg]	TA 100 per µmole	TA 100 per dose [col/µg]	TA 1535 per µmole	TA 1535 per dose [col/µg]	TA 1537 per µmole	TA 1537 per dose [col/µg]
1)	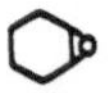	< 0.6	27/3300	41	980/3300	39	925/3300	< 0.3	6/3300
2)	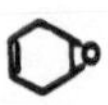	< 0.6	27/3400	43	1420/3400	48	1325/3400	< 0.3	12/3400
3)	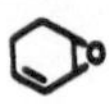	< 0.6	20/3350	115	1300/3350	58	730/3350	< 0.3	10/3350
4)	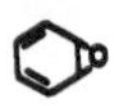	< 0.9	13/2000	< 2	78/2000	< 0.9	22/2000	< 0.5	10/2000
		< 1	21/1600	< 2	94/1600	< 1	25/1600	< 0.6	5/1600
5)	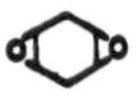 cis/trans	< 0.3	27/8000	5	362/8000	7	338/8000	< 0.2	7/8000
6)	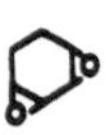 cis/trans	< 0.3	20/8000	8	390/8000	9	343/8000	< 0.2	8/8000
7)	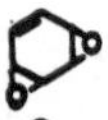	3.1	47/1000	78	840/2000	69	368/1000	< 1	8/1000
8)	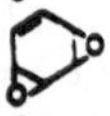	1.4	74/4000	95	1600/4000	99	1475/4000	< 0.3	11/4000
9)	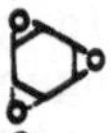	< 0.3	21/8000	2	258/8000	2	159/8000	< 0.2	13/8000
10)	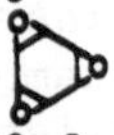	< 0.6	16/4000	< 1	107/4000	< 0.6	28/4000	< 0.3	4/4000
11)	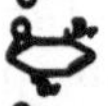	128	173/ 300	635	970/ 300	107	153/ 300	< 9	13/ 300
12)	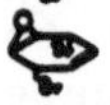	126	128/ 300	587	662/ 300	285	217/ 300	< 9	9/ 300
13)	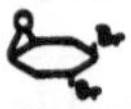	< 3	17/2000	18	221/2000	7	49/2000	< 1	10/2000
14)	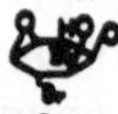	< 0.7	29/8000	< 1	120/8000	< 0.7	25/8000	< 0.3	7/8000
15)	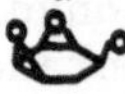	< 1	19/2000	2.6	150/2000	2	49/2000	< 0.6	5/2000
16)	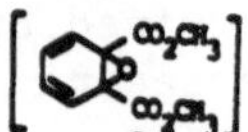	< 4	13/1000	< 8	87/1000	< 4	5/1000	< 2	8/1000
17)	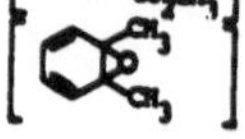	< 2	16/1000	< 4	84/1000	< 2	4/1000	< 1	3/1000

Fig. 1. Mutagenicity and structure of benzene and congeners. Revertants per µmol: revertants minus spontaneous rate of mutation per µmol, taken from the linear region of the dose-response curve. Revertants per dose: maximal number of revertants including spontaneous revertants per plate and corresponding dose. From (16); reprinted by permission of Elsevier/North-Holland, Biomedical Press, Amsterdam.

study included partially and fully hydrogenated derivatives as well as simple and multiple epoxides derived from the benzene structure (16). Bacterial mutagenicity was used as an analytical tool to indirectly visualize the electrophilically reactive derivatives. Cyclohexene oxide, a congener of benzene oxide in which both of its double bonds are hydrogenated, shows a relatively low mutagenic effect on the strain TA 100. If one double bond is introduced in formal conjugation with the oxirane ring (1,3-cyclohexadiene oxide), the mutagenicity increases 2- to 3-fold. This is chemically understandable because the double bond which is in formal conjugation with the oxirane ring activates the oxirane ring which will, therefore, react more easily with nucleophilic constituents. The same applies for the diepoxide where, when a double bond is introduced, irrespective of the geometry of the two oxirane rings (trans or cis), the mutagenicity is dramatically increased (about 10-fold). To get an increase of mutagenicity by introduction of a double bond it is also necessary that the double bond is in formal conjugation with the oxirane ring. Thus, no increase in mutagenicity is observed when 1,4-cyclohexadiene oxide is compared with cyclohexene oxide. If additionally, a halogen atom is introduced at the carbon atom vicinal to the oxirane ring, a very dramatic increase and a qualitative change in the mutagenicity occurs. Strain TA 98, which was only marginally mutated by any of the other derivatives, is now also very susceptible towards mutagenicity corresponding with the fact that a chemically new group is introduced in the compound (16).

Thus, one level of control is provided by the chemistry of the compound. This is largely system-independent. It will be similar in different test-systems because it depends on the chemistry of the compound. It is important to realize that it is dependent on the chemistry of the reactive metabolite and not on that of the mother compound. Thus, structure-activity-relationship studies, where the chemical structure of a group of compounds is compared, taking into account only the parent compounds, can lead to misinterpretation in the case where not the compound itself but rather a metabolite is responsible for the toxic effect.

This is the first level of control which is linked to the chemistry of the reactive metabolite and is therefore dependent on the compound. A second important level of control is the enzymatic control of the formation and of the further metabolism of these reactive metabolites. This second level of control is largely dependent on the test system because the mother compounds have to be metabolized to the reactive metabolites and the metabolizing systems are highly different in different systems.

RELATIVE IMPORTANCE OF SEVERAL ENZYMES WHICH CONTROL THE CONCEN-
TRATION OF ACTIVE METABOLITES DERIVED FROM AROMATIC COMPOUNDS

Many endomembranes of mammalian cells possess monooxygenase
activities capable of transforming these relatively unreactive
aromatic compounds into reactive epoxides (17). There is a set
of further enzymes which are capable of metabolizing these epoxides (Fig. 2): for example, epoxide hydrolases, which transform
these epoxides to chemically unreactive trans-dihydrodiols (1,3,
4,12-14,18); glutathione-S-transferases, which open the epoxide
ring by adding the elements of glutathione (1,3,4,10,13); epoxide
reductases, which convert the derivative back to the mother compound (19,20). Also non-enzymic isomerizations of the intermediate epoxides can occur (1,3,4). The enzymes are present in multiple forms which differ from each other in their substrate preferences. In larger molecules they have their preferential site of
attack which will lead to various sets of reactive mtabolites
which are toxicologically different. The benzo(a)pyrene molecule,

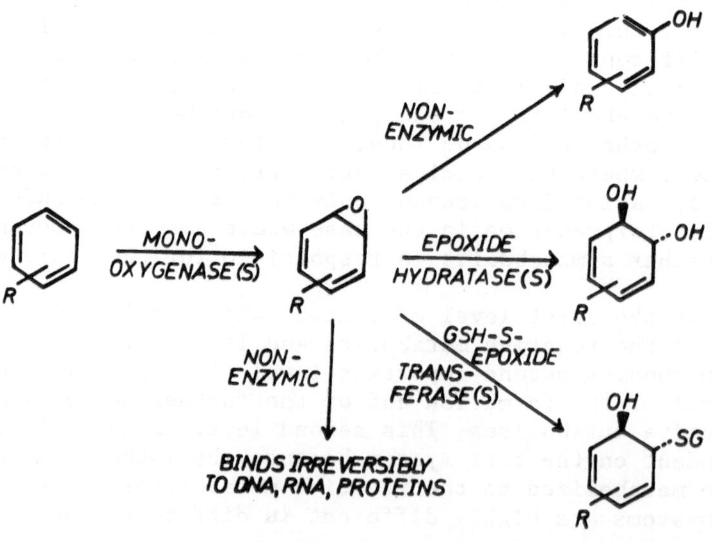

Fig. 2.   Biological formation and further metabolism
           of epoxides. From (12); reprinted by permis-
           sion of Springer Verlag, Heidelberg.

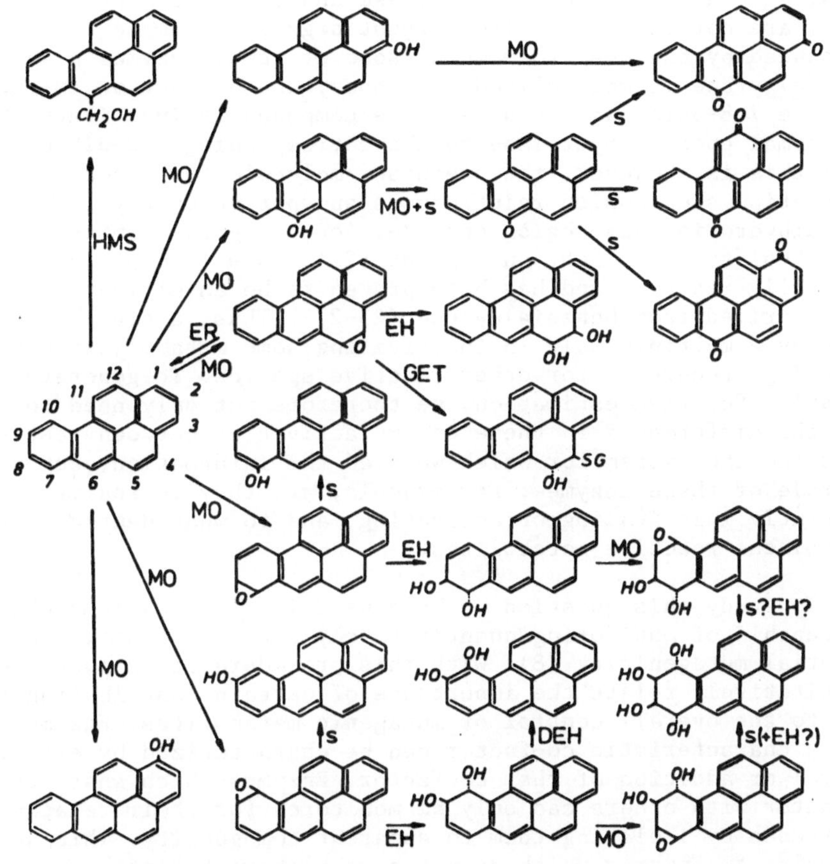

Fig. 3. Some pathways of aromatic hydrocarbon metabolism: exemplified with benzo(a)pyrene: DEH, dihydrodiol dehydrogenase; EH, epoxide hydrolase;
ER, epoxide reductase; GET, glutathione S-trans-
ferase; HMS, 6-hydroxymethylbenzo(a)pyrene synthetase; MO, monooxygenase; S, spontaneous reaction. From H.R. Glatt, Ph.D. thesis, University
of Basel, 1976.

taken as an example, has exclusively aromatic rings and, therefore, no other metabolism is possible except aromatic metabolism.
Yet, it is sufficient to create a complicated pattern of metabolites as shown in Fig. 3, which does not even show the scheme of
the whole metabolism, since the sequestrating conjugating reactions, such as glucuronyl transferase and sulfotransferase reactions, are not indicated. The largest degree of complexity is
introduced by the dual role which some of these enzymes play (21).
Benzo(a)pyrene is metabolized by monooxygenase reaction to the
reactive 7,8-oxide and this reactive compound is inactivated by
microsomal epoxide hydrolase to the corresponding 7,8-dihydro-
diol; this is, however, the precursor molecule for a second mono-
oxygenation step, which reintroduces an epoxide moiety leading
to a dihydrodiol bay-region epoxide. According to chemical quantum calculations by Lehr and Jerina (22), this is especially
chemically reactive and has been proven to be an ultimate carcinogen derived from benzo(a)pyrene (23-27). Thus, a single enzyme
can play a multiple role in inactivating some metabolites but
producing precursors for other reactive species. To generate information for risk estimation, we therefore not only need to
know the differences in these enzyme activities between test systems and the system for which we need the information, but also
the role of these enzymes. For example, are they in reality predominantly inactivating or activating, and to what degree do they
control the reactive metabolites.

To study this question we have used in vitro systems which
are capable of monitoring quantitatively a toxic effect, e.g.
bacterial mutagenicity (8). With this procedure it is possible to
quantitatively relate the importance of certain contributing factors to the overall control of mutagenic metabolites. Enzymes
with a characteristic co-factor can be characterized by either
removal or addition of that co-factor. Enzymes which share their
co-factor with others can only be monitored for their relative
importance by isolating them to apparent homogeneity. This applies also to enzymes which do not have a characteristic co-factor,
such as epoxide hydrolase, which merely adds the elements of water (1,18).

Table 1 shows the isolation procedure of microsomal epoxide
hydrolase which, after solubilization from the microsomal membrane in active form, was purified with a few standard enzyme purification steps until a mixture of constituents of the microsomal
membrane was obtained which were all very hydrophobic (28,29).
When attempting to isolate them in pure form one usually removes
the more hydrophilic species, leaving the hydrophobic constituents which stick very tightly together in the aqueous environment
of the buffer. At this point hydrophobic chromatography was introduced; the hydrophilic column material being used has hydro-

Table 1. Purification of rat liver epoxide hydrolase

Purification step	Volume (ml)	Total protein (mg)	Total units	Specific activity[a]	Relative purification	Yield %
10 000 g supernatant (fraction 1)	1660	49 800	82 557	1.67	1	100
Solubilised microsomes (fraction 2)	1660	11 454	102 107	8.91	5.3	124
Ammonium sulphate precipitate (fraction3)	360	5 184	99 270	19.15	11.5	120
DEAE-cellulose effluent (fraction 4)	500	740	69 300	93.8	56	84
Conc. cellulose phosphate effluent (fraction 5)	6	80	24 000	300	179	29
Butyl-Sepharose effluent (fraction 6)	50	21	14 500	690	415	17.7
Final preparation (fraction 7)	4.8	15.7	8 100	516	310	9.8

[a]Specific activity expressed as nmol styrene glycol per mg protein per min. From (28); reprinted by permission of North-Holland Publishing Company, Amsterdam.

phobic arms attached to it. As a side-chain the n-butyl-side chain
proved optimal in that it retained epoxide hydrolase, let pass all
other components and allowed epoxide hydrolase to be eluted in active form (28,29). This step led to an apparently homogeneous preparation (28,30). It is important to make sure that one has pure
enzymes, to monitor their exact role. To find out if the end product was pure several independent methods were applied, which
showed the apparent homogeneity of the preparation (28,30).

    Bacterial mutagenicity was then used as one of the tests
for monitoring reactive metabolites (8). What produces bacterial
mutagenicity will in many, although not all cases, also produce
chemical carcinogenicity (31,32). The system proved to be a very
useful analytical tool to monitor for reactive metabolites which
chemically cannot be quantitated because they are too reactive
(8). The system consists of giving on an agar plate, a chemical
compound, bacteria as tester strains, and an activating system,
e.g., liver microsomal preparation with the required co-factor
for monooxygenase activity, NADPH, that creates the reactive
metabolites. If the reactive metabolites on the agar plate have
to travel from the microsomal vesicles to the bacteria, the system could be envisaged as being biased for the less interesting
metabolites, i.e. those which are less reactive and can survive
the trip from the microsomal vesicles to the bacteria. We, therefore, studied electron microscopically, the interaction between
the microsomal vesicles and the bacteria. We could show that for
physicochemical reasons, the microsomal vesicles bind tightly to
the surface of the bacterium (33), so that reactive metabolites
can reach the bacterium surface by lateral diffusion within the
lipid matrix of the microsomal vesicle, and can then migrate to
the bacterium DNA. This is in analogy to the situation in a eucaryotic cell where the majority of the reactive metabolites are
produced in the endoplasmic reticulum, part of which is in con-
tiguous contact with the nuclear envelope. The metabolite can
then reach the nuclear membrane by lateral diffusion through the
lipid matrix, and from there the nuclear DNA.

    Frequently several reactive metabolites are involved in a
given toxic response. They are toxicologically different from
one another and since they are reactive and short-lived it is
difficult and in many cases impossible to quantitate them chemically. Therefore, we monitored with various strains of bacteria,
their preferences to be mutated by certain reactive metabolites
which we had chemically synthesized in pure form. The preference
of a certain strain for a certain metabolite, depends on the
particular section of the DNA within the bacterium where the

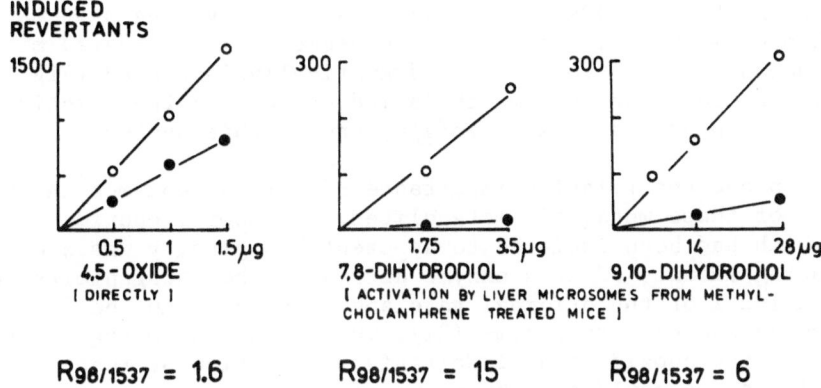

Fig. 4.   Differential susceptibility of various
Salmonella typhimurium strains for the mutagenic action of various benzo(a)pyrene derivatives.

mutation occurs. When we monitored the chemically synthesized
K-region epoxide, benzo(a)pyrene 4,5-oxide, with TA 98 and TA 1537,
we noticed that the strain 98 was more efficiently mutated. The
difference between the two strains, however, was small, a characteristic and reproducible factor of 1.6 (Fig. 4). After in situ
bioactivation of the chemically synthesized 7,8-dihydrodiol to
the corresponding dihydrodiol bay-region epoxide, the strain
TA 98 was much more efficiently reverted than is TA 1537, reproducibly by a factor of about 15. This ratio is again different
from that observed after in situ bioactivation of the 9,10-di-
hydrodiol etc. So for various reactive metabolites which are
derived from the same mother compound there is a characteristic
ratio of how various strains of bacteria are reverted. This can
be used to monitor in a complex metabolic situation which reactive metabolites have been predominantly responsible for the effect, which is then quantitated by counting the number of the reverted colonies.

The spontaneous mutation rate is not increased when benzo-(a)pyrene is added to the bacterial strains with no metabolically activating system present. If liver microsomes and the required cofactor NADPH are added, as metabolically activating systems (in this experiment it was liver microsomes from untreated mice), the spontaneous mutation rate is dramatically increased (Fig. 5). This is the mutation rate which is induced by all the reactive metabolites produced from benzo(a)pyrene in this system.

To probe the relative importance of various enzymes in the control of these mutagenic metabolites, microsomal epoxide hydrolase which had been isolated to apparent homogeneity was added. Increasing amounts of this enzyme decreased the mutagenicity to between 1-2 % of the original rate and this could not be further reduced by adding more enzyme (21). This remaining mutagenicity is due to the epoxide hydrolase-resistant portion of reactive metabolites. We could show by means of the ratios of various strains that the K-region 4,5-oxide was mainly responsible for the major (i.e. epoxide hydrolase-sensitive) portion of the mutagenic effect under these conditions. The situation was completely different when liver microsomes from mice pre-treated with 3-methylcholanthrene were used, producing a different pattern of monooxygenase isoenzymes. These create a different pattern of primary reactive metabolites and in this situation epoxide hydrolase has first a weak but activating effect (21). This is because now dihydrodiol epoxides are predominantly responsible for the mutagenic effect. The microsomes used for creating the metabolites do themselves possess epoxide hydrolase and can generate dihydrodiol epoxides, but addition of more epoxide hydrolase leads to an (small but significant) increase of the mutagenicity, since more of these dihydrodiol epoxides are produced. If the amount of epoxide hydrolase is further increased a small decrease and then a small increase of the mutagenicity is observed (21); this effect is multiphasic because many metabolites and many enzymes with different K_m-values are measurably contributing to the control of the mutagenic metabolites.

In this bioactivation of benzo(a)pyrene by 3-methylcholanthrene-induced monooxygenases, microsomal epoxide hydrolase has a very weak and multiphasic effect (21). It is conceivable that when dihydrodiol epoxides are the species predominantly contributing to the observed mutagenic effect, there exists an alternative enzyme which now takes over the control where microsomal epoxide hydrolase obviously is very inefficient. We assumed that one major reason why the second monooxygenase step works so efficiently on benzo(a)pyrene-7,8-dihydrodiol is because monooxygenase works as an electrophile in that it adds the oxygen atom to a portion of the molecule which is relatively electron-rich. Because of

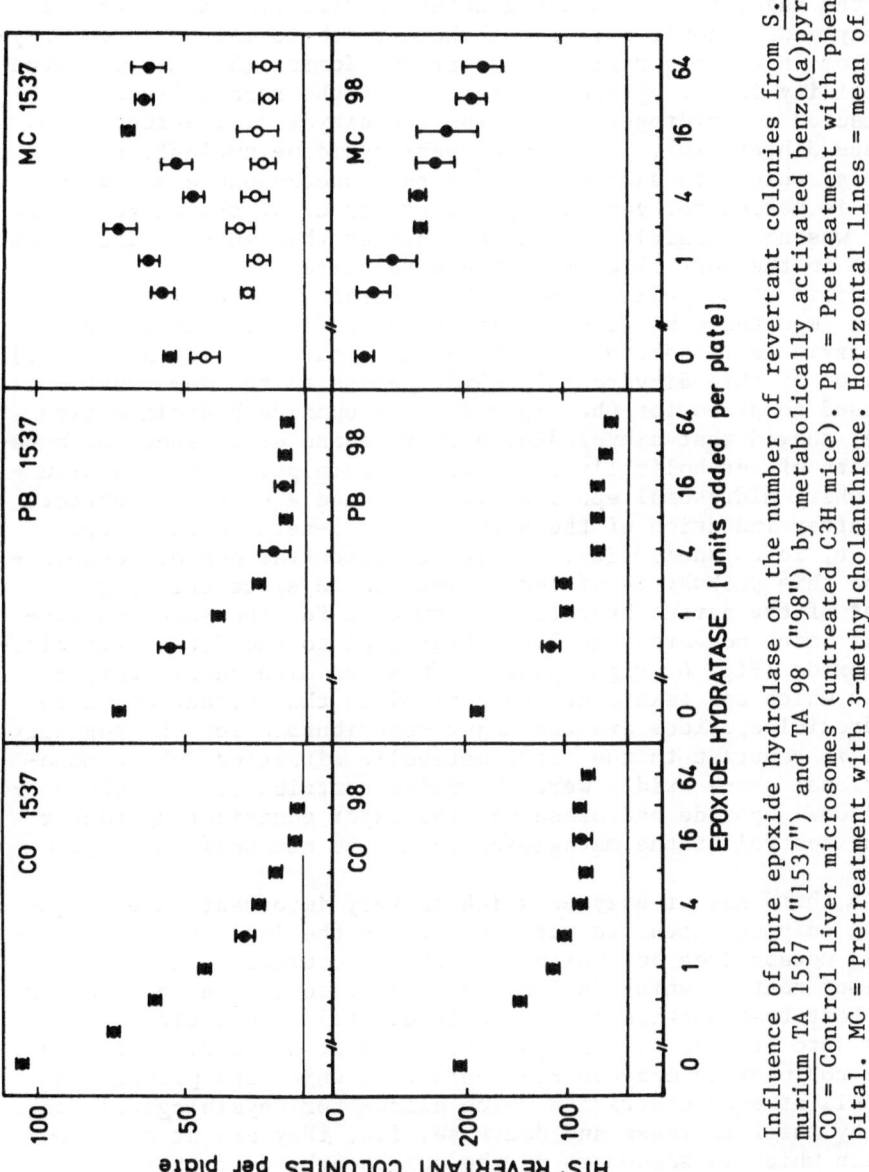

Fig. 5.   Influence of pure epoxide hydrolase on the number of revertant colonies from S.typhi-
murium TA 1537 ("1537") and TA 98 ("98") by metabolically activated benzo(a)pyrene.
CO = Control liver microsomes (untreated C3H mice). PB = Pretreatment with phenobarbital. MC = Pretreatment with 3-methylcholanthrene. Horizontal lines = mean of spontaneous mutations. From (12); reprinted by permission of Springer Verlag, Heidelberg.

interruption of the aromaticity of the angular benzo-ring by the
dihydrodiol structure an olefinic double bond is present in the
7,8-dihydrodiol. An enzyme capable of removing the two hydrogen
atoms of the dihydrodiol moiety thereby reintroducing aromaticity
into the angular ring should generate a situation in which the
monooxygenase should have a much harder job to introduce the oxygen atom in the bay region. Ayengar and Tomida (34) had observed
an activity in the cytosolic fraction of the rabbit liver which
abstracted two hydrogen atoms from the dihydrodiol structure of
benzene dihydrodiol. The enzyme needs pyridine nucleotide cofactors, which are also needed for the monooxygenase activity
which is needed for generating the precursor of the dihydrodiol.
So it was not possible to monitor whether this enzyme also plays
a role in the control of reactive metabolites derived from dihydrodiols of polyclic aromatic hydrocarbons and what is its relative importance by simply removing or adding the cofactors.
The enzyme was, therefore, purified to apparent homogeneity (35).
Addition of this dihydrodiol dehydrogenase to the same system as
was used to probe for the importance of epoxide hydrolase (see
above) showed that dihydrodiol dehydrogenase diminished the mutagenicity of metabolically activated benzo(a)pyrene in the situation where microsomal epoxide hydrolase had a very weak effect,
i.e. after induction of the animals with 3-methylcholanthrene
(Fig. 6, left panel) (36). At higher concentrations of benzo(a)-
pyrene this pathway is of lesser importance since the large
amount of the parent hydrocarbon competes for the same monooxygenase which converts the 7,8-dihydrodiol to the 7,8-dihydrodiol-
9,10-oxide (Fig. 6, right panel). Thus, an alternative enzyme
exists which can take over the control in that situation where
dihydrodiol epoxides are the major contributors for the toxicity
(36), in contrast to the first metabolic situation, where mono-
functional arene oxides were the major contributors and where
microsomal epoxide hydrolase was the major contributing factor
in the control of the mutagenically active metabolites (21).

A third set of enzymes which is very important, are conjugating enzymes which are not involved in the inactivation of reactive metabolites but which sequester precursors. This is a
level of control which is frequently overlooked. In the standard
Ames test that portion of metabolic control is practically not
taken into account. Yet it is a very important level of control.
These conjugating enzymes need cofactors which are present in
the cell at a concentration which allows for physiological control by their increase and decrease, i.e. they are at a concentration which is somewhere in the neighbourhood of their K_m-
values. On the plate on which the test is performed, there is
an enormous dilution so that these cofactors are now present
in concentrations which are orders of magnitude below their K_m-
values, so that these conjugating reactions proceed very slowly

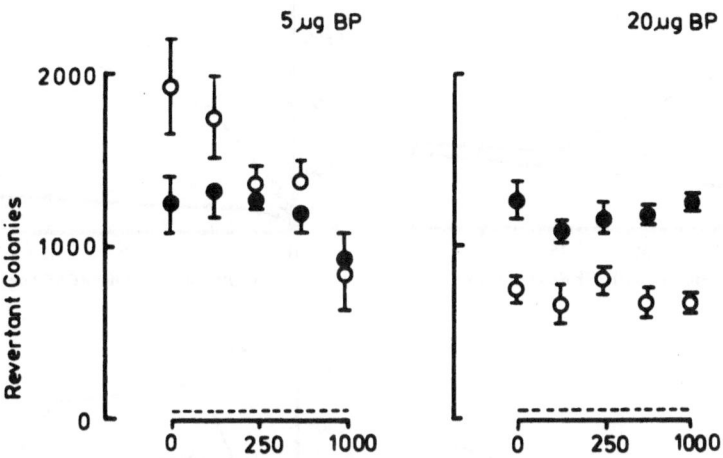

Fig. 6.   Effect of dihydrodiol dehydrogenase upon the
mutagenicity of benzo(a)pyrene activated by
microsomes from 3-methylcholanthrene-treated
mice. Salmonella typhimurium TA 98 were incubated with a low (5 µg BP) or higher (20 µg BP)
concentration of benzo(a)pyrene in the presence (•) or absence (o) of the epoxide hydrolase inhibitor 1,1,1-trichloropropene oxide
(1 mM). Colonies (his$^+$ revertants) were counted after two days. Values represent means $\pm$
S.D. Horizontal dashed lines represent the
mean of spontaneous mutations in the absence
of benzo(a)pyrene. From (12); reprinted by
permission of Springer Verlag, Heidelberg.

or practically not at all. This makes the test more sensitive.
For some purposes that may be desirable, but in order to have
the real picture one needs to take into account that a cell possesses control enzymes which remove precursors for secondary
reactive metabolites. The major intermediates in benzo(a)pyrene
metabolism, 9-hydroxybenzo(a)pyrene, 3-hydroxybenzo(a)pyrene,
the 7,8- and 9,10-dihydrodiol of benzo(a)pyrene were, therefore,

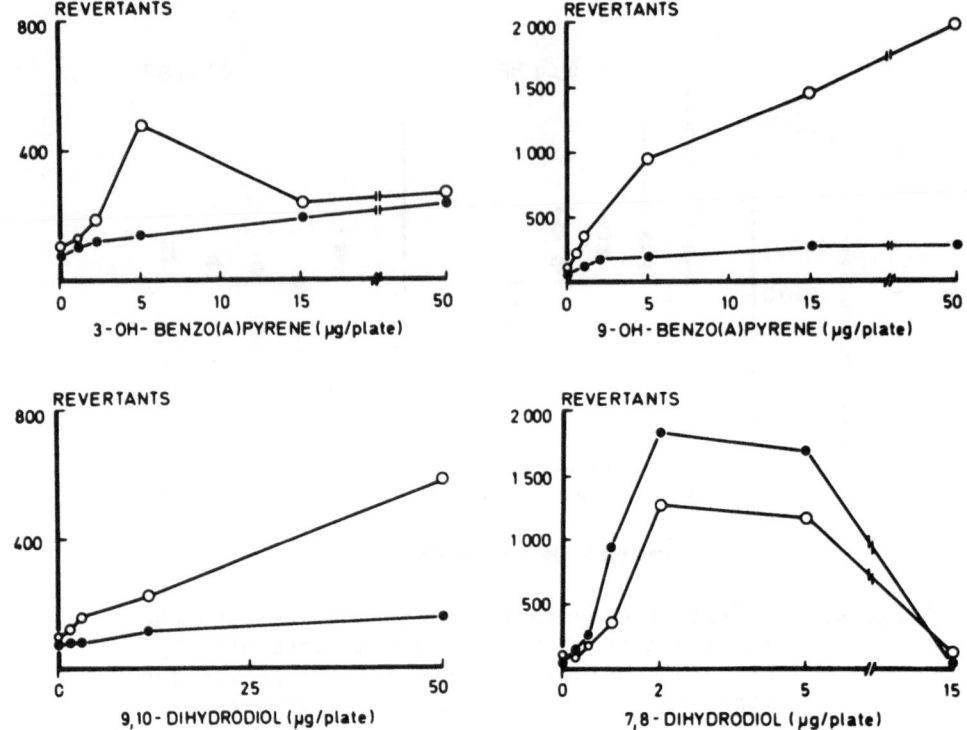

Fig. 7.   Mutagenicity of BP metabolites in S. typhi-
          murium TA 100, directly (▲) or in the pre-
          sence of intact hepatocytes (●), homogenized
          hepatocytes (□), or homogehized hepatocytes
          and a NADPH-generating system (o). The NADPH-
          generating system consisted of 2 mM NADP and
          2.5 mM glucose 6-phosphate. Values are means
          of 3 incubations. The coefficient of varia-
          tion was always smaller than 0.1. From (37);
          reprinted by permission of Cancer Research,
          Inc., Philadelphia.

tested for their bacterial mutagenicity (Fig. 7) (37) and this
was compared with the known whole animal carcinogenicity of these
intermediates, which revealed an enormous discrepency. In the
carcinogenicity tests the 9-hydroxy- and the 3-hydroxybenzo(a)-
pyrene and the 9,10-dihydrodiol proved to be either fully inactive or exceedingly weak (25). In the standard Ames test, however, all three were very potently mutagenic (37). Now we compared this with a situation of the metabolic activation not by the
homogenate of the cells but using whole cells, isolated hepatocytes, because these contain the cofactors for these conjugating

enzymes at their usual cellular concentration. Under these conditions all three derivatives were very weak doubtful mutagens (37) closely reflecting the situation in the whole animal carcinogenicity test. However, the 7,8-dihydrodiol is the precursor for the dihydrodiol bay region epoxide and is, together with that the most active derivative of benzo(a)pyrene in the whole animal carcinogenicity (23-27,38). Using whole cells for metabolic activation the 7,8-dihydrodiol is the only one of the tested derivatives which is highly active, even slightly more active than it is with the homogenate (37); in other words the conjugating enzymes are not capable of efficiently removing the 7,8-dihydrodiol in the whole cell and a very marked mutagenicity results in line with its potent carcinogenicity in the whole animal test (24,38).

Thus, three sets of enzymes are critical in the control of reactive metabolites, and interpretation and extrapolation of results require - contrary to usual practice - that all three are taken into account; activating enzymes, inactivating enzymes and sequestering enzymes.

DIFFERENCES IN THESE ENZYMES BETWEEN ANIMAL SPECIES AND BETWEEN TEST SYSTEMS RELATED TO DIFFERENCES IN TOXIC EFFECTS AND TEST RESULTS

In the metabolic situation which was first discussed in the preceeding chapter (liver microsomes from untreated mice) microsomal epoxide hydrolase played a simple inactivating role and could remove about 98 % of the total mutagenicity (Fig. 5). In this control situation one would, therefore, anticipate that differences in microsomal epoxide hydrolase activity are very decisive for the toxic effect.

When bioactivation of benzo(a)pyrene by two different microsomal systems, taken from the liver of two different animal species, the rat and the mouse, were compared the resulting mutagenicity was indeed very different (Fig. 8) (8). With liver microsomes from rats which had not been pretreated with inducers a very weak increase of maximally 1.7-fold the spontaneous mutation rate was observed.However, a very high mutagenicity resulted when liver microsomes from untreated mice were used. The mice have, compared to rats a higher monooxygenase activity (with most substrates about 2-fold), and a lower activity of microsomal epoxide hydrolase by a factor between 6 and 7 (8). 1,1,1-Trichloropropene oxide when used at a concentration of about 0.3 mM inhibits microsomal epoxide hydrolase without affecting the activity of monooxygenase or of any other microsomal enzyme investigated (41-44). In the experiment shown in Fig. 9 rat liver microsomes were used. Inhibition of microsomal epoxide hydrolase resulted in a large

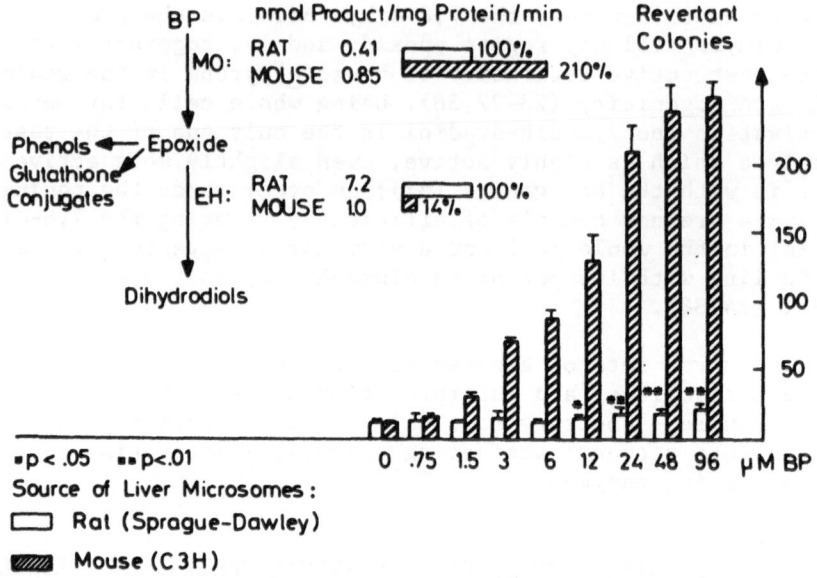

Fig. 8.   Activation of benzo(a)pyrene to a mutagen:
           Microsomes from species with different monooxy-
           genase and epoxide hydrolase activities. Benzo-
           (a)pyrene (BP) was incubated in the presence of
           S. typhimurium TA 1537 with microsomes from male
           Sprague Dawley rats or female C3H mouse liver,
           and the his⁺ revertant colonies were counted
           after 48 h. Microsomal monooxygenase (MO) acti-
           vity was determined with benzo(a)pyrene as sub-
           strate (39) and microsomal epoxide hydolase (EH)
           activity was determined with 7-³H-styrene oxide
           as substrate (40). Values represent means; bars
           represent the standard error of the mean. From
           (8); reprinted by permission of the International
           Agency for Research on Cancer, Lyon.

increase in the mutagenicity (8), very similar to that observed
when mouse liver microsomes were used (Fig. 8). This indicates a
causal relationship between the difference in activity of microsomal epoxide hydrolase and the vastly different degree of accumulation of mutagenic metabolites derived from benzo(a)pyrene.

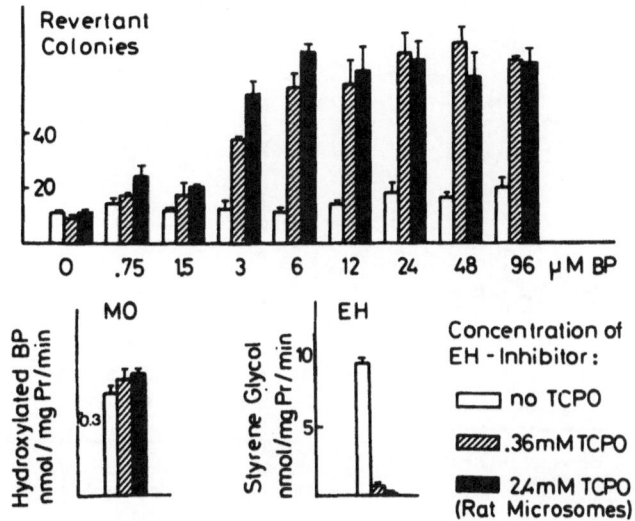

Fig. 9. Activation of benzo(a)pyrene to mutagen: Po-
tentiation by inhibition of epoxide hydrolase.
Benzo(a)pyrene (BP) was incubated with microsomes from male Sprague-Dawley rat liver and
S. typhimurium TA 1537 bacteria in the presence
or absence of 1,1,1-trichloropropene oxide
(TCPO). Concentrations indicated are calculated with respect to the top agar. Microsomal
monooxygenase (MO) and epoxide hydrolase (EH)
were assayed as described (39,40). Values represent means + standard error. From (8); reprinted by permission of the International
Agency for Research on Cancer, Lyon.

Phenanthrene is a compound which, as one of its reactive
metabolites, produces the K-region, 9,10-epoxide (45). The direct
mutagenicity of the synthetic K-region epoxide proved to be high
(46). We also proved by radiotracer trapping technique that this
metabolite was formed by the microsomal preparation which was
used for the mutagenicity test. The mutagenicity test of the
metabolically activated phenanthrene was, however, negative (Fig. 10) (46). We attributed the lack of mutagenicity to

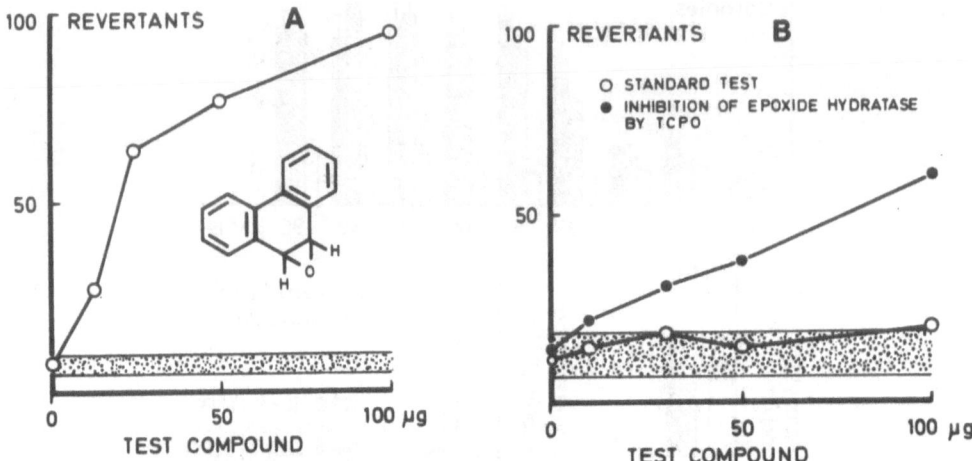

Fig. 10.   Dose dependency of (a) the direct mutagenic effect
            of phenanthrene 9,10-oxide and of (b) the mutagenic
            effect of phenanthrene after activation with liver
            microsomes from mice induced with Aroclor 1254
            (500 mg/kg) for Salmonella typhimurium TA 1537 in
            presence or absence of the epoxide hydrolase inhib-
            itor 1,1,1-trichloropropene oxide (0.6 μl in 10 μl
            dimethylsulfoxide). The horizontal lines indicate
            the range of numbers of colonies on plates without
            test compound (n = 8). Data from (46); reproduced
            by permission of Elsevier/North-Holland Biomedical
            Press, Amsterdam.

the fact that the 9,10-epoxide is a very good substrate of microsomal epoxide hydrolase activity (1,3). Inhibition of microsomal
epoxide hydrolase by 1,1,1-trichloropropene oxide by about 95 %
led indeed to a significant mutagenic activity. Thus lowering
the activity of microsomal epoxide hydrolase by a factor of about
20 converted the apparent non-mutagen phenanthrene to a clear
mutagen because the reactive metabolite can accumulate. By what
factors do these enzyme activities differ in nature? A study on

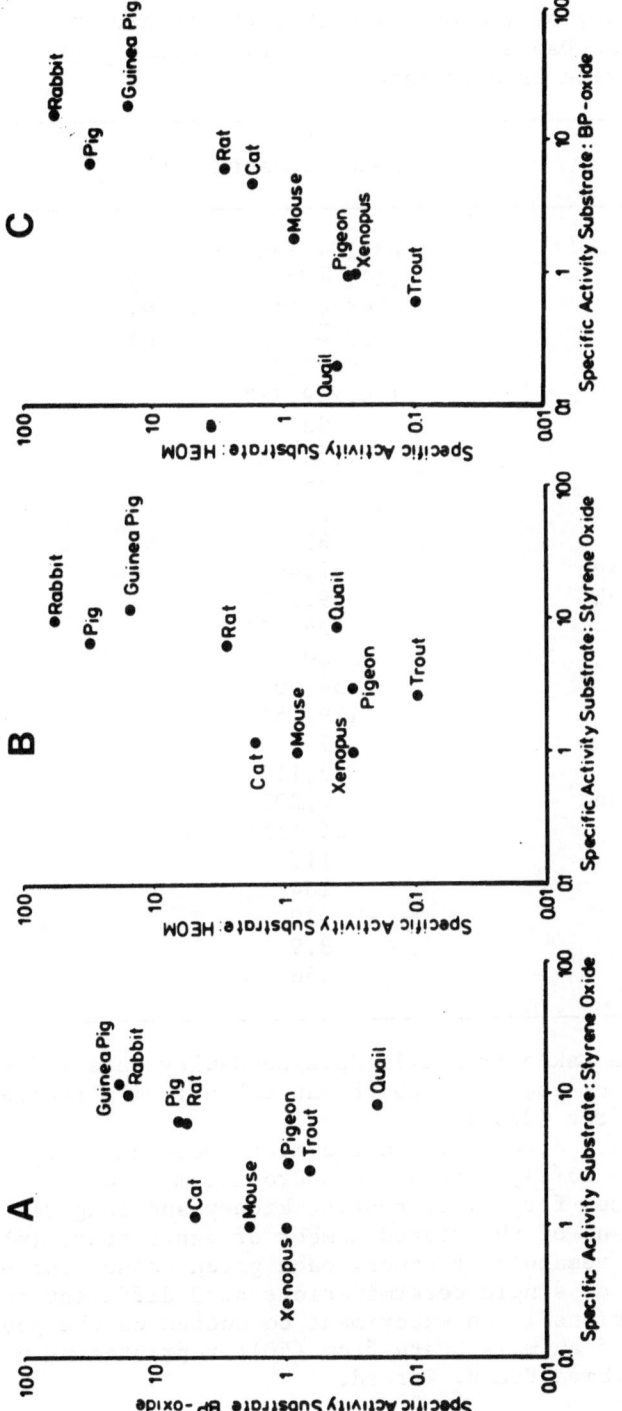

Fig. 11. Comparison of epoxide hydrolase in different species measured with three different substrates. All values are expressed as specific activities in nmol diol product/min per mg protein. The correlation coefficients were (A) benzo(a)pyrene 4,5-oxide: styrene oxide, 0.76; (B) HEOM: styrene oxide, 0.55; (C) HEOM: benzo(a)pyrene 4,5-oxide, 0.70. From (47); reprinted by permission of Elsevier/North-Holland, Bio-medical Press, Amsterdam.

Table 2. Activity of microsomal epoxide hydrolase in
          Sprague-Dawley rats measured with benzo(a)pyrene
          4,5-oxide as substrate

Organ[a]	Specific activity[b]
Liver	6391 $\pm$ 636 (n = 8)
Testis	1472 $\pm$ 247 (n = 7)
Kidney	705 $\pm$ 118 (n = 8)
Lung	362 $\pm$ 46 (n = 10)
Adrenal gland	196,322
Fat (Kidney)	179,249,367
Bladder	90
Prostate gland	41,52,72
Trachea	166
Tongue	59
Oesophagus	87
Membranous stomach	37,49
Glandular stomach	59,90
Small intestine	95,125,158
Caecum	80
Colon	54,60
Epidermis	129,156
Cutis	57,66
Subcutis	82,115
Submaxillary gland	240,293
Spleen	125,155
Thymus	111
Brain	104
Heart	20
Triceps muscle	8,9
Ovary	556

[a]The organs were taken from male Sprague-Dawley rats (220-
280 g) except for the ovary which was taken from a female
Sprague-Dawley rat (270 g).
[b]The sp. act. were determined using microsomes and are given in pmol benzo(a)pyrene 4,5-dihydrodiol mg protein^{-1}
min^{-1}. The values for liver, testis, kidney and lung represent the means of the stated number of experiments (n)
$\pm$ S.D. For the remaining tissues, each given value represents the mean of single determinations at 3 different protein concentrations in an experiment conducted on the pooled organs of 3-5 animals. Data from (50); reprinted by permission of Pergamon Press, Oxford.

the phylogenetic development of hepatic microsomal epoxide hydrolase activity within vertebrate species showed roughly that the
higher the vertebrates were developed the higher was the specific
activity (Fig. 11) (47). Most interestingly, the range in activities of hepatic microsomal epoxide hydrolase within the vertebrates is more than 1000-fold, humans not included (Fig. 11).
We have recently also included primates and humans, and found
that the range of hepatic microsomal epoxide hydrolase activities becomes then about 5000-fold (48). In Table 2 differences
between organs are shown. A very sensitive epoxide hydrolase
assay was developed (49), which allowed determination of the
activity of microsomal epoxide hydrolase in all 26 organs of the
rat that were investigated. In all the organs epoxide hydrolase
activity was present. However, there were enormous differences
in specific activity (50). There was a 1000-fold difference between the highest activity in the liver and the lowest activity
in muscle. So even within a given animal species differences in
activity of microsomal epoxide hydrolase activity are up to
1000-fold (Table 2).

Thus nature provides differences in these enzyme activties
which by far exceed those shown in test systems to be sufficient
to convert a potent mutagen to an apparent non-mutagen.

SUMMARY

Many different enzymes are involved in the formation or disposition of reactive metabolites. Especially well studied is the
important group of enzymes responsible for the control of reactive epoxides. Aromatic compounds can be transformed to epoxides
by microsomal monooxygenases present in many mammalian organs.
By virtue of their electrophilic reactivity such epoxides may
spontaneously react with nucleophilic centers in the cell and
thus covalently bind to DNA, RNA and protein. Such alterations
of critical cellular macromolecules may disturb the normal biochemistry of the cell and lead to cytotoxic, allergenic, mutagenic and/or carcinogenic effects. Whether such effects will be
manifested depends on one hand on the chemical reactivity as well
as other properties (geometry, lipophilicity) of the epoxide in
question.

On the other hand, enzymes controlling the concentration of
such epoxides are an important contributing factor. Several microsomal monooxygenases exist differing in activity and substrate
specificity. With respect to large substrates, some monooxygenases preferentially attack at one specific site different from
that attacked by others. Some of these pathways lead to reactive
epoxides, others are detoxification pathways. Enzymes metaboliz-

ing such epoxides represent a further determining factor. These enzymes include epoxide hydrolases and glutathione S-transferases. These enzymes do not play a pure inactivating role but can in some cases also act as coactivating enzymes. A further set of enzymes sequester precursors of reactive metabolites into pathways leading to less toxic or untoxic metabolites, such as UDP-glucuronyltransferases and sulfotransferases. With some substrates, these can also play multiple roles. Some enzymes can combine sequestring and inactivating roles such as dihydrodiol dehydrogenase which can sequester dihydrodiols and inactivate dihydrodiol epoxides.

Enzymes involved in the control of epoxides and other reactive metabolites differ in quantity and sometimes also in substrate specificity betwen organs, developmental stages, sexes and animal species. They, therefore, represent one important contributing factor to differences in susceptibilities between organs, animal species and test systems.

ACKNOWLEDGEMENTS

The author thanks his collaborators for their work quoted in this article. This work was supported by a grant from the Stiftung Volkswagenwerk.

REFERENCES

1. Oesch, F. (1973) Xenobiotica 3, 305-340.
2. Miller, E.C. & Miller, J.A. (1974) in Molecular Biology of Cancer, ed. Busch, H. (Academic, New York), pp. 377.
3. Jerina, D.M. & Daly, J.W. (1974) Science 185, 573-582.
4. Sims, P. & Grover, P.L. (1974) Adv. Cancer Res. 20, 165-274.
5. Heidelberger, C. (1975) A. Rev. Biochem. 44, 79-121.
6. Nebert, D.W., Robinson, J.R., Niwa, A., Kumaki, K. & Poland, A.P. (1975) J. Cell Physiol. 85, 393-414.
7. Wood, A.W., Wislocki, P.G., Chang, R.L., Levin, W., Lu, A.Y.H., Yagi, H., Hernandez, O., Jerina, D.M. & Conney, A.H. (1976) Cancer Res. 36, 3358-3366.
8. Oesch, F. & Glatt, H.R. (1976) in Screening Tests in Chemical Carcinogenesis, eds. Montesano, R., Bartsch, H. & Tomatis, L. (IARC Scientific Publications No. 12, Lyon), pp. 255-295.
9. Jerina, D.M., Lehr, R.E., Yagi, H., Hernandez, O., Dansette, D.M., Wislocki, P.G., Wood, A.W., Chang, R.L., Levin, W. & Conney, A.H. (1976) in In Vitro Metabolic Activation in Mutagenesis Testing, eds. de Serres, C.F.J., Fouts, J.R., Bend, J.R. & Philpot, R.M. (North Holland Biochemical Press, Amsterdam), pp. 159-177.

10. Arias, I.M. & Jakoby, W.B. (1976) Kroc Foundation Series 6, Raven Press, New York.

11. Ullrich, V., Hildebrandt, A., Roots, I., Estabrock, R.W. & Conney, A.H. (1977) Microsomes and Drug Oxidation, Pergamon Press, Oxford.

12. Oesch, F. (1979) in Mechanism of Toxic Action on Some Target Organs, eds. Chambers, P.L. & Günzel, P. (Springer-Verlag, Heidelberg), pp. 215-227.

13. Oesch, F. (1980) in Quantitative Aspects of Risk Assessment in Chemical Carcinogenesis, eds. Clemmesen, J., Conning, D.M., Henschler, D. & Oesch, F. (Springer Verlag, Heidelberg), pp. 179-194.

14. Guenthner, T.M. & Oesch, F. (1981) in Polycyclic Hydrocarbons and Cancer, eds. Gelboin, H. & Ts'o, P.O.P. (Academic Press, New York), pp. 183-212.

15. Guenthner, T.M. & Oesch, F. (1981) TIPS 2, 129-132.

16. Jung, R., Beermann, D., Glatt, H.R. & Oesch, F. (1981) Mutat. Res. 81, 11-19.

17. Stasiecki, P., Oesch, F., Bruder, G., Jarasch, E.D. & Franke, W.W. (1980) Eur. J. Cell Biol. 21, 79-92.

18. Oesch, F. (1979) in Progress in Drug Metabolism, eds. Bridges, J.W. & Chasseaud, L.F. (John Wiley, Chichester, England), Vol. 3, pp. 253-301.

19. Booth, J., Hewer, A., Keysell, G.R. & Sims, P. (1975) Xenobiotica 5, 197-203.

20. Sugiura, M., Yamazoe, Y., Kamataki, T. & Kato, R. (1980) Cancer Res. 40, 2910-2914.

21. Bentley, P., Oesch, F. & Glatt, H.R. (1977) Arch. Toxicol. 39, 65-75.

22. Lehr, R.E. & Jerina, D.M. (1977) Arch. Toxicol. 39, 1-6.

23. Kapitulnik, J., Wislocki, P.G., Levin, W., Yagi, H., Jerina, D.M. & Conney, A.H. (1978) Cancer Res. 38, 354-358.

24. Kapitulnik, J., Wislocki, P.G., Levin, W., Yagi, H., Thakker, D.R., Akagi, H., Koreeda, M., Jerina, D.M. & Conney, A.H. (1978) Cancer Res. 38, 2661-2665.

25. Levin, W., Wood, A.W., Wislocki, P.G., Chang, R.L., Kapitulnik, J., Mah, H.D., Yagi, H., Jerina, D.M. & Conney, A.H. (1978) Polycycl. Hydrocarb. Cancer 1, 189-202.

26. Slaga, T.J., Bracken, W.J., Gleason, G., Levin, W., Yagi, H., Jerina, D.M. & Conney, A.H. (1979) Cancer Res. 39, 67-71.

27. Slaga, T.J., Viaje, A., Bracken, W.M., Berry, D.L., Fischer, S.M., Miller, D.R. & Leclerc, S.M. (1977) Cancer Lett. 3, 23-30.

28. Bentley, P. & Oesch, F. (1975) FEBS Lett. 59, 291-295.

29. Guenthner, T.M., Bentley, P. & Oesch, F. (1981) Methods Enzymol. 77, 344-349.

30. Bentley, P. & Oesch, F. (1975) FEBS Lett. 59, 296-299.

31. McCann, J., Choi, E., Yamasaki, E. & Ames, B.N. (1975)
     Proc. Nat. Acad. Sci. USA 72, 5135–5139.
32. Glatt, H.R., Schwind, H., Zajdela, F., Croisy, A., Jacqui-
     gnon, P.C. & Oesch, F. (1978) Mutat. Res. 66, 307–328.
33. Glatt, H.R. & Oesch, F. (1977) Arch. Toxicol. 39, 87–96.
34. Ayengar, P.K., Hayaishi, O., Nakajima, M. & Tomida, I.
     (1959) Biochim. Biophys. Acta 33, 111–119.
35. Vogel, K., Bentley, P., Platt, K.L. & Oesch, F. (1980)
     J. Biol. Chem. 255, 9621–9625.
36. Glatt, H.R., Vogel, K., Bentley, P. & Oesch, F. (1979)
     Nature 277, 319–320.
37. Glatt, H.R., Billings, R., Platt, K.L. & Oesch, F. (1981)
     Cancer Res. 41, 270–277.
38. Kapitulnik, J., Levin, W., Conney, A.H., Yagi, A.H. &
     Thakker, D.R. (1977) Nature 266, 378–380.
39. Nebert, D.W. & Gelboin, H.V. (1968) J. biol. Chem. 243,
     6242–6249.
40. Oesch, F., Jerina, D.M. & Daly, J. (1971) Biochim. Biophys.
     Acta 227, 685–691.
41. Oesch, F., Kaubisch, N., Jerina, D.M. & Daly, W. (1971)
     Biochemistry 10, 4858–4866.
42. Oesch, F. & Daly, J. (1972) Biochem. Biophys. Res. Commun.
     46, 1713–1719.
43. Oesch, F., Jerina, D.M., Daly, J.W. & Rice, J.M. (1973)
     Chem.-Biol. Interact. 6, 189–202.
44. Oesch, F. (1974) Biochem. J. 139, 77–88.
45. Grover, P.L., Hewer, A, & Sims, P. (1971) FEBS Lett. 18,
     76–80.
46. Bücker, M., Glatt, H.R., Platt, K.L., Avnir, D., Ittah, Y.,
     Blum, J. & Oesch, F. (1978) Mutat. Res. 66, 337–348.
47. Walker, C.H., Bentley, P. & Oesch, F. (1978) Biochim. Bio-
     phys. Acta 539, 427–434.
48. Glatt, H.R., Lorenz, J., Fleischmann, R., Remmer, H.,
     Ohnhaus, E.E., Kaltenbach, E., Tegtmeyer, F., Rüdiger, H.
     & Oesch, F. (1980) in Microsomes, Drug Oxidations and
     Chemical Carcinogenesis, eds. Coon, M.J., Conney, A.H.,
     Estabrook, R.W., Gelboin, H.V., Gillette, J.R. & O'Brian,
     P.J. (Academic Press, New York), Vol. II, pp. 651–654.
49. Schmassmann, H.U., Glatt, H.R. & Oesch, F. (1976) Anal.
     Biochem. 74, 94–104.
50. Oesch, F., Glatt, H.R. & Schmassmann, H. (1976) Biochem.
     Pharmacol. 26, 603–607.

N-SUBSTITUTED AROMATIC COMPOUNDS

Charles M. King

Department of Chemical Carcinogenesis
Michigan Cancer Foundation
Detroit, Michigan 48201

INTRODUCTION

Aromatic compounds that have nitrogen atoms attached to their ring carbons have a potential for eliciting a variety of adverse cytotoxic, mutagenic and carcinogenic responses. The actual biological effects produced by these agents are dependent on their structure, the ability of the host organism to metabolize the compound and the response of the organism to the metabolites that are generated. Although this group of compounds is most often referred to as aromatic amines, the term N-substituted aromatic compounds is more appropriate since it is sufficiently broad to include both nitrocompounds that may be converted metabolically to aromatic amines, as well as metabolites of amines, e.g. hydroxamates, amides and nitroso derivatives, that have quite different chemical properties. This report is intended to provide insight into the carcinogenic potential of these compounds and the mechanisms by which they are believed to effect this activity.

The reader is directed to earlier reviews for additional details and alternative perspectives on the epidemiology (Parkes, 1976), structure activity relationships (Clayson and Garner, 1976) and mechanisms of action (Miller, 1978; and Irving, 1979) of aromatic amines.

HISTORICAL PERSPECTIVE

With the advent of synthetic organic chemistry in the 19th century, the production of synthetic dyes led to the recognition that bladder tumors were occurring in men engaged

25

in this industry years after their first exposure. Although
these tumors were called "aniline cancers", evidence
concerning the identity of the compounds responsible for these
tumors came only in the 1930s when Hueper demonstrated that
the administration of 2-naphthylamine to dogs resulted in the
development of bladder cancer. Earlier the induction of liver
tumors in rats by o-aminoazotoluene had given the first
indication of carcinogenic potential by a compound other than
a polycyclic aromatic hydrocarbon. Since that time the
greater understanding of the requirements for demonstration of
carcinogenicity in experimental animals, increased efforts in
this area and more detailed records concerning human exposure
have led to the identification of a wide variety of
N-substituted aromatic compounds that can induce cancer in man
and animals. The structures, names and potential sources of
exposure of carcinogens representative of this class are shown
in Figure 1. Each have been shown to induce tumors in humans
and/or experimental animals, save for the potent mutagen,
1-nitropyrene (Wang et al, 1980), which is only now being
studied for determination of carcinogenic potential. Evidence
of carcinogenicity in man has been obtained for
4-aminobiphenyl, benzidine, 2-naphthylamine, chlornaphazin and
phenacetin, all of which can induce urinary bladder cancer
(Parkes, 1976; Clayson & Garner, 1976). Phenacetin causes
tumors of the renal pelvis as well (Bengtsson et al., 1978).

The criteria used to assess the carcinogenicity of these
agents are those commonly applied in experimental
carcinogenesis studies, i.e. an increase in the percentage of
tumor-bearing animals, a decrease in the latent period for the
development of tumors, and an increase in the number of tumors
per animal. For example, a recent study of men engaged in
benzidine production disclosed that 13 of 25 developed bladder
tumors 15 to 20 years after their first exposure (Zavon et
al., 1973). Their average age at the time of diagnosis was
47, approximately 20 years younger than the usual age at which
men develop this disease. The frequent recurrences of bladder
tumors can be regarded as an increased number of tumors per
animal. In general, those compounds known to be carcinogenic
in humans have induced tumors in experimental animals when
adequately tested. To use the case of benzidine again, rats
treated with a total dose as low as 8 mg developed both
mammary and Zymbal gland tumors (Morton et al., 1981).

Prior to the late 1970s, it was believed that the
structural requirements for an aromatic amine to be a
carcinogen were that it contain at least 2 rings and that the
position para to the nitrogen be occupied, or blocked, by an
atom other than hydrogen. As the results of the massive
National Cancer Institute tests for carcinogenicity have

become available over the past several years, it has become
clear that single ring compounds without blocked para
positions (e.g. o-anisidine) are carcinogenic (National Cancer
Institute 1978a). In fact, the prolonged exposure of adequate
numbers of animals has now shown that the simplest of these
compounds, aniline, can induce tumors of the spleen in rats
(National Cancer Institute 1978b). These revelations serve to
warn those who might prematurely judge a compound inactive on
the basis of limited data, and to prompt those who wish to
define structure-activity relationships to seek more rigorous
data than has generally been available.

EXPOSURE

The earliest information on the carcinogenicity of
aromatic amines came from what must be assumed to be extreme
industrial exposure to a relatively uncommon class of
compounds that resulted in the development of tumors
infrequently observed in the general public. Consequently,
most who were aware of the carcinogenicity of this class of
compounds have tended to regard them only as a potential
occupational hazard. This idea is readily dispelled by
recognition that individuals are likely to be exposed to these
compounds in a variety of ways. In fact, aromatic amine
derivatives to which we might be exposed are either
synthesized intentionally for some specific commercial use, or
they are byproducts of processes involving exposure of organic
materials to high temperatures.

Aromatic amine derivatives are employed in the
manufacture of dyes, antioxidants, polymers, explosives,
pesticides and pharmacological agents. The manufacture of
these compounds carries with it the potential for exposure of
the workers engaged directly in the manufacturing process, as
well as the exposure of the general populace through the
release of waste into the environment. In some cases the
products themselves may be intended for consumption, as with
the pharmacological agents, but most are apparently destined
for uses where human exposure would be inadvertent.

In contrast to the often-times large scale industrial
synthesis of aromatic amine derivatives, these compounds are
produced unintentionally in low concentration as byproducts of
processes where organic materials are exposed to elevated
temperature. Aromatic amine derivatives may be produced in
these processes by two different mechanisms. The partial
combustion or pyrolysis of nitrogen-containing organic
materials can result in the production of both
azaheterocyclics and arylamine compounds as exemplified by the
detection of 2-naphthylamine in cigarette smoke (Hoffmann and

Structure	Name	Use/Occurrence
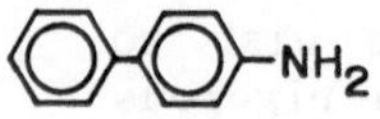	4-Aminobiphenyl	Antioxidant
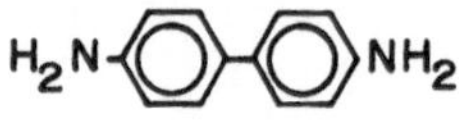	Benzidine	Dye Intermediate
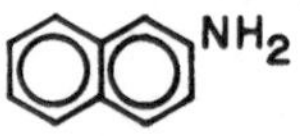	2-Naphthylamine	Antioxidant
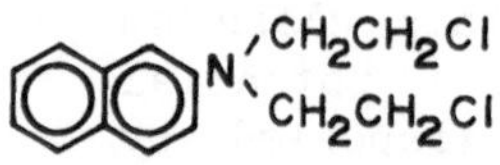	Chlornaphazin	Pharmacological Agent
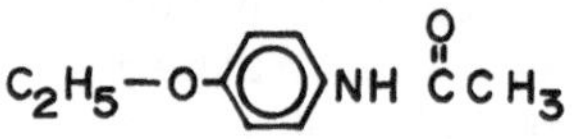	Phenacetin	Analgesic
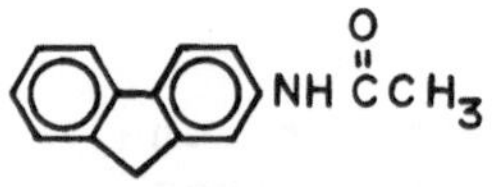	2-Acetylaminofluorene	Insectide (Never marketed)
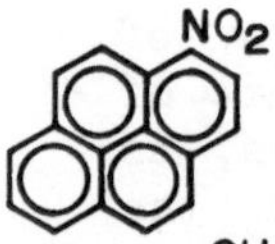	1-Nitropyrene[a]	Combustion Product
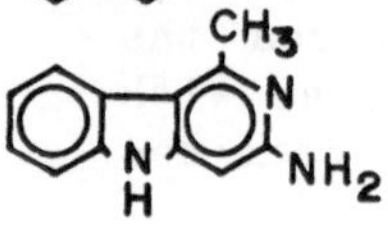	"Trp-P-2"	Food Pyrolysis

[a] The carcinogenic potential of this potent mutagen is now being determined.

Fig. 1. Representative carcinogenic N-substituted aromatic compounds.

Wynder, 1976), amino-substituted carbolines (e.g. Trp-P-2, Figure 1) in amino acid pyrolysates (Kosuge et al 1978) and indirect mutagens believed to be primary aromatic amines in synthetic fuels (Epler et al., 1980).

A second more indirect mechanism for the production of amines is seen in the formation of nitroaromatic compounds as a consequence of combustion processes. In this case, polycyclic aromatic hydrocarbons can be nitrated by nitrogen oxides formed at high temperatures from atmospheric nitrogen. While these compounds may be formed during or immediately after the combustion process, their subsequent photochemical formation has not been excluded. Indirect evidence for the formation of nitrated aromatics as byproducts of the combustion process comes from two sources. The model studies of Pitts and his collaborators (1978) demonstrated that polycyclic aromatic hydrocarbons were readily nitrated by levels of nitrogen oxides that might be expected in the atmosphere. The second line of evidence comes from analysis of the mutagenicities of particulates collected from internal combustion engines (Claxton and Huisingh, 1980), and the atmosphere (Wang et al., 1980). The mutagenicities of these materials in Salmonella typhimurium are decreased if tested in strains that are deficient in the ability to be reverted to prototrophy by arylnitro compounds. Rosenkranz and his collaborators (Mermelstein et al, 1981) have shown that the nitropyrene derivatives detected in carbon black and xerographic toners are among some of the most potent mutagens yet identified. Even though the carcinogenicity of these nitro derivatives has not been established, their potent genotoxicity and probable conversion to reactive species by reduction in mammalian systems strongly suggest that they will be found carcinogenic when tested adequately.

TISSUE SUSCEPTIBILITY

Although aromatic amines are known to induce urinary bladder cancer in man, bladder tumors and other tumors develop in some experimental animals exposed to these compounds. These agents are unusual in that they have the potential for causing neoplasms in a wide range of tissues. A particularly interesting example of tissue specificity has emerged from the extensive study of 2-acetylaminofluorene. This compound and its metabolites have been shown to induce tumors in tissues of the species shown in Table 1. Two significant points have emerged from these studies. The tumors do not always develop at the site of application of the carcinogen, and each species responds in a characteristic manner.

A further demonstration of specificity is to be seen in the change in tissue susceptibility that occurs with relatively minor alterations in the structures of carcinogen, as shown in Table 2. The biphenyl and fluorene nuclei differ only by one carbon, but yet the fluorene is a more potent carcinogen. In comparing the two orthomethoxyfluorene derivatives, only the isomer which carries a substituent adjacent to the methylene bridge is active.

Table 1
THE MOST COMMON TUMORS INDUCED BY
2-ACETYLAMINOFLUORENE (AAF) DERIVATIVES

TISSUE	RAT	HAMSTER	RABBIT	GUINEA PIG	MOUSE	CHICKEN	DOG	CAT
Liver	+	+			+		+	
Kidney						+		
Stomach	+	+						
Small Intestine	+	+		+				
Lung								+
Mammary Gland	+							
Ear Duct	+							
Bladder	+	+			+		+	
Uterus			+					

Compiled from the following sources:

Clayton and Garner, 1976.
Weisburger and Weisburger, 1958.
Miller et al., 1964.
Coogan et al., 1978.

METABOLISM

Most investigators feel that the tissue specificities of the aromatic amines result from differences in the metabolic disposition of the agents. In spite of their insolubility, these compounds are readily absorbed through biological

membranes, including skin, and are then transported
systemically. The metabolism is extensive and rapid by the
pathways depicted in Figure 2. While little or no methylation
of aromatic amines occurs, they are acylated by an acetyl
CoA-dependent N-acetyltransferase in all mammalian species
except the dog (Weber, 1973). This reaction can be reversed
by hydrolysis of the N-acetyl moiety, primarily by microsomal
enzymes (Irving, 1966, Jarvinen et al., 1971). Both the free
amine and the acetamide can be oxidized by cytochrome P450
systems at either the carbon or nitrogen atoms (Thorgeirsson
et al, 1977). Although the N-oxidized derivatives can be
reduced easily by mammalian enzymes, the phenolic oxidation
products are rarely reduced. While not shown in Figure 2,
enzymatic C-oxidation of the acetyl group can yield
glycolamides, a class of metabolites that have not been
implicated in carcinogenicity (Shirai, et al, 1981a). The
phenolic, N-hydroxy, and amine functions can be conjugated
enzymatically to yield more polar compounds that are more
easily excreted. Additionally, compounds such as the nitroso
and quinoneimine derivatives are sufficiently reactive that
they can combine nonenzymatically with protein, but not with
nucleic acids (King and Kriek, 1965, King and Phillips, 1969,
King et al., 1976).

As with other xenobiotics, it is believed that the higher
the molecular weight the more likely the aromatic amine
metabolite will be excreted in the bile. The majority of the
excretion of aromatic amines usually occurs within 48 hours
after their adminstration, with metabolites appearing more
quickly in the urine than in the feces. Glucuronate and
sulfate conjugates are the most commonly encountered urinary
metabolites of aromatic amines. Few conjugates are expected
in the feces due to hydrolysis by the flora of the gut; the
N-oxidized compounds will be reduced. Freed of their polar
moieties, these deconjugated metabolites will then be subject
to reabsorption via the portal system. It is unusual to
detect more than a minor fraction of the parent amine or amide
as an excretion product.

METABOLIC ACTIVATION

The tissue specificities described above imply that the
metabolism of these agents by the host and/or the target
tissue somehow plays a crucial role in tumor development. In
the late 1940s, the Millers and their collaborators observed
that N,N-dimethyl-4-aminoazobenzene formed covalent adducts
with protein of rat liver through an unknown metabolic
pathway. This observation gave impetus to the idea that
carcinogens might act by altering tissue macromolecules after
being metabolized to reactive derivatives, i. e., "metabolic

activation". They subsequently identified N-hydroxy-2-acetyl-aminofluorene as an N-oxidized urinary metabolite of 2-acetylaminofluorene (Cramer et al., 1960), and then demonstrated it to be a more potent carcinogen than the parent amide (Miller et al., 1961). Although N-hydroxy-2-acetylamino-fluorene was not reactive per se, it focused attention on the role of N-oxidized intermediates in the carcinogenic process and provided a substrate which would later be shown to be activated by a single further metabolic reaction. After Kriek (1965) found that the hydroxylamine could react with nucleic

Table 2
THE MOST FREQUENTLY INDUCED TUMORS IN THE RAT BY STRUCTURALLY RELATED AROMATIC AMINES

	ORGAN						
COMPOUND	LIVER	KIDNEY	SMALL INTESTINE	EAR DUCT	BREAST	BLADDER	PANCREAS
2-naphthyl-amine						+	
4-amino-biphenyl					+		
'4-fluoro-4-amino-biphenyl	+	+	+				+
4-amino-stilbene				+	+		
2-amino-fluorene	+		+	+	+		
1-methoxy-2-amino-fluorene	+		+				
3-methoxy-2-amino-fluorene							

Compiled from Clayson & Garner, 1976.

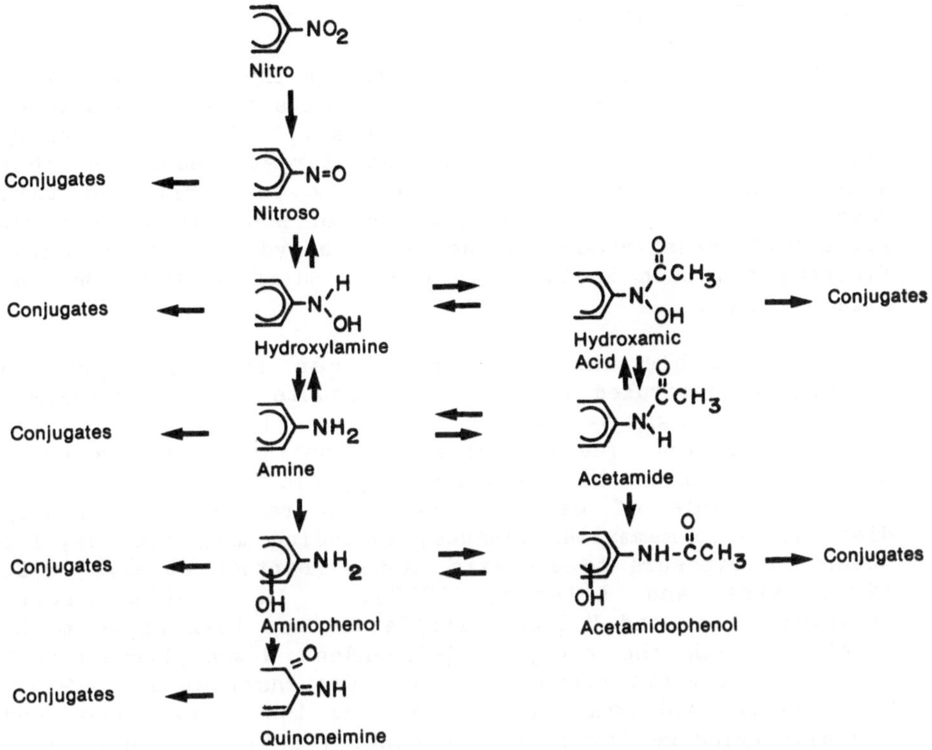

Conjugations with glucuronic acid, sulfate, lipids and amino acids have been observed.

Fig. 2. Metabolism of N-substituted aromatic compounds.

acids in acidic media, he and the Millers (Kriek et al., 1967) then showed that an ester of N-hydroxy-2-acetylaminofluorene could react at neutrality with carbon-8 of guanine derivatives.

Evidence of the enzymatic activation of N-hydroxy-2-ace-tylaminofluorene was shown (King and Philips 1968, DeBaun et al., 1970) in experiments in which labeled N-hydroxy-2-acetyl-aminofluorene was incubated with an enzyme preparation from the target tissue (i.e., male rat liver) in the presence of nucleic acid that had been added to trap the putative reactive metabolite. Two reactions were observed to be carried out by cytosolic enzymes. Conjugation with sulfate yielded arylacet-amide-substituted adducts (Figure 3).   The second reaction took place in the absence of cofactors with loss of the N-acetyl moiety. Subsequent studies demonstrated that both active derivatives combined with the C-8 position of guanine (Figure 4)(King and Philips, 1969), the position at which

N-acetoxy-2-acetylaminofluorene reacts (Kriek et al., 1967).

Further studies showed that although the sulfotransferase that was capable of activating arylhydroxyamic acids was found in the liver of the rat (DeBaun et al., 1970), the mammary gland and Zymbal gland of the rat and target tissues in other species had essentially no capacity to carry out this reaction, (Irving et al., 1971). One of possibly several rat liver sulfotransferases that activates N-hydroxy-2-acetylamino fluorene has been isolated in highly purified form (Wu and Straub, 1976).

The soluble enzyme of rat liver that can produce arylamine-substituted nucleic acid adducts from N-hydroxamic acids was shown by Bartsch et al. (1972) to involve N,O-acyltransfer. The crucial metabolite is believed to be an N-acyloxyarylamine that ionizes to yield a nitrenium ion. Enzymes capable of carrying out this reaction are widely distributed in mammalian tissues, including many that develop tumors on exposure to aromatic amines (Bartsch et al., 1972, 1973; King and Allaben, 1980). In rabbit liver, arylhydroxamic acid N,O-acyltransferase has been shown to be identical with the acetyl CoA-dependent N-acetyltransferase that can acetylate aromatic amines (Glowinski et al., 1980). The aromatic hydroxamic acid serves as the acetyl donor and the hydroxylamine formed in the donor reaction then acts as the acetyl acceptor. Such relationships have not yet been established for other species.

Enzymatic deacetylation of arylhydroxamic acids can yield arylhydroxylamines that have little reaction with nucleic acids at neutrality. In contrast, deacylation of their glucuronide conjugates can yield a reactive O-glucuronide (Cardona and King, 1976), but enzymes capable of carrying out this reaction are apparently confined to the microsomes of the liver of only a few species.

Recently, it has been recognized that there are additional microsomal deacylases that are clearly distinguishable from the cytosolic acyltransferase by virtue of their inhibition by organotriphosphate inhibitors. However, these enzymes appear to activate arylhydroxamic acids by an analogous mechanism (Shirai et al., 1981a, Glowinski et al., 1981). As with the cytosolic enzymes, these microsomal acyltransferases are found in a wide variety of tissues.

Peroxidation was first shown to activate arylhydroxamic acids by producing N-acetoxy-2-acetylaminofluorene which could then react with nucleic acid to give arylacetamide-substituted polynucleotides (Bartsch and Hecker, 1972). More recently

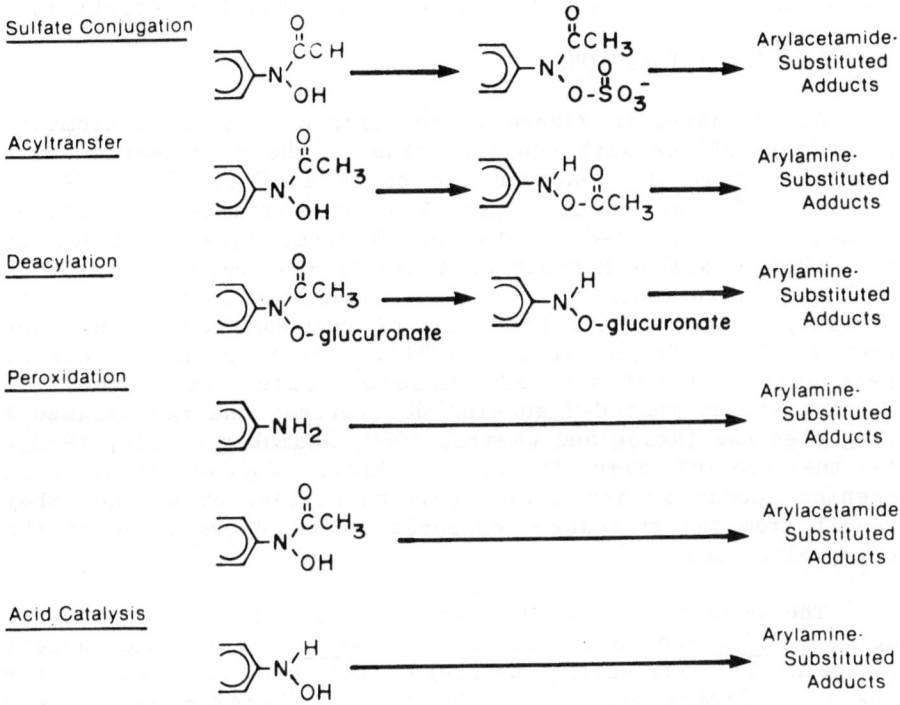

Fig. 3.   Pathways of nucleic acid adduct formation.

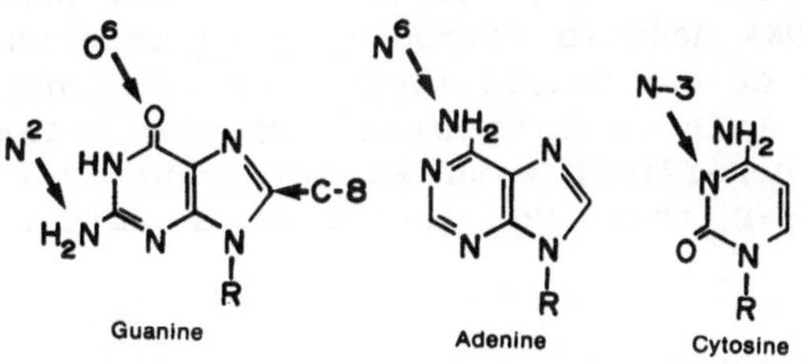

Fig. 4.   Sites of reaction with nucleic acid.

(Zenser et al., 1980) have shown that benzidine can be activated on peroxidation by prostaglandin synthetase to yield arylamine-substituted nucleic acids. Little is known of the potential of susceptible tissues to actually carry out the reactions necessary for this pathway of metabolic activation.

NUCLEIC ACID ALTERATIONS

As indicated in Figure 4, reaction of activated aromatic amine derivatives with nucleic acids or their monomeric units has shown that the reaction can occur at C-8, N^6 or O^6 of guanine, N^6 of adenine and N-3 of cytidine derivatives (Kadlubar et al., 1980, Kriek and Westra, 1979, Scribner et al., 1978). Although chain cleavage of RNA occurs on reaction with arylhydroxlamines in acidic media, evidence that this lability is due to the formation of phosphotriesters has not been obtained (Vaught et al., 1981). Further indications of secondary alterations of nucleic acids come from the demonstrations that C-8 guanine derivatives undergo imidazole ring cleavage (Kriek and Westra, 1980, Kadlubar et al., 1980). At the present time it is not known whether these ring openings occur in the intact polynucleotide, or whether they result from the procedures employed in the degradation of the polynucleotide.

The adducts formed between aromatic amines and nucleic acids in vivo and in intact cells in vitro reflect the variety of metabolic activation pathways that are responsible for their formation. Both arylacetamide- and arylamine-substituted adducts are formed (Kriek and Westra, 1979). Thus, rat liver cells exposed to tritiated N-hydroxy-2-acetyaminofluorene contain DNA and RNA adducts that previously had been identified in cell-free systems by use of sulfotransferase, acyltransferase and synthetic procedures (Howard et al., 1981). A pattern that emerges from the study of DNA adducts formed in vivo is that the majority of the adducts do not retain their N-acetyl group. Therefore, they are arylamine-substituted adducts whose pathway of formation is consistent with an acyltransfer or deacylation mechanism rather than one involving a sulfate conjugation (Figure 3).

GENETICS

The belief that carcinogen-induced genetic changes are crucial to the initiation of tumors has prompted efforts in two areas. One aim has been to try to determine how the host organism attempts to repair damage induced by the carcinogen. A second goal has been to determine what changes in function result from the modification of the genome by the carcinogen.

The repair of carcinogen-induced genomic lesions has been approached by application of both specific and non-specific techniques. On one hand, the investigator may determine the time-dependent loss of a specific carcinogen lesion. Of necessity, this has generally meant the loss of a covalent adduct between the carcinogen and the nucleic acid component. For example, Howard et al. (1981) have attempted to relate the rate of removal of specific N-hydroxy-2-acetyla-minofluorene-induced adducts from hepatocytes to the structure of those adducts. Their data show that C-8-2-acetylaminofluo-rene-substituted guanine adducts are removed more rapidly than either the C-8-2-aminofluorene or the N-acetylaminofluorene adducts.

An alternative approach has been to determine the extent of unscheduled DNA synthesis that has been stimulated by the carcinogen, a technique that is not agent specific. This approach has also been criticized by some because it deals only with lesions that the cell is able to repair and not those that may be of greater importance because the cell cannot repair them. Despite these observations, unscheduled DNA synthesis may play a useful role in attempts to determine, for example, what metabolic pathways are responsible for the generation of lesions that are recognized by the repair system (Shirai and King, 1981b).

An important goal in the area of genetic effects will be the identification of the actual modifications in codes that result from carcinogen-induced changes. While some information has been obtained by treating DNA of known sequence with N-acetoxy-2-acetylaminofluorene and then subjecting the product of transcription of this polynucleotide to sequential analysis (Moore and Strauss, 1979), it seems likely that definitive answers await the use of site-specific modifications of DNA that can be used as templates in vitro and in vivo. Such molecular biological techniques are now becoming available (Bhanot et al., 1979). Coupled with the recent structural studies described above and newer methods of synthesis (Lee and King, 1981) more rapid progress in this area should be possible.

In the absence of these site-specific experiments, it has been possible to amply demonstrate that the metabolites of aromatic amines can be mutagenic. The transforming DNA system employed by Maher et al., (1968) showed clearly that the attachment of arylamine derivatives to DNA could induce mutations. Subsequently, there has been a wide spread use of Salmonella typhimurium for the detection of mutagenic aromatic amine derivatives. This method is simple to use, and it responds to arylhydroxylamines, possibly because of a bacterial activation system. However, it does not detect the reactive sulfate ester of N-hydroxy-acetylaminofluorene or the metabolites from the acyltransferase activation that are capable of reacting with nucleic acids (Weeks et al., 1978, 1980; Wirth and Thorgeirsson, 1980). A further idiosyncrasy of the use of these organisms is that they contain nitroreductases which can reduce unreactive nitro aromatic compounds so as to produce mutations from them without the addition of an external metabolic activation system.

The use of mammalian cells for mutagenicity and transformation studies has been complicated because of the general emphasis on the need for stable cell lines. This has lead to the development of systems that employ target cells that are relatively ineffective in the metabolic activation of aromatic amines. This deficiency has resulted in the use of external metabolic activation systems that may not provide that the most active metabolites, in which there is greatest interest, will play a role.

RELATIONSHIP OF METABOLIC ACTIVATION TO TUMOR DEVELOPMENT

More information is available on the metabolic activation and carcinogenicity of aromatic amines in the rat than in any other species. Table 3 indicates, in a qualitative fashion, the capacities of a number of rat organs to metabolically activate N-hydroxy-2-acetylaminofluorene, as well as their susceptibility to this compound. Clearly, no one pathway of metabolic activation can be correlated directly with the carcinogenicity of this compound in the rat.

Most investigators would probably agree that aromatic amines exert their carcinogenic effects on cells as a consequence of their metabolic activation and alteration of the target cells' genetic apparatus. Yet these two factors alone will not inevitably lead to tumor development. The carcinogenic process is complicated by both sequence and time, the details of which have not yet been clarified. Thus, attempts to elucidate the role of metabolic activation of aromatic amines in the induction of tumors must take into account anatomical, biochemical, and biological factors that moderate the carcinogenic process. A factor of obvious importance is that the systemic distribution of appropriate substrates must be accomplished so that the carcinogen can be activated in the target cells. Since the most reactive of the aromatic amine metabolites are by definition unstable, the distance through which they are likely to excert their carcinogenic properties is limited. Conversely, it is probable that the final metabolic activation takes place in the tissue in which tumors are induced.

N-Oxidized derivatives, that are most probably formed in the liver, can be transported by the blood, urine, or bile to the tissues in which a terminal metabolic activation can occur. The extent to which the compound is excreted in the bile or urine may determine in part whether tumors are formed in the urinary or gastrointestinal tract. For example, in the rabbit, metabolites of 2-acetylaminofluorene are excreted in the urine but not in the bile (Irving et al., 1967). Not surprisingly, tumors are induced in the rabbit bladder by 2-acetylaminofluorene and not in the gastrointestinal tract even though the small intestine has rather high levels of acyltransferase (King and Allaben, 1980).

Although both the distribution of carcinogen and metabolic activation capacity may be adequate for the formation of DNA adducts, tumors may not result. The binding of N,N-dimethyl-4-aminostilbene to DNA of rat liver is linear over a wide dose range, but yet does not induce tumors or other lesions in this organ (Neumann, 1980). Such damage may not be expressed because the rate of DNA synthesis is sufficiently slow and the rate of DNA repair is fast enough to correct these lesions before the altered template must be copied and, thereby, fixed through the misincorporation of bases. Rat liver tumors are generally induced by aromatic amines only if the carcinogen-derived arylhydroxamic acid is activated by conjugation with

Table 3

RELATIONSHIP OF METABOLISM TO THE CARCINOGENICITY OF
N-HYDROXY-2-ACETLYAMINOFLUORENE IN THE SPRAGUE-DAWLEY RAT

ORGAN	METABOLIC CAPACITY			CARCINOGENIC RESPONSE
	SULFOTRANS-FERASE	ACYLTRANS-FERASE	DEACYLASE	
Liver				
Male	+	+	+	+
Female	—	+	+	—
Mammary Gland	—	+	—	+
Small Intestine	—	+	+	+
Zymbal Gland	—	+	+	+

sulfate so that it elicits a hepatotoxic response. The hepatotoxicity may serve to stimulate the replication of cells that are resistant to the toxic effects of the carcinogen because they do not conjugate the arylhydroxamic acids with sulfate. DNA adducts in these resistant cells, when used as a template for DNA synthesis, would result in genetic changes that eventually lead to tumor formation.

Evidence in support of this hypothesis has been obtained in experiments with N-hydroxy-4-acetylaminobiphenyl. This compound, which is not normally a hepatocarcinogen in the rat, is bound to rat liver nucleic acid by metabolic pathways that are independent of sulfate conjugation, possibly by an acyltransferase mechanism (King et al., 1976). The animals were female Sprague-Dawley-derived rats which, 1) have little if any capacity to activate arylhydroxamic acids by sulfate conjugation, 2) do not develop liver tumors on treatment with arylhydroxamic acids that are carcinogenic for their male counterparts, and 3) do not exhibit hepatotoxicity on treatment with these compounds (Gutmann et al., 1972). Partial hepatectomy of these animals prior to adminstration of a single dose of N-hydroxy-4-aceylaminobiphenyl and subsequent treatment with phenobarbital resulted in the formation of neoplastic nodules and foci of gammaglutamyltranspeptidase-containing cells (Shirai et al.,1981c). Thus neoplastic lesions from a single dose of an arylhydroxamic acid in the absence of sulfate conjugation, could be induced by forcing the liver to undergo regeneration at the time of challenge with carcinogen and then administering phenobarbital, a non-carcinogenic compound known to augment the formation of liver tumors if given subsequent to carcinogen administration. These studies strongly suggest that the induction of rat liver tumors by aromatic amines may be the combined results of a gene-altering event that is independent of sulfate conjugation, followed by secondary hepatotoxicity. The toxicity may result from reactive sulfate conjugates of arylhydroxamic acids that leads to cell replication which fixes and amplifies genetic alterations by stimulating the growth of resistant but altered cells (Farber et al., 1976).

The mechanisms of metabolic activation involved in the induction of tumors in the mammary gland of the rat by aromatic amines may be better understood than those of any other organ. A single direct application of N-hydroxy-2-acetylaminofluorene to the mammary gland of an immature Sprague-Dawley female rat results in the induction of tumors whereas the related acetamide and hydroxylamine derivatives were less active (Malejka-Giganti and Gutmann, 1975). The gland has an acyltransferase, but neither sulfotransferase nor deacylase has been demonstrated in this organ (Shirai et al.,1981a;

Irving et al., 1971; Irving, 1979). The RNA adducts formed in vivo in this organ are compatible with their formation via acyltransfer (King et al., 1979). Administration of a series of arylhydroxamic acids that differed in their capacity for activation by mammary gland acyltransferase showed that tumor formation was greatest with those compounds that could be activated by one of the acyltransferases of this tissue (Shirai et al., 1981a). These data strongly support the idea that the cytosolic, paraoxon-insensitive acyltransferase of the mammary gland of the rat is associated with tumor induction in this tissue.

The development of tumors by aromatic amine derivatives in the mammary gland and liver of rat appear to be closely linked to arylhydroxamic acids. In contrast, dogs may not be able to form these compounds since they can not acetylate aromatic amines (Weber, 1973). Nevertheless, dogs readily develop bladder tumors when treated with aromatic amines (Clayson and Garner, 1976). Thus, in this species, bladder tumor induction is independent of acetylated derivatives.

FUTURE PROSPECTS

These observations support the conclusion that tumors may be induced by a variety of metabolic activation pathways and that not all metabolic activation leads to tumor formation. An important goal of future studies will be to define, in molecular terms, how and what genetic lesions are induced by carcinogenic aromatic amines so that the functional consequences of these modifications can be determined.

A second aim should be to attempt to utilize more circumscribed experimental protocols that employ brief or single treatments with doses that are as small as possible for tumor induction. Success in this area would facilitate our approach to the problem of resolving the carcinogenic process into more discrete steps than is now possible.

ACKNOWLEDGEMENT

The studies in this report from the A. Alfred Taubman facility were supported by grant CA 23386 from the National Cancer Institute, and an institutitional grant from the United Foundation of Detroit. I wish to thank Debbie Scarborough for her assistance in the preparation of this manuscript.

REFERENCES

Bartsch, H. and Hecker, E., 1971, On the metabolic activation of N-hydroxy-N-2-acetylaminoflourene. III. Oxidation with horseradish peroxidase to yield 2-nitrosofluorene and

N-acetoxy-N-2-acetylaminofluorene,   Biochim.   Biophys.
Acta., 237:567-578.
Bartsch, H., Dworkin, M., Miller, J.A., and Miller, E.C.,
1972, Electrophilic N-acetoxyaminoarenes derived from
carcinogenic N-hydroxy-N-acetylaminoarenes by enzymatic
deacetylation and transacetylation in liver, Biochim.
Biophys. Acta., 286: 272-298.
Bartsch, H., Dworkin, C., Miller, E.C., and Miller, J.A.,
1973, Formation of electrophilic N-acetoxyarylamines in
cytosols from rat mammary gland and other tissues by
transacetylation   from   the   carcinogen
N-hydroxy-2-acetylaminobiphenyl, Biochim. Biophys. Acta.,
304: 42-55.
Bengtsson, U., Johansson, S., and Angervall, L., 1978,
Malignancies of the urinary tract and their relation to
analgesic abuse, Kidney Internatl., 13: 107-113.
Bhanot, O.S., Khan, S.A., and Chambers, R.W, 1979, A new
system for studying molecular mechanisms of mutation by
carcinogens, J. Biol. Chem., 254: 12684-12693.
Cardona, R.A. and King, C.M., 1976, Activation of the
O-glucuronide of the carcinogen N-hydroxy-2-fluorenyl-
acetamide by enzymatic deacetylation in vitro: formation
of fluorenylamine - tRNA adducts, Biochem. Pharmacol.,
25: 1051-1056.
Clayson, D.B., and Garner, R.C., 1976, Carcinogenic aromatic
amines and related compounds, in: "Chemical Carcinogens,"
C.E. Searle, ed., American Chemical Society, Washington,
D.C.
Claxton, L. and Husingh, J., 1980, Characterization of the
mutagens associated with diesel particle emissions, 11th
Annual Meeting Environmental Mutagen Society, March
16-19, p. 54.
Coogan, P.S., H.T. Maganini, J.J. Newton, Jr., and G.M. Hass,
1978, Progesterone inhibition of 2-AAF induction of
urogenital tumors in rabbits, Lab. Investigations, 38:
339.
Cramer, J.W., Miller, J.A., and Miller, E.C., 1960,
N-Hydroxylation: a new metabolic reaction observed in
the rat with the carcinogen 2-acetylaminofluorene, J.
Biol. Chem., 235: 885-888.
DeBaun, J.R., Miller, E.C., and Miller, J.A., 1970,
N-Hydroxy-2-acetylaminofluorene sulfotransferase: its
probable role in carcinogenesis and in protein-(methion-
S-yl) binding in rat liver, Cancer Res., 30: 577-595.
Epler, J.L., Rao, T.K., and Larimer, F.W., 1980, Isolation and
identification of mutagenic polycyclic aromatic amines in
synthetic crude oils. 11th Annual Meeting, Environmental
Mutagen Society, March 16-19, p. 54.
Glowinski, I.B., Weber, W.W., Fysh, J.M., Vaught, J.B., and
King, C.M., 1980, Evidence that arylhydroxamic acid

N,O-acyltransferase and the genetically polymorphic N-acetyltransferase are properties of the same enzyme in rabbit liver, J. Biol. Chem., 255: 7883-7890.

Glowinski, I.B., Savage, L., King, C.M., 1981, Relationship between metabolic activation and deacylation of arylhydroxamic acids by liver microsomes of several species, Proc. Am. Can Res., 22:102.

Gutmann, H.R., Malejka-Giganti, D., Barry, E.J., and Rydell, R.E, 1972, On the correlation between the hepatocarcino-genicity of the carcinogen, N-2-fluorenylacetamide, and its metabolic activation by the rat, Cancer Res., 31: 1554-1561.

Hoffman, D. and Wynder, E.L., 1976, Environmental respiratory carcinogenesis, in: "Chemical Carcinogens, ACS Monograph 173," C.E. Searle, ed., American Chemical Society, Washington, D.C.

Howard, P.C., Casciano, D.A., Beland, F.A., and Shaddock, J.G., Jr., 1981, The binding of N-hydroxy-2-acetylamino-fluorene to DNA and repair of the adducts in primary rat hepatocyte cultures, Carcinogenesis., 2: 97-102.

Irving, C.C., 1966, Enzymatic deacetylation of N-hydroxy-2-acetylaminofluorene by liver microsomes, Cancer Res., 26: 1390-1396.

Irving, C.C., 1979, Species and tissue variations in the metabolic activation of aromatic amines, in: "Carcinogens: Identification and Mechanisms of Action," Griffin, A.C. and Shaw, C.R., eds., Raven Press, New York.

Irving, C.C., Janss, D.H., and Russell, L.T., 1971, Lack of N-hydroxy-2-acetylaminofluorene sulfotransferase activity in the mammary gland and Zymbal's gland of the rat, Cancer Res., 31: 387-391.

Irving, C..C., Wiseman, R., Jr., and Hill, J.T., 1967a, Biliary excretion of the O-glucuronide of N-hydroxy-2-acetylaminofluorene by the rat and rabbit, Can Res., 27-2309-2317.

Jarvinen, M., Santti, R.S.S., Hopsu-Havu, V.K., 1979, Partial purification and characterization of two enzymes from guinea pig liver microsomes that hydrolyze carcinogenic amides, 2-acetylaminofluorene and N-hydroxy-2-acetyl-aminofluorene, Biochem. Pharm., 20: 2971-2982.

Kadlubar, F.F., Unruh, L.E., Beland, F.A., Straub, K.M., and Evans, F.A., 1980, In vitro reaction of the carcinogen, N-hydroxy-2-naphthyamine, with DNA at the C-8 and N^2 atoms of guanine and at the N^6 atom of adenine, Carcinogenesis, 1: 139-150.

King, C.M., Allaben, W.T., 1980, Arylhydroxamic acid acyl-transferase, in: "Enzymatic Basis of Detoxication, Vol. II," W. Jakoby, ed., Academic Press, Inc.

King, C.M., and Kriek, E., 1965, The differential reactivity of the oxidation products of o-aminophenols towards protein and nucleic acid. Biochim. Biophys. Acta., 111: 147-153.

King, C.M., and Phillips, B. 1968, Enzyme-catalyzed reactions of the carcinogen N-hydroxy-2-fluorenylacetamide with nucleic acid. Science, 159: 1351-1353.

King, C.M., and Phillips, B., 1969, N-Hydroxy-2-fluorenylacetamide. Reaction of carcinogen with guanosine, ribonucleic acid, deoxyribonucleic acid, and protein following enzymatic deacetylation or esterification, J. Biol. Chem., 244.

King, C.M., Traub, N.R., Cardona, R.A., and Howard, R.B., 1976, Comparative adduct formation of 4-aminobiphenyl and 2-aminofluorene derivatives with macromolecules of isolated liver parenchymal cells, Can. Res., 36: 2374-2381.

King, C.M., Traub, N.R., Lortz, Z.M.,and Thissen, M.R., 1979, Metabolic activation of arylhydroxamic acids by N-O-acyltransferase of rat mammary gland, Can Res., 3369-3372.

Kosuge, T., Tsuji, K., Wakabayashi, K., Okamoto, T., Shudo, K., Iitaka, Y., Itai, A., Sugimura, T., Kawachi, T., Nagao, M., Yahagi, T., and Seino, Y., 1978, Isolation and structural studies of mutagenic principles in amino acid pyrolysates, Chem. Pharm. Bull., 26: 611-619.

Kriek, E., 1965, On the interaction of N-2-fluorenylhydroxylamine with nucleic acids in vitro. Biochem. Biophys. Res. Commun., 20: 793-799.

Kriek, E., Miller, J.A., Juhl, U., and Miller, E.C., 1967, 8-(N-2-Fluorenylacetamido)guanosine, an arylamidation reaction product of guanosine and the carcinogen N-acetoxy-N-2-fluorenylacetamide in neutral solution, Biochemistry, 6: 177.

Kriek, E., and Westra, J.G., 1979, Metabolic activation of aromatic amines and amides and interactions with nucleic acids , in: "Chemical Carcinogens and DNA, Vol. II," Grover, P.L., ed., CRC Press, Inc., Boca Raton, FA.

Lee, M.S., and King, C.M., 1981, New syntheses of N-(guanosin-8-yl)-4-aminobiphenyl and its 5'-monophosphate, Chem. Biol. Interactions, 34: 239-248.

Lofroth, G., 1978, Mutagenicity assay of combustion emissions, Chemosphere, 7: 791-798.

Maher, V.M., Miller, E.C., Miller, J.A., and Szybalski, W., 1968, Mutations and decreases in density of transforming DNA produced by derivatives of the carcinogens 2-acetylaminofluorene and N-methyl-4-aminoazobenzene, Mol. Pharm, 4: 411-426.

Malejka-Giganti, D., and Gutmann, H.R., 1975, N-Hydroxy-2-fluorenylacetamide, an active intermediate of the mammary carcinogen N-hydroxy-2-fluorenylbenzenesulfonamide

(38980), Proc. Soc. Expl. Biol. Med., 150: 92-97.

Mermelstein, R., Kariazides, D.K., Butler, M., McCoy, E.C., and Rosenkranz, H.S., 1981, The extraordinary mutagenicity of nitropyrenes in bacteria, Mutation Res, 89: 187-196.

Miller, E.C., 1978, Some current perspectives on chemical carcinogenesis in humans and experimental animals: presidential address, Cancer Res., 38: 1479-1496.

Miller, E.C., Miller, J.A.., and Hartman, H.A., 1961, N-hydroxy-2-acetylaminofluorene: A metabolite of 2-acetylaminfluorene with increased carcinogenic activity in the rat, Cancer Res., 31: 815-824.

Moore, P., and Strauss, B.S., 1979, Sites of inhibition of in vitro DNA synthesis in carcinogen-and UV-treated φ X174 DNA, Nature, 278: 664-666.

Morton, K.C., Wang, C.Y., Garner, C.D., and Shirai, T., 1981, Carcinogenicity of benzidine, N,N'-diacetylbenzidine, and N-hydroxy-N-N'-diacetylbenzidine for female CD rats, Carcinogenesis, 2: 747-752.

National Cancer Institute, 1978a Bioassay of aniline hydrochloride for possible carcinogenicity, CAS No. 142-04-1, NIC-CG-TR-130.

National Cancer Institute, 1978b Bioassay of o-Anisidine hydrochloride for possible carcinogenicity, CAS NO. 134-29-0, NCI-CG-TR-89.

Neumann, H.G., 1980, On the significance of metabolic activation and binding to nucleic acids of aminostilbene derivatives in vivo, Natl. Cancer Inst. Monogr., in press.

Parkes, H.G., 1976, "The epidemiology of the aromatic amine cancers in: Chemical carcinogens, C.E. Searle, ed., Am. Chem. Soc., Washington, D.C.

Pitts, J.A., Jr., Van Cauwenberghe, K.S., Grosjean, D., Schmid, J.P., Fitz, D.R., Belser, W.L., Jr., Knudson, G.B., and Hynds, P.M., 1978, Atmospheric reactions of polycyclic aromatic hydrocarbons: facile formation of mutagenic nitro derivatives, Science, 202: 515-519.

Scribner, D.L., and McCloskey, J.A., 1978, Deamination of 1-methylcytosine by the carcinogen N-acetoxy-4-acetamido stilbene: Implications for hydrocarbon carcinogenesis, J. of Organic Chem, 43: 2085.

Shirai, T., Fysh, J.M., Lee, M.S., Vaught, J.B.,and King, C.M., 1981a, N-hydroxy-N-acylarylamines: relationship of metabolic activation to biological response in the liver and mammary gland of the female CD rat, Cancer Res: 41: 4346-4353.

Shirai, T., and King, C.M., 1981b, Relationship of H-thymidine incorporation to the metabolic activation of arylhydroxamic acids by rat hepatocytes, Proc. Am Assoc. Can Res: 22: 99.

Shirai, T., Lee, M.S., Wang, C.Y., King, C.M., 1981c, Effects of partial hepatectomy and dietary phenobarbital on liver and mammary tumorigenesis by two N-hydroxy-N-acylamino-biphenyls in female CD rats, Cancer Res., 41: 2350-2456.

Thorgeirsson, S.S., Wirth, P.J., Nelson, W.L., and Lambert, G.H., 1977, Genetic regulation of metabolism and mutagenicity of 2-acetylaminofluorene and related compounds in mice, in: "Origins of Human Cancer,"Hiatt, Watson, Winsten, eds., Cold Spring Harbor, NY.

Vaught, J.B., Lee, M.S., Shayman, M.A., Thissen, M.R., and King, C.M, 1981, Arylhydroxylamine-induced ribonucleic acid chain cleavage and chromatographic analysis of arylamine ribonucleic acid adducts, Chem. Biol Interactions, 34: 109-124.

Wang, C.Y., Lee, M.S., King, C.M., and Warner, P.O., 1980, Evidence for nitroaromatics as direct-acting mutagens as airborne particulates, Chemosphere, 9: 83-87.

Weber, W.W., 1973, Acetylation of drugs, in: "Metabolic conjugation and metabolic hydrolysis", W.H. Fishman, ed., Academic Press, New York.

Weeks, C.E., Allaben, W.T., Louie, S.C., Lazear, E.J., and King, C.M., 1978, Role of arylhydroxamic acid acyltransferase in the mutagenicity of N-hydroxy-N-2-fluorenylacetamide in Salmonella typhimurium, Cancer Res., 38: 613-618.

Weeks, C.E., Allaben, W.T., Tresp, N.M., Louis, S.C., Lazear, E.J., and King, C.M., 1980, Effects of structure of N-acyl-N-2-fluorenylhyroxylamines on arylhydroxamic acid acyltransferase, sulfotransferase and deacylase activities, and on mutations in Salmonella Typhimurium TA 1538, Cancer Res., 40: 1204-1211.

Wirth, P.J., and Thorgeirsson, S.S., 1980, Mechanism of N-hydroxy-2-acetylaminofluorene mutagenicity in the Salmonella test system, role of N-O-acyltransferase and sulfotransferase from rat liver, Mol. Pharm: 19: 337-344.

Wu, S-C.G., and Straub, K.D., 1976,. Purification and characterization of N-hydroxy-2-acetylaminofluorene sulfotransferase from rat liver, J. Biol. Chem., 251: 6529-6536.

Zavon, M.R., Hoegg, R., and Bingham, E., 1973, Benzidine exposure as a cause of bladder tumors, Arch. Environ. Health, 27: 1-7.

Zenser, T.V., Mattammal, M.B., Armbrecht, H.J., and Davis, B.B., 1980, Benzidine binding to nucleic acids mediated by the peroxidative activity of prostaglandin endoperoxide synthetase, Can Res., 40: 2839-2845.

METABOLIC EPOXIDATION OF AFLATOXIN B_1 AND ITS METABOLITES: PATTERNS OF DNA ADDUCT FORMATION AND REMOVAL IN RELATION TO BIOLOGICAL EFFECTS

John M. Essigmann, Robert G. Croy[1]
Richard A. Bennett[2] and Gerald N. Wogan

Laboratory of Toxicology
Department of Nutrition and Food Science
Massachusetts Institute of Technology
Cambridge, MA 02139

[1] Present Address: Sidney Farber Cancer Institute
Harvard Medical School, Boston, MA 02144

[2] Present Address: Milton S. Hershey Medical Center
Hershey, PA 17033

INTRODUCTION

Aflatoxin B_1 (AFB_1) is the most toxic and carcinogenic member of a family of difuranocoumarins produced as secondary metabolites by strains of <u>Aspergillus flavus</u> and related fungi[1]. Exposure to aflatoxin is a public health hazard in technologically developing areas of the world, where AFB_1-producing fungi are distributed widely and where food production and storage conditions are conducive to mold spoilage and consequent mycotoxin production. In most animals, the main target for the biological effects of AFB_1 is the liver, although the relative sensitivity of different animal species varies markedly; the rat, rainbow trout and duck are highly sensitive whereas the mouse is resistant. The liver is also apparently a target in humans, in that a high incidence of hepatocellular carcinoma has been observed in chronically exposed populations[2]. Additional factors may act in concert in initiating the putative carcinogenic effects of AFB_1 in humans; these include abnormal nutritional status or concomitant pathological conditions such as viral hepatitis.

In recent years we have been examining the metabolism and macromolecular-binding characteristics of AFB_1 with the objective of determining how these factors relate to its biological effects in animals and humans. We have emphasized studying the interactions of metabolically activated forms of carcinogens with DNA, an approach engendered by the key role of this macromolecule as the cellular repository of genetic information. Thus, it represents an inherently reasonable site at which chemical damage by carcinogen-DNA adduct formation can be fixed biologically. In a mechanistic sense, the presence of adducts could lead to temporary alteration in the regulation of gene function, or it could abnormally affect the fidelity of transcription or replication. Alternatively, structural modification of DNA by covalent adduct formation might cause gene rearrangement or result in the induction of an error-prone repair process and thus indirectly cause fixation of the molecular lesion. It is our working hypothesis that aflatoxin adducts somehow alter the functional properties of DNA, most likely by mechanisms initiated by somatic cell mutation. Ultimately, these initiating events may result in transformation of normal cells into cancer cells, albeit by processes that are not well understood at present.

This review summarizes the current status of our efforts toward developing an understanding of the molecular mechanisms underlying the biological effects of AFB_1. We will describe the biochemical pathways through which aflatoxin is activated and becomes bound to DNA, with the specific objective of relating the qualitative, quantitative and kinetic features of binding to initiating events in carcinogenesis.

PATHWAYS OF METABOLIC ACTIVATION OF AFLATOXIN B_1 AND FORMATION OF DNA ADDUCTS

Metabolism is required to convert AFB_1 to chemically reactive, DNA-binding forms that presumably are responsible for its potent biological effects. (Known transformations of AFB_1 are summarized in Fig. 1.) The predominant AFB_1 metabolite that binds to DNA in animal and human tissues is the AFB_1-2,3-oxide[3-8]. The stereochemistry of this epoxide was determined through in vitro studies[5], and it is evident that the mixed function oxidase activity that biotransforms AFB_1 stereoselectively produces the β or exo isomer. The epoxide possesses such a high degree of reactivity that it has never been isolated, despite numerous attempts to do so in this laboratory and others. Its structure was established mainly on the basis of indirect evidence, including identification of the AFB_1-2,3-dihydrodiol as an acid degradation product of AFB_1-modified RNA and DNA[3,4], and identification of the absolute structure of the primary adduct that the epoxide forms upon interaction with guanyl residues in DNA[5,6].

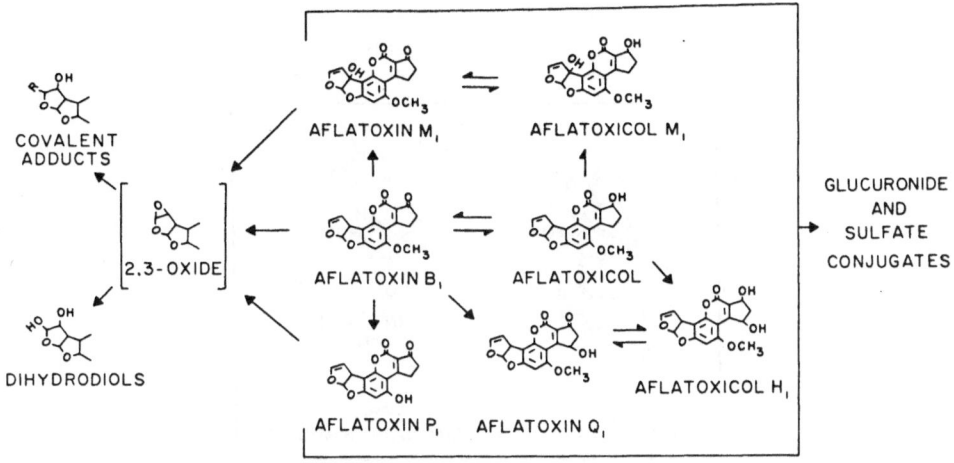

Fig. 1.   Pathways of metabolism of aflatoxin B₁.

The major aflatoxin-DNA adduct that forms in vivo in liver or other tissues of animals, and in vitro in the presence of DNA and a metabolic activation system is 2,3-dihydro-2-(N^7-guanyl)-3-hydroxy-aflatoxin B₁ (AFB₁-N^7-Gua; [5-9]).   The absolute structure of this adduct has been established unambiguously (Fig. 2).   An important analytical tool used to isolate and identify this and other aflatoxin adducts is high-pressure liquid chromatography (HPLC), and Fig. 3 depicts an HPLC separation of hydrolysis products isolated from the liver of a rat injected with [³H]-AFB₁ (0.6 mg/kg) and killed 2 hr later.

The various peaks in the chromatogram account for more than 99% of the radioactivity covalently bound to DNA, and the AFB₁-N^7-Gua product comprises approximately 80% of the DNA adducts that are present.

Recent investigations have resulted in complete structural identification of the second most abundant adduct in DNA, the adduct denoted as peak G in Fig. 3.   This adduct is 2,3-dihydro-2-(N^5-formyl)-2',5',6'-triamino-4'oxo-N^5-pyrimidyl-3-hydroxyaflatoxin B₁ (AFB₁-formamidopyrimidine), a derivative of AFB₁-N^7-Gua that forms in the intracellular environment.   It constitutes approximately 7% of the AFB₁-derived radioactivity in Fig. 3.   The formation of this adduct is attributed to the positive charge that exists in the imidazole ring of AFB₁-N^7-Gua in DNA (Fig. 4).   Our early work on this DNA adduct showed that the charged structure resulted in a destabilized deoxyglycosidic bond, which was highly susceptible to hydrolysis[5].   It was later discovered by Lin et al.[6]

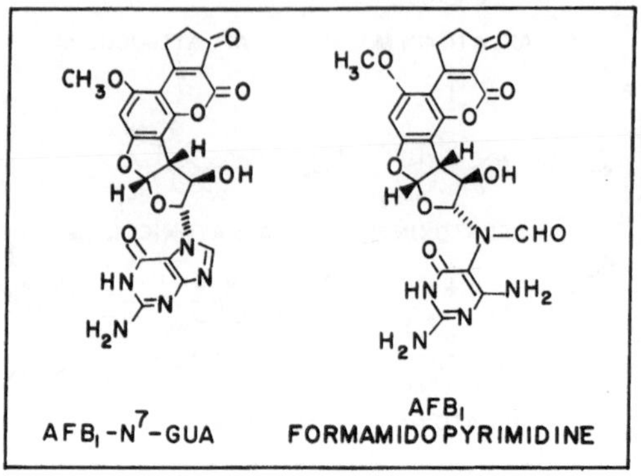

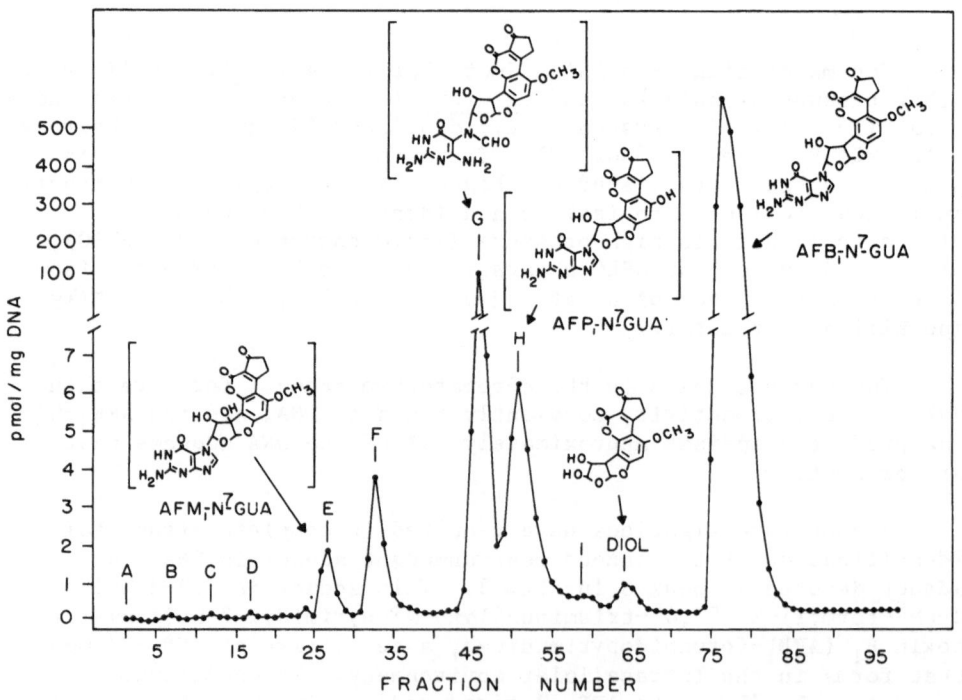

Fig. 2.   Absolute structures of aflatoxin-DNA component adducts.

Fig. 3.   DNA adducts formed from AFB$_1$ in rat liver.

that this structure also rendered the charged imidazole ring of guanine susceptible to attack by hydroxide ion at C-8, resulting initially in a carbinolamine derivative that ultimately rearranged through imidazole ring opening to an AFB_1-formamidopyrimidine structure. On the basis of NMR, mass spectral and other data we recently have assigned the absolute structure of adduct G as shown in Fig. 2. We therefore establish the structure postulated by the Millers and co-workers[6]. One of the interesting consequences of imidazole ring opening is the fact that the bond linking the AFB_1-formamidopyrimidine to the deoxyribose of the DNA backbone becomes chemically stabilized, a property of potentially great biological significance. On purely chemical grounds, one would expect this adduct to be stable in DNA, whereas AFB_1-N^7-Gua would have a tendency to depurinate. This in fact was found to be the case as will be shown in a later section where the rates of formation and removal of individual adducts are described.

A total of 12 peaks containing AFB_1-derived radioactivity can

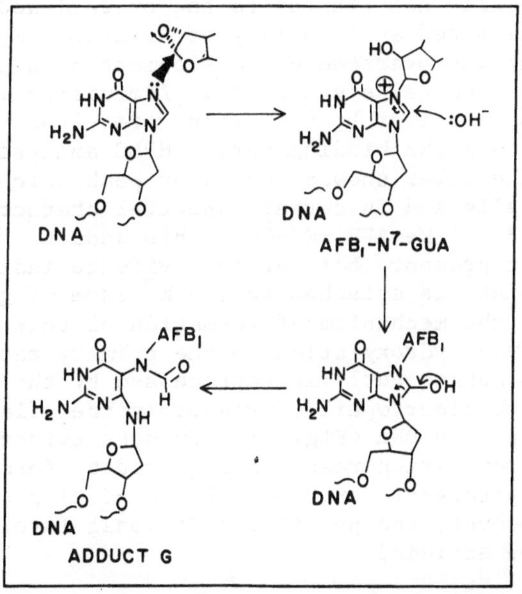

Fig. 4. Mechanism of conversion of the major AFB_1-DNA adduct, AFB_1-N^7-Gua, to its formamidopyromidne derivative, adduct G.

be identified in Fig. 3. As indicated above, the AFB_1-N^7-Gua and AFB_1-formamidopyrimidine (peak G) adducts are the major components, and only these adducts have been unambiguously characterized. However, a considerable amount of evidence drawn from several related lines of investigation enables us to make reasonable structural proposals for nearly all of the remaining DNA-bound derivatives of AFB_1. This evidence, which will be published in full elsewhere, can be summarized as follows.

Peak H in Fig. 3 has properties consistent with those of an adduct formed by metabolic activation of aflatoxin P_1, a known metabolite of AFB_1 that results from O-demethylation (Fig. 1). Aflatoxin P_1 previously was thought to represent a polar detoxification product of AFB_1, but this conclusion must now be reevaluated in light of present evidence that it can undergo further metabolism to a DNA-binding form. Preliminary structural data on this adduct are consistent with a structure formed by attack of the N^7 atom of guanine on the aflatoxin $P_1-2,3$-oxide. Thus, this adduct provisionally has been identified as 2,3-dihydro-2-$(N^7$-guanyl)-3-hydroxyaflatoxin AFP_1 (AFP_1-N^7-Gua).

Similarly, another well-characterized hydroxylated AFB_1 metabolite, aflatoxin M_1, possesses an epoxidizable double bond and thus potentially contributes to the overall adduct pattern. The problem of limited availability of aflatoxin M_1 for metabolic studies recently was overcome by development of a procedure for its large-scale chemical synthesis[10]. Administration of racemic aflatoxin M_1 to rat liver by perfusion[11] resulted in its bio-transformation to a DNA-binding form. HPLC analysis of DNA isolated from the liver showed one major peak which was identical chromatographically and in certain spectral characteristics to peak E in Fig. 3. Like AFP_1-N^7-Gua, this adduct is incompletely characterized at present, but current evidence indicates that the aflatoxin M_1 moiety is attached to the N^7 atom of guanine. We have postulated that the mechanism of formation of this adduct from AFB_1 initially involves hydroxylation to the primary metabolite, afla-toxin M_1, which subsequently is reprocessed by the liver to generate a highly reactive electrophile, presumably the aflatoxin $M_1-2,3$-oxide, which binds to DNA (Fig. 1). Present evidence indicates that the initial hydroxylation reaction required to form 2,3-dihydro-2-$(N^7$-guanyl)-3-hydroxyaflatoxin M_1 (AFM_1-N^7-Gua) probably occurs in the liver[11]; however, the possible additional involvement of other organs cannot be excluded.

Two hours after the rat is dosed with AFB_1, the putative AFM_1-N^7-Gua and AFP_1-N^7-Gua adducts represent 2.2 and 3.8%, respectively, of the total DNA adducts in liver DNA (peaks E and H in Fig. 3). The discovery that formation of these adducts involved substitution of guanine at N^7, with concomitant introduction of a

positive charge into the imidazole ring, provided a clue as to
the structure of two additio'al adducts. Imidazole ring-opening
mediated by hydroxide ion attack on these guanine adducts would
be expected by a mechanism analogous to that postulated in Fig. 4
for formation of adduct G from AFB_1-N^7-Gua. This was confirmed
by treating DNA containing AFM_1 and AFP_1 adducts with alkali.
Subsequent chromatographic analyses of the DNA hydrolysates indicated that the AFM_1-N^7-Gua and AFP_1-N^7-Gua adducts had been almost
quantitatively converted to more polar derivatives that comigrated
with products formed in vivo; these products eluted in the region
of peaks A-E (Fig. 3).

The structure of peak F presently is unknown, although Lin
et al.[6] recently suggested that it may be an AFB_1-N^7-Gua derivative
with an hydroxylated imidazole ring, i.e., the carbinolamine
derivative shown in Fig. 4. Our structural data are insufficient
to differentiate this possibility from others. However, we have
observed that incubation of a purified preparation of peak G at
room temperature resulted in formation of an equilibrium mixture
of both peaks G and F. Similarly incubated peak F produced
exactly the same relative amounts of peaks G and F. Thus, these
adducts are in equilibrium. The same equilibrium relationship has
been established for the putative formamidopyrimidine derivatives
of the AFM_1-N^7-Gua and AFP_1-N^7-Gua adducts, and two other polar
peaks in the A-E region of Fig. 3.

Collectively, therefore, unambiguous or tentative structural
data are available for most of the DNA adducts that form in the
livers of rats injected with AFB_1. This information strongly supports the generalization that the N^7 atom of guanyl residues is
the principal (if not exclusive) target in DNA for metabolically
activated AFB_1 or its metabolites. Furthermore, the main biochemical event leading to production of DNA bound forms of aflatoxin
is epoxidation of the vinyl bond in the terminal furan ring.

DNA ADDUCTS AND ORGANOTROPISM IN THE RAT

Following identification of the major AFB_1-DNA adducts and
with the availability of sensitive analytical methodology to
detect and quantify minor DNA-bound AFB_1 derivatives, we have
applied this experimental approach in evaluating possible relationships between qualitative and quantitative features of adduct
formation and organotropic effects of AFB_1 in rats[12]. Among the
noteworthy features of AFB_1 carcinogenesis in rats is the high
degree of specificity with which it induces tumors and toxic
lesions in the liver. In marked contrast, over a period of many
years we have observed neither tumors nor other treatment-related
histopathologic changes in the kidneys of large numbers of Fischer

rats treated with AFB_1. Therefore, it seemed justifiable to compare liver and kidneys as representative of target and non-target tissues in this rat strain.

[^{3}H]-AFB_1 was injected into male Fischer rats at a dose of 1 mg/kg body weight, and the animals were killed two hr later. Nuclei were isolated from livers and kidneys, and nucleic acids were in turn isolated from the nuclei and total DNA-bound radioactivity was determined. DNA was hydrolyzed, analyzed by HPLC and the distribution of radioactivity in components of the chromatogram was determined. A typical chromatogram for liver DNA is shown in Fig. 3, and that for kidney was qualitatively very similar.

Levels of individual adducts present in the kidney DNA were only about 10% of their levels in liver, as indicated by the maximal concentration of AFB_1-N^7-Gua, i.e., 120 µmole/mg DNA x 10^{-7}. Six of the ten minor peaks identified in the liver (E, F, G, H, I and diol) have been quantified in the kidney. These products represented a higher proportion of the adducts in the kidney (30%) than the liver (20%) with peak H (AFP_1-N^7-Gua) increasing in the largest amount. Thus, it appears that virtually the same spectrum of DNA adducts is produced from AFB_1 in the non-target (kidney) as in the target tissue (liver). However, the total level of binding, and therefore of each of the adducts, was greatly reduced in the non-target tissue.

SPECIES SUSCEPTIBILITY AND AFB_1-DNA ADDUCT PATTERNS

A similar approach was used for investigating DNA adducts formed in tissues of the Swiss mouse, a species with a high level of resistance to the hepatocarcinogenic effects of AFB_1[1]. [^{3}H]-AFB_1 was injected into adult male Swiss mice at a dose of 12 mg/kg of body weight. This dose presents an acute toxicity that is approximately equal to that produced by the 1 mg/kg dose given in the rat experiment described above. As in the rat experiment, DNA was isolated from liver and kidneys, hydrolyzed and subjected to HPLC analysis.

The chromatogram of mouse liver DNA in its main features was qualitatively similar to that of rat liver, in that the major components (AFB_1-N^7-Gua and peaks F, G, and H) were prominently represented. The most striking feature of the adduct pattern, however, was the very low level at which even the major adducts were present. The major component, AFB_1-N^7-Gua, had a concentration of only about 12 µmoles/mg DNA x 10^{-7}, in the order of 0.1% of the level of the same adduct in rat liver DNA. The other adducts were proportionately reduced. These results indicate that mouse liver activates AFB_1 essentially through the same

pathways as rat liver and either has a very limited capacity for
activation or possesses a very efficient pathway for removal of
adducts that form as a result of activation.

The adduct pattern seen in mouse kidney was also very similar
in character to that of rat kidney, differing principally in the
absence of several of the minor peaks. However, the concentration
of the major adducts was significantly higher in mouse kidney than
in mouse liver. The major adduct attained a concentration
approaching 80 μmoles/mg DNA x 10^{-7}, of comparable magnitude to
the level of the same component in rat kidney (120 μmoles/mg
DNA x 10^{-7}).

The main quantitative features of these experiments relating
to tissue specificity and species responsiveness can be summarized
as follows: in terms of total AFB_1 binding levels in DNA, the
greatest difference occurred in adduct levels in rat and mouse
liver. Rat liver DNA contained adducts at a total level of 114
AFB_1 residue per 10^6 nucleotides whereas the comparable value for
mouse liver was 2 per 10^6. DNA from kidneys of the two species
contained adducts at more similar concentrations, 13 AFB_1 per 10^6
nucleotides in the rat, and 7 per 10^6 in the mouse.

When these total binding levels are fractionated to take into
account the levels of individual adducts in accordance with the
HPLC data, the range of levels for individual components is very
large, as illustrated in the data in Table 1. The extremes of the
range are indicated by the maximum concentration of AFB_1-N^7-Gua in
the rat liver (91 adducts per 10^6 nucleotides) and the maximum
level of peak D in mouse liver (0.03 AFB_1 residue per 10^6 nucleotides). At this time, evidence is insufficient to postulate
whether any of these adducts have greater functional significance
than others.

In summarizing these observations relating adduct formation
to tissue specificity and species difference in response, differential ability to activate AFB_1 to its ultimate DNA binding form,
the 2,3-oxide, may play a role in determining the known tissue
specificity for toxicity and carcinogenicity in the Fischer rat.
Liver, the target tissue, and kidney, the non-target tissue,
produced qualitatively similar patterns of DNA adducts, although
there is difference in total binding level in the two tissues of
about 10-fold.

A comparable conclusion is supported by the experiments
in mice. The great resistance of mouse liver to the toxic and
carcinogenic effects of AFB_1 cannot be attributed to a lack of
metabolic competence for AFB_1 activation, since the spectrum of
DNA adducts produced in mouse liver and kidney is generally simi-

Table 1. Quantitative Relationships Among Acid Hydrolysis
Products of DNA Modified by AFB_1 in vivo

AFB_1 Residues per 10^6 Bases[a]

HPLC Peak	Liver[b]		Kidney[c]	
	Rat	Mouse	Rat	Mouse
A	0.2	--	--	--
B	0.2	--	--	--
C	0.2	0.06	--	--
D	0.4	0.03	--	--
E	2.3	0.03	0.2	--
F	3.7	0.1	0.2	0.3
AFB_1-FAPY	7.7	0.2	0.6	0.2
H,I	6.7	0.3	2.3	--
Diol	1.6	0.2	0.2	0.08
AFB_1-N^7-Gua	91.0	1.0	9.1	6.6
TOTAL	114	2	13	7

[a]Binding level determined 2 hr after dosing with AFB_1 at levels of
1 (rats) or 12 (mice) mg/kg.

[b]Mean of 3 determinations.

[c]Mean of 2 determinations.

lar to that present in rat tissues. However, in this case, the differential in total binding levels is very large (> 100-fold) compared to the rat.

KINETICS OF DNA ADDUCT FORMATION IN RAT LIVER FOLLOWING A SINGLE AFB₁ DOSE

With the availability of sensitive analytical methodology to detect and quantify minor DNA-bound AFB_1 derivatives, it was of interest to apply this experimental approach in studying relationships between the kinetics of adduct formation and removal in rat liver under conditions of dosing which produce well-characterized biological or biochemical effects in this tissue[13]. Initial experiments examined the population of DNA adducts present at various times after a single sublethal dose of AFB_1 (0.6 mg/kg).

$[^3H]$-AFB_1 was injected into male Fischer rats and groups of animals were killed 2, 4, 12, 24, 48, and 72 hr later. Nuclei were isolated from the livers, DNA was in turn isolated from the nuclei and total DNA-bound radioactivity was determined. DNA was hydrolyzed, and the hydrolysate was analyzed by HPLC.

The earliest sampling point (2 hr after dosing) was chosen on the basis of numerous previous investigations indicating that most biochemical effects induced by AFB_1 are maximal at this time. Animals killed at 2 hr showed the following pattern of binding. In quantitative terms, the total level of binding was one AFB_1 residue per 11,000 nucleotides, and AFB_1-N^7-Gua, the major adduct, was present at a level of one adduct per 14,000 nucleotides. The next most abundant adducts were peaks G (1 per 160,000) and F (1 per 350,000). Peak B was the least abundant, with a frequency of one adduct per 1.3×10^8 nucleotides, a level which represents approximately the limit of sensitivity of the analytical methodology under conditions applied in these experiments.

Liver DNA of animals killed at later time points revealed marked alterations in relative adduct levels, as shown in Fig. 5. AFB_1-N^7-Gua levels declined rapidly with an apparent half-life of 7.5 hr from an initial value of about 22,000 µmoles/mg DNA x 10^{-8} at 2 hr to 26 at 72 hr; these levels represent more than 90% and less than 1% of total bound radioactivity, respectively. Peaks H (the putative AFP_1-N^7-Gua) and E (AFM_1-N^7-Gua) declined with similar kinetics. In contrast, peaks G (the imidazole ring-opened derivative of AFB_1-N^7-Gua) and the related F remained at relatively constant levels after an initial increase during the 4- to 12-hr period. Thus, the greater stability predicted for the ring-opened form of the AFB_1-N^7-Gua adduct is substantiated by these observations.

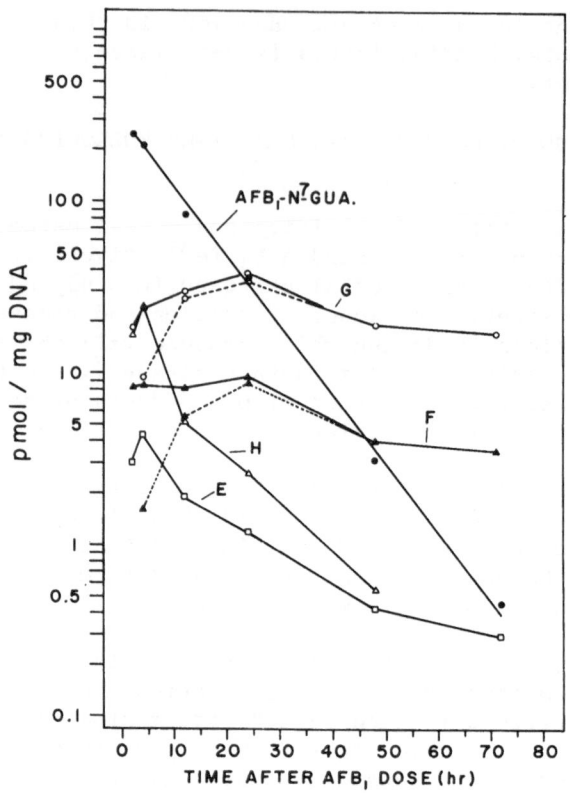

Fig. 5. DNA adduct levels in rat liver following a single dose of
0.125 mg AFB_1/kg body weight.

RAT LIVER ADDUCT PATTERNS FOLLOWING REPEATED AFB_1 DOSING

        It is well established that a single AFB_1 dose is not an
efficient carcinogenic regimen so the relevance of the findings
discussed above to initiating events in carcinogenesis is uncertain.
However, a dosing regimen of small repeated doses can effectively
induce hepatocellular carcinoma in every animal treated with
appropriate total dose levels. We therefore investigated DNA
adduct formation in livers of rats dosed according to a schedule
known to be an effective carcinogenic regimen.

        During a 14-day period, 25 µg of [^{3}H]-AFB_1 (0.125 mg/kg) was
administered i.p. in 25 µl of DMSO to rats on days 0, 1, 2, 3, 4,
7, 8, 9, 10, and 11 (no AFB_1 was given on days 5, 6, 12, and 13).
Two rats were sacrificed each day 24 hr after dosing, and the DNA
of their livers isolated, hydrolyzed, and analyzed chromatographi-

cally. With the exception of day 0, animals were not administered
AFB_1 on the day of sacrifice.

Figure 6 shows the chromatographic profile of AFB_1-DNA
hydrolysis products in rat liver, 2 hr after the injection of the
initial 25 μg dose of AFB_1 (day 0). This chromatogram is similar
to Fig. 3, where rats were treated with 0.6 mg/kg. In quantitative terms, the levels of each peak ranged from 1.9×10^{-5}
modifications/base (50,000 bases/modification) for AFB_1-N^7-Gua to
4.0×10^{-9} modifications/base (25×10^{-7} bases/modification), for
peak D which represented less than 0.1% of the covalently bound
material. After the 2-hr period, 7.3×10^{-5} moles of AFB_1 were
covalently bound per milligram of DNA. Assuming 12 mg of DNA per
liver, a total of 8.8×10^{-4} moles of AFB_1 was covalently associated with liver DNA 2 hr after dosing. This is approximately 1%
of the administered dose of 8.0×10^{-2} moles of AFB_1.

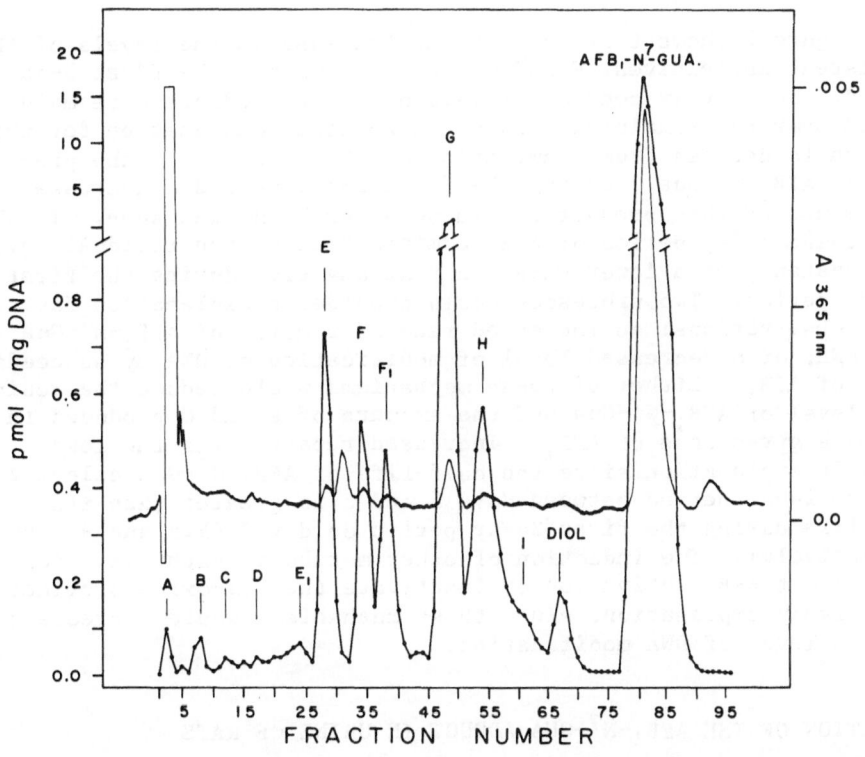

Fig. 6. HPLC chromatogram of AFB_1-DNA adducts 2 hr after a single
dose of 0.125 mg AFB_1/kg body weight. Upper curve A_{365}; lower [³H].

highest concentration in DNA and attained a relatively constant
level of 1.8×10^{-5} μmoles/mg DNA at the end of the first 5-day
dosing period. Its level did not significantly change with cessation of dosing on days 5 and 6, or during the second dosing
period, days 7 through 11. A similar behavior was seen with peak
F, at a lower level of modification.

The amount of AFB_1-N^7-Gua remaining 24 hr after the AFB_1
administration showed a gradual decline during the first 5-day
period. On day 6, 48 hr after cessation of dosing, a precipitous
decline in the residual level was seen, which was further apparent
on day 7, 72 hr after the last AFB_1 dose. Resumption of treatment
on day 7, for a second 5-day period, resulted in an increase on
day 8 to approximately 10 times the level seen on day 7. This
level remained constant during this period until day 13, when
dosing was again stopped and a second sharp decline in the residual
amount of AFB_1-N^7-Gua occurred.

The level of peak E and other minor products, B, C, D, E, I,
and diol, remained relatively constant throughout the entire period.

Figure 7 shows that most of the increase in the levels of the
persistent derivatives, F and G, occurred within the first 5-day
period. Relatively constant levels of these products were maintained over the remaining 9 days. A possible explanation for this
pattern is derived from examination of the kinetics of the precursor, AFB_1-N^7-Gua. During the first 5-day period a decrease in
the amount of this product remaining after 24 hr was seen. In the
subsequent 5-day period of AFB_1 administration, the residual level
was constant, at a lower value than at any time during the first
dosing period. Two processes could provide an explanation for
these observations: an increased rate of removal of AFB_1-N^7-Gua
from DNA; or a decreased level of modification of DNA by succeeding
doses of AFB_1. Either of these mechanisms would reduce the residual level of AFB_1-N^7-Gua and the amounts of F and G produced in
DNA by a given dose of AFB_1. Increased repair seems the less
probable explanation since the half-life of AFB_1-N^7-Gua calculated
for the 24-hr period between days 5 and 6 is greater than its
half-life during the first 24-hr period on day 0 (5.5 and 9.0 hr,
respectively). The induction of other metabolic pathways which
would limit AFB_1 activation or inactivate the 2,3-oxide provides a
more likely explanation, since these mechanisms would decrease the
initial level of DNA modification.

EXCRETION OF THE AFB_1-N^7-GUA ADDUCT IN URINE OF RATS

In the beginning of this review an assumption was made that
the nucleic acid interactions described herein bear some relevance

The kinetics of removal of this material during the first
24-hr period were similar to those described previously for a 0.6
mg/kg body weight dose. After 24 hr, 88% of the covalently bound
AFB_1 had been removed from DNA. The remaining 12% was found primarily in 3 peaks, F, G and AFB_1-N^7-Gua, containing 11, 51, and
34% respectively of this residual material. The remaining 4% was
distributed among 7 other peaks containing 1% or less in each.
During the 2-week period the three major peaks accounted for
greater than 90% of the AFB_1 derivatives hydrolyzed from DNA.

Figure 7 shows the levels of G, F and AFB_1-N^7-Gua hydrolyzed
from rat liver DNA during the 2-week period. Peak E (the putative
AFM_1-N^7-Gua) is included in this figure to be representative of
the relative levels of the minor AFB_1 hydrolysis products in
relation to the three major adducts. Peak G was present at the

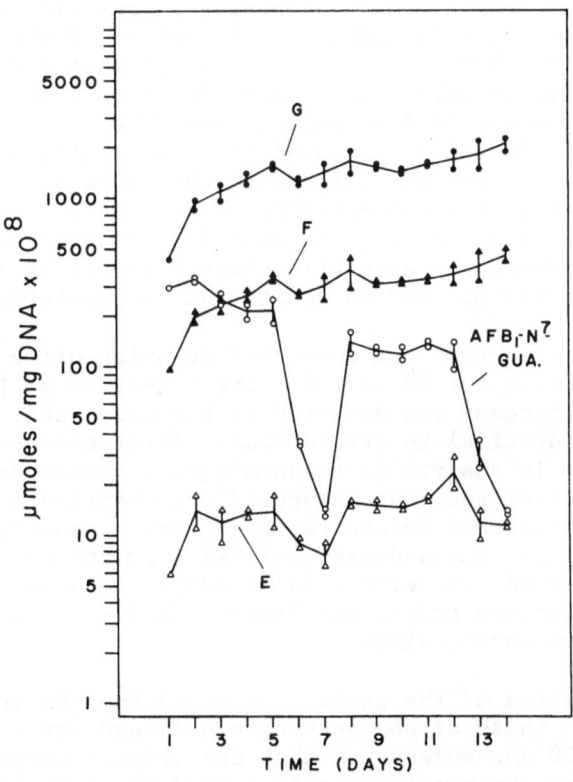

Fig. 7.   DNA adduct levels in liver of rats repeatedly dosed with
AFB_1 (0.125 mg/kg) on days 0-4 and 7-11. Animals were killed 24 hr
after dosing.

to the carcinogenic effects of AFB_1. Indeed, the data on adduction in animal tissues presented in the preceding sections appear to support this hypothesis. As a first step toward extending this approach to risk assessment in human populations, we have begun to adapt our analytical strategy, developed originally for adducted DNA analysis, to search for the products of adduct removal from nucleic acids in easily accessible body fluids. In view of the rapid kinetics of removal of the major DNA adduct from rat liver DNA, we began this line of research by exploring the possibility that AFB_1-N^7-Gua was excreted in the urine. If excreted and measurable, quantification of this adduct could provide the basis for a non-invasive method for assessment of AFB_1 body-burden as well as information on metabolic activation and DNA repair capability. A suitably sensitive and quantitative method would have potential application for monitoring human populations for aflatoxin exposure.

A method for isolation of AFB_1-N^7-Gua from urine was developed and subsequently applied to monitoring the excretion of this adduct from AFB_1-treated rats[14]. Rigorous evaluation of the method for recovering AFB_1-N^7-Gua from rat urine showed that the method was applicable for accurately quantifying adduct in samples containing 50 ng adduct or more; smaller amounts could be determined semi-quantitatively. At the 50 ng level of sensitivity, quantification of AFB_1-N^7-Gua in urine was based upon the spectral properties of the adduct and not upon the presence of a radioactive label. Therefore, the method does not require administration of radioactive carcinogen, an obviously essential characteristic in a procedure that eventually may be used to monitor human populations.

A preliminary study was conducted in which urine was collected from rats for 48 hr following injection of $[^{14}C]-AFB_1$. A radioactive compound was detected in the urine that was chromatographically identical to AFB_1-N^7-Gua. After necessary refinements were made in analytical methodology, a chromatographic procedure was developed that separated the putative adduct from potentially interfering UV-absorbing urinary compounds (Fig. 8). Subsequently, this compound was isolated from the combined urines of 15 rats injected i.p. with 1 mg/kg AFB_1. An estimated total of 3.6 µg of putative adduct was isolated and submitted to an abbreviated structure analysis.

The UV spectra of the urinary compound in both acid and base were similar to those of the authentic compound for wavelengths greater than 300 nm, suggesting that the urinary compound contained aflatoxin. This observation was in accordance with the appearance of radiolabel in this compound following the injection of labeled AFB_1. The lack of a bathochromic shift in alkali indicated that the putative urinary adduct was not a 2-hydroxyaflatoxin derivative.

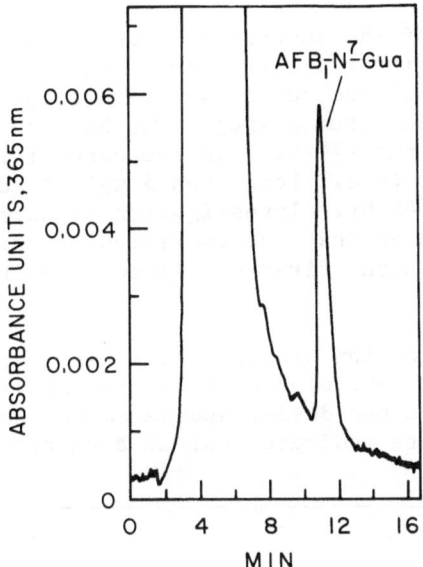

Fig. 8. Chromatogram showing the final purification of AFB_1-N^7-Gua from the urine of a rat injected with AFB_1.

The presence of guanine in the putative urinary adduct was demonstrated by methylation of the adduct and subsequent perch-loric acid hydrolysis of the methylated product. The methylation was performed under conditions which afford selective methylation of the imidazole nitrogen atoms of guanine, and the only detec-table methylated guanine derivative formed from either authentic or putative urinary adduct was 9-methylguanine. This result is consistent with the assumption that the urinary compound con-tained guanine and that the guanine was substituted by the afla-toxin moiety at the 7-position at the time of methylation[5].

Taken together, the results of the methylation and the spectral analyses argue strongly that the urinary compound contains an AFB_1

derivative covalently bound to the N^7 atom of guanine. Thus, the urinary compound is identical to authentic AFB_1-N^7-Gua by these criteria.

Determination of the amounts of adduct excreted by rats at various times following i.p. AFB_1 administration indicated that at a 1 mg/kg dose, 80% of the total excretion of adduct occurred during a 48-hr period after dosing. The balance of adduct excretion occurred between 48 and 144 hr. In the case of a 0.25 mg/kg dose, no detectable levels (i.e., less than 5 ng) of adduct were observed at times later than 48 hr. Investigation of adduct excretion at shorter times indicated that the excretion of this compound occurred to an equal extent in the first and second days following AFB_1 administration.

Because the excretion of adduct was nearly complete in 48 hr, the amounts of adduct excreted by this time at various dose levels were used to generate the dose-response curve shown in Fig. 9. These preliminary data indicate that an accurate dose-excretion

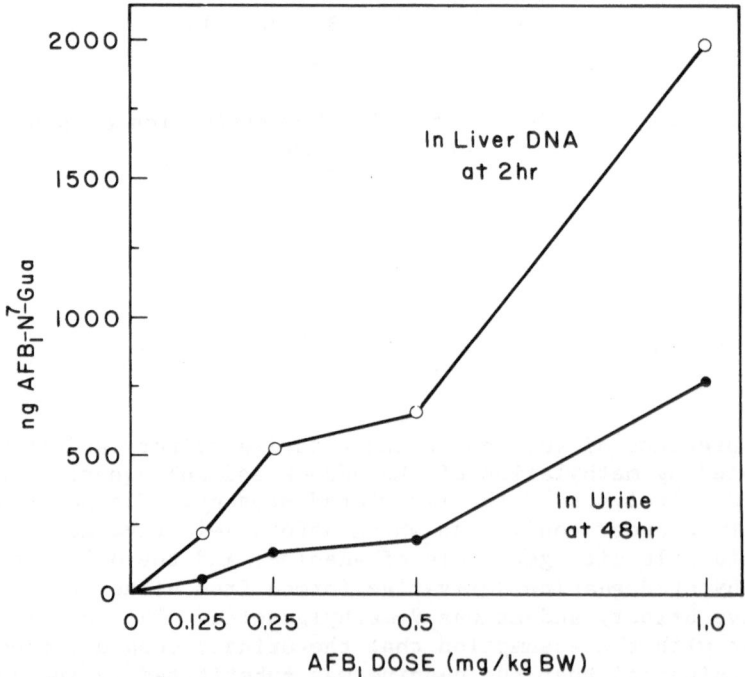

Fig. 9. Dose-response relationships in 48-hr urinary excretion of AFB_1-N^7-Gua, and the corresponding levels of this adduct in liver DNA 2 hr after dosing of rats.

plot could be constructed through which the level of exposure
could be estimated reliably. It is of interest that the amount
of adduct excreted represented a relatively constant fraction
(30-40%) of the maximum amount of adduct present in liver DNA.
Thus, it is possible under the conditions used here to apply the
method for estimation of AFB_1 body burden in the rat. This method
in its present form, however, probably is not sufficiently sensitive to be applicable to human population studies. We currently
are exploring ways to improve the analytical technology of adduct
detection in order to attain the necessary levels of sensitivity.

REFERENCES

1. G. N. Wogan, Aflatoxin carcinogenesis, in: "Methods in Cancer
    Research, Vol. III," H. Busch, ed., Academic Press, New
    York, 1973, pp. 309-344.
2. G. N. Wogan, The induction of liver cell cancer by chemicals,
    in: "Liver Cell Cancer," H. M. Cameron, D. A. Linsell, and
    G. P. Warwick, eds., Elsevier/North-Holland Biomedical
    Press, Amsterdam, The Netherlands (1976).
3. D. H. Swenson, E. C. Miller, and J. A. Miller, Aflatoxin B_1-
    2,3-oxide: Evidence for its formation in rat liver in vivo
    and by human liver microsomes in vitro, Biochem. Biophys.
    Res. Commun., 60:1036 (1974).
4. D. H. Swenson, J. K. Lin, E. C. Miller, and J. A. Miller,
    Aflatoxin B_1-2,3-oxide as a probable intermediate in the
    covalent binding of aflatoxin B_1 and B_2 to rat liver DNA
    and ribosomal RNA in vivo, Cancer Res., 37:172 (1977).
5. J. M. Essigmann, R. G. Croy, A. M. Nadzan, W. F. Busby, Jr.,
    V. N. Reinhold, G. Buchi, and G. N. Wogan, Structural
    identification of the major DNA adduct formed by aflatoxin
    B_1 in vitro, Proc. Natl. Acad. Sci. USA, 74:1870 (1977).
6. J. K. Lin, J. A. Miller, and E. C. Miller, 2,3-dihydro-2-
    (guan-7-yl)-3-hydroxyaflatoxin B_1, a major acid hydrolysis
    product of aflatoxin B_1-DNA or -rRNA adducts formed in
    hepatic microsome mediated reactions and in rat liver in
    vivo, Cancer Res., 37:4430 (1977).
7. R. G. Croy, J. M. Essigmann, V. N. Reinhold, and G. N. Wogan,
    Identification of the principal aflatoxin B_1-DNA adduct
    formed in vivo in rat liver, Proc. Natl. Acad. Sci. USA,
    75:1745 (1978).
8. H. Autrup, J. M. Essigmann, R. G. Croy, B. F. Trump, G. N.
    Wogan, and C. C. Harris, Metabolism of aflatoxin B_1-DNA and
    identification of a major aflatoxin B_1-DNA adduct formed
    in cultured human bronchus and colon, Cancer Res., 39:694
    (1979).
9. C. N. Martin and R. C. Garner, Aflatoxin B_1-oxide generated by
    chemical or enzymatic oxidation of aflatoxin B_1 causes

guanine substitution in nucleic acids, Nature, 267:863 (1977).

10. G. H. Buchi, M. A. Francisco, J. M. Liesch, and P. F. Shuda, A new synthesis of aflatoxin M_1, J. Am. Chem. Soc., 103: 3497 (1981).

11. J. M. Essigmann, P. R. Donahue, D. L. Story, G. N. Wogan, and H. Brunengraber, Use of the isolated perfused rat liver to study carcinogen-DNA adduct formation from aflatoxin B_1 and sterigmatocystin, Cancer Res., 40:4085 (1980).

12. R. G. Croy and G. N. Wogan, Quantitative comparison of covalent aflatoxin-DNA adducts formed in rat and mouse livers and kidneys, J. Natl. Cancer Inst., 66:761 (1981).

13. R. G. Croy and G. N. Wogan, Temporal patterns of covalent DNA adducts in rat liver after single and multiple doses of aflatoxin B_1, Cancer Res., 41:197 (1981).

14. R. A. Bennett, J. M. Essigmann, and G. N. Wogan, Excretion of an aflatoxin-guanine adduct in urine of aflatoxin B_1-treated rats, Cancer Res., 41:650 (1981).

PROBLEMS ASSOCIATED WITH THE USE OF CHEMICAL CLASS CONTROLS IN

ABSENCE OF INFORMATION ON THE UNDERLYING MECHANISM

Franz Oesch

Department of Toxicology
Institute of Pharmacology and Toxicology
University of Mainz
D-6500 Mainz, FRG

It is simply not possible to test all chemicals in adequately performed whole animal carcinogenicity tests. Short-term tests are, therefore, frequently used as a substitute. None of these short-term tests give results which correspond in all cases to the results obtained in whole animal carcinogenicity tests. Certain short-term tests have a notoriously poor predictibility for whole animal carcinogenicity for certain classes of chemicals. Therefore, if a chemical, whose carcinogenicity is unknown, is tested in a short-term test, frequently related compounds of known carcinogenicity are also tested simultaneously as chemical class controls.

One important contributing factor, which largely determines whether a given short-term test system is adequate for testing a given chemical is the presence and appropriate activity of enzymes which control the reactive metabolites of the compound in question. However, the data which will be presented below, show that a given enzyme can play roles in the control of reactive metabolites which are opposite for various members of a chemical class, even if these members are very closely related.

The influence of apparently homogeneous microsomal epoxide hydrolase (1,2) and dihydrodiol dehydrogenase (3) on the bacterial mutagenicity of the 12 isomeric monomethylbenzo(a)anthracenes, metabolically activated by liver postmitochondrial fraction from Aroclor 1254-treated C3H mice, was very different for the individual compounds (Table 1) (4). The addition of dihydrodiol dehydrogenase had only a significant effect on 3 of the deriva-

Table 1.   Effect of apparently homogeneous epoxide
hydrolase and dihydrodiol dehydrogenase on
the mutagenicity of benzo(a)anthracenes

Test compound	% Change in mutants above solvent control by		
	EH	DH	EH + DH
Benz(a)anthracene	− 17*	− 8	− 22*
1-MBA	− 48*	− 2	− 51*
2-MBA	− 94*	− 1	− 95*
3-MBA	− 29*	+ 7	− 30*
4-MBA	− 73*	− 4	− 73*
5-MBA	+ 116*	± 0	+ 89*
6-MBA	+ 209*	− 2	+ 205*
7-MBA	− 36*	−18*, −15*[a]	− 57*
8-MBA	− 22*	− 9	− 22*
9-MBA	− 50*	− 10	− 51*
10-MBA	− 47*	+ 6	− 41*
11-MBA	− 79*	− 8	− 82*
12-MBA	− 16*	−26*, −22*[a]	− 51*
7,12-DMBA	+ 8	−29*, −26*[a]	− 36*

The compounds (20 µg/plate) were tested for mutagenicity
with S. typhimurium TA 100 in the presence of 21 or
42 µl liver postmitochondrial fraction from Aroclor
1254-treated C3H mice and an NADPH-generating system.
Pure microsomal epoxide hydrolase (EH, 50 units) and/or
pure cytosolic dihydrodiol dehydrogenase (DH, 1 unit)
was added to some incubations. Statistically significant
(p < 0.05) effects are marked with an asterisk. Data
from (4); reprinted by permission of IRL Press, Oxford.
[a]Values obtained in a repeat experiment.

tives. Interestingly, the three were also very active carcinogens
(for references see 4). This indicates that for these active carcinogens dihydrodiol epoxides play an important role. With 2-
methylbenz(a)anthracene the epoxide hydrolase can practically eliminate the mutagenicity. But with 7,12-dimethylbenz(a)anthracene
there is practically no effect. With 5-methyl and 6-methylbenz(a)-
anthracene the epoxide hydrolase markedly increases the mutagenicity. So, if these enzymes have effects which are opposite for individual members of this series of closely related compounds, we
could say, we don't understand anything anymore at all. Let's go

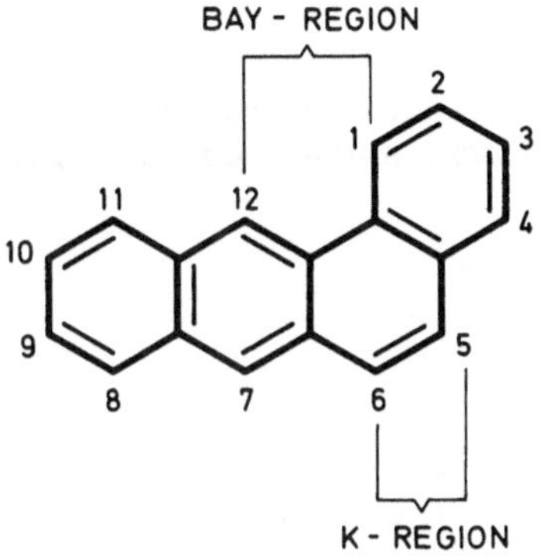

Fig. 1. Structural elements of benzo(a)anthracene.

back to blind testing and forget about the molecular mechanisms, they are far too complicated. But that is exactly the wrong reaction. The situation is not so complicated as not to be understandable at all. In the series of the 12 isomeric monomethylbenzo(a)-anthracenes microsomal epoxide hydrolase significantly lowers the mutagenicity of all isomers except for the 5-methyl and 6-methyl-benzo(a)anthracene where it increases the mutagenicity (Table 1). These two derivatives are the two K-region substituted derivatives (Fig. 1). Therefore, metabolism in the K-region is reduced or blocked. With these isomers little or no K-region epoxide will be formed, and other epoxides play the major role in the mutagenic effect. These can, after hydrolysis by microsomal epoxide hydrolase produce vicinal dihydrodiol epoxides (5-7) which is in agreement with the increase of mutagenicity after addition of apparently homogeneous epoxide hydrolase (Table 1). If the relatively electron-rich K-region is not substituted, a large proportion of the total epoxidation can occur there and microsomal epoxide hydrolase can inactivate these epoxides (8,9). This results in a decrease in mutagenicity after addition of microsomal epoxide hydrolase to all these isomers (Table 1).

Thus, twofold caution is required. First, the frequently adopted method which uses related compounds as chemical class controls can be misleading if the underlying mechanism of control is unknown. Variations in the activity of a given enzyme may have effects on the result which are opposite, even for such closely related compounds as simple positional isomers (Table 1) (frequently compounds are taken as "closely related chemical class controls" which differ from each other much more than that).

Second, apparent complications can often be resolved by considering which is the reactive metabolite responsible for the toxic response under investigation and how is it controlled enzymically.

ACKNOWLEDGEMENTS

    The author thanks his collaborators for their work quoted in
this article. This work was supported by a grant from the Stiftung
Volkswagenwerk.

REFERENCES

1.   Bentley, P. & Oesch, F. (1975) FEBS Lett. $\underline{59}$, 291-295.
2.   Bentley, P., Oesch, F. & Tsugita, A. (1975) FEBS Lett. $\underline{59}$,
     296-299.
3.   Vogel, K., Bentley, P., Platt, K.-L. & Oesch, F. (1980)
     J. Biol. Chem. $\underline{255}$, 9621-9625.
4.   Glatt, H.R., Vogel, K., Bentley, P., Sims, P. & Oesch, F.
     (1981) Carcinogenesis $\underline{2}$, 813-821.
5.   Bentley, P., Oesch, F. & Glatt, H.R. (1977) Arch. Toxicol.
     $\underline{39}$, 65-75.
6.   Wood, A.W., Levin, W., Lu, A.Y.H., Yagi, H., Hernandez, O.,
     Jerina, D.M. & Conney, A.H. (1976) J. Biol. Chem. $\underline{251}$,
     4882-4890.
7.   Sims, P., Grover, P.L., Swaisland, A., Pal, K. & Hewer, A.
     (1974) Nature $\underline{252}$, 326-328.
8.   Bentley, A., Schmassmann, H.R., Sims, P. & Oesch, F. (1976)
     Eur. J. Biochem. $\underline{69}$, 97-103.
9.   Jerina, D.M., Dansette, P.M., Lu, A.Y.H. & Levin, W. (1977)
     Mol. Pharmacol. $\underline{13}$, 342-351.

DISCUSSION

Dr.Taylor: You mentioned a sex-difference in response to carcinogens. Did you take into account that hormones could be involved in this?

Dr.King: Yes. DeBaun,working with the Millers,had shown that hormone manipulation would alter sulfotransferase levels.Male rats generally had higher levels than females.In our experiments,female Charles River rats with low levels of sulfotransferase developed both liver and mammary lesions after partial hepatectomy and/or administration of phenobarbital.Even males will develop mammary tumor under certain conditions;they also have N-O-acyltransferase in this tissue.On the other hand,female Fischer rats rarely develop mammary tumors on treat ment with aromatic amines even though they do respond to MNU.Thus,one must take into account the strain,sex,exposure to proper substrate, metabolic activation capability and hormonal promotion factors.

Dr.Taylor: There is not much known about hormonal patterns.It may be a naive way of expressing it but,to me it seems that you have to have c receptor for the carcinogen in the carcinogenic process.It may be the alteration in the receptor,wherever it may be located in the cell; then,.the hormones may be affecting the receptors rather than the carcinogenic process.

Dr.King: I may be biased but there are no conclusive data available to substantiate the involvement of receptors in the carcinogenic process.Our supposition is that phenobarbital may change the metabolism of endogenous hormones and alter their promotional activity.

Dr.Meerman: It is known that the ratio of deacetylated to acetylated adducts to DNA is higher than it is for RNA or cytosolic protein.Can this be due to the shorter half-life of the reactive sulfate-ester oj N-hydroxy-2-acetylamino-fluorene,which is responsible for the forma- tion of acetylated DNA-adducts,compared to the reactive species that are formed by N-O-acetyltransferase so that most of the reactive N-O- sulfate ester is already decomposed before it can reach the DNA insid the nucleus?Or can it be that the reactive species that are respons- ible for the formation of deacetylated DNA adducts are formed more ir the vicinity of DNA,for instance,in the nuclear membrane?

Dr.King: On one hand,the sulfate ester of N-OH-AAF is polar and charged.So if it is generated in the cytosolic milieu,it may not be able to be transported to the nucleus,because of that problem.Maybe this is one reason why the ribosomal RNA is much more highly acetyl- ated than is the DNA in rat liver.This is also consistent with Thor- geirsson's work in which they found that purified sulfotransferase cannot generate a mutagen that is recognized by the Salmonella system. On the other hand,we do not know about the intracellular location of the acetyltransferase.This could be nuclear.It is relatively small with a molecular weight of about 30,000.So,I think that even in the case of hepatocytes some of this material may leak out.This is evi- dent in the work of Howard,Casciano and Beland who have found that there were relatively fewer of the deacetylated arylamine adducts in DNA than in the intact animal.If you compare the sulfotransferase ac- tivities with the acetyl-transferase activities in isolated hepato- cytes and liver,the latter activity is about the same,but the sulfo- transferase activity is about three times higher in isolated hepato- cytes than in liver.This is one of the technical problems we have to worry about:translocation or even loss.For example,in our liver slices,in which cells are ruptured,microsomal deacylase activity is not lost because the microsomal components are held in place,while sulfotransferase activity is lost.The question of how the acetylamine adducts with DNA are formed is a very appropriate one,and from all the indication we have so far,I think one can say that it is probably as the consequence of acetyltransferase,but that does not preclude the possibility of other mechanisms.

Dr.Schulte-Hermann: There may be initiated cells after AFB-treatment even in mouse livers which are not promoted due to lack of necrogenic effects of AFB.Has anybody tried to promote the effect of AFB in mice after short initial treatment by compounds such as phenobarbital?

Dr.Wogan: These experiments have not been done,but would be logical ways to investigate the effects of modulation of adduct levels on initiation.

Dr.Cerutti: How much of the AFB_1-N^7-Gua excreted by rats originates from RNA?

Dr.Wogan: We do not know the exact proportions.Much of it probably comes from RNA,possibly the majority.However,it is not an import- ant factor in the use of this parameter as a dosimeter of aflatoxin exposure.Indeed,it may improve the sensitivity of the measurement of body-burden.

Dr.King: Has any attempt been made to use partial hepatectomy to try to resolve the question of whether the N^7-AFB,or the ring opened adduct is important in initiation?

Dr.Wogan: It is technically difficult to do these types of studies due to the toxicity of aflatoxin in partially hepatectomized animals.How- ever,we are now investigating the effects on tumor incidence of par- tial hepatectomy after the stable ring-opened product has been produced at high levels by multiple dosing.

Dr.Rueff: Is it possible to extrapolate the animal data on hepatocarcin ogenesis caused by aflatoxins to man?There are claims that rule out the role of aflatoxins as hepatocarcinogens in man,in favor of hepatitis B virus.In fact,areas in which hepatoma is endemic coincide with areas in which aflatoxin exposure and hepatitis virus infection are maximal.

Dr.Wogan: The observational data are as you just described.In many, though not all,areas where the incidence of liver cancer is high, there is simultaneous exposure to both agents.We have just initiated a project to determine aflatoxin exposure in Greece where the incidence of hepatitis B is high.We do not yet know about the aflatoxin exposure,but there is no reason to expect it to be high.However, a large amount of earlier data are available on the subject.When data from several studies are pooled together,a very convincing linear relationship emerges between afltoxin intake(calculated on a mg/kg body weight basis)and hepatocellular carcinoma incidence.Unfortunately,hep atitis B infection was not simultaneously investigated in those studies.It would have been very instructive regarding this possible interaction.

Dr.Nicolini: It is unclear to me how,in your experimental design, you are able to discriminate between effects and chemical modifications due to cancer induction and those changes related mainly to induced cell proliferation or induced cell toxicity/death.Could you please elaborate on this?

Dr.Wogan: We can not dissociate the parameters of cell death and regeneration from initiation.The data presented are purely observational. They can,however,be useful in formulation of experimental models capable of discriminating.

Dr.Taylor: First does a difference of 10 to $100/10^6$ labelled bases have any statistical significance?Secondly,are female rats more or less susceptible (tumor incidence) than male rats?

Dr.Wogan: Assuming that the experimental data are reproducible,as they appear to be,even the relatively small adduct levels and the difference between them,i.e. 10 vs 100,would be meaningful.Female are much less susceptible;tumor incidence in females is approximately 50-60% of the incidence in males at the dose level used in these experiments

Dr.King: Have you established that the 8-OH-N-7 adduct is a precursor of the ring-opened product?Does the ring opening appear to be non-enzymatic or may this be an enzyme-mediated reaction?

Dr.Wogan: It has not been rigorously established that the 8-OH-N-7 adduct is a precursor of AFB_1-FABY.However,collectively,our experiments suggest that the two exist in an equilibrium state in which the ring-opened product is present at a level approximately twice that of the putative 8-OH derivative.There is no evidence to suggest any enzymatic involvement in ring opening of the AFB_1-N^7-Gua adduct in DNA.

Dr.Lutz: You mentioned that carbohydrates are nucleophilic targets for electrophilic carcinogen metabolites.What carbohydrates or carcinogens were you thinking of?

Dr.Oesch: Beside nucleic acid and proteins,the oxygen atoms in carbohydrates,which are of course nucleophilic,are attacked by active electrophilic metabolites.For example,it is known that methyliodide will bind to carbohydrates.This is,however,not thoroughly investigated because most of the attention is focused on DNA.

Dr.Taylor: A naive question: Is it known if free radicals are produced from polycyclic hydrocarbons during epoxide formation?If such radicals are formed might they be involved in the carcinogenic step(s)?

Dr.Oesch: The way by which cytochrome P450-dependent monooxygenases activate oxygen is not fully established,but all evidence points towards the existence of an enzyme-bound oxene,i.e. and oxygen atom with 6 electrons,and the enzyme operates as an oxene transferase.This implies that the reactive oxygen species responsible for the epoxidation catalyzed by microsomal monooxygenases,is not a radical.However it is known that during the whole reaction cycle,at least,in vitro,there is side production of radicals,in that oxygen is reduced to superoxide radicals,which eventually lead to hydroxyl radicals.This may be an important mechanism of damage to the cell,including damage to the DNA. This damage to DNA represents damage that cannot be analyzed by monitoring for adducts formed,yet this mechanism could play a role in the loss of control over cell proliferation.

Dr.Friedman: What is the definition of expression time in the case of a long exposure to a carcinogen,and for exposure to procarcinogens versus ultimate carcinogens?

Dr.Oesch: The word "expression" per se is used in this context to indicate that a primary damage caused by the carcinogen is expressed as something which can be observed in the test in question.In the case of a long exposure to a carcinogen,this expression starts already during the exposure time.Also,during the exposure to a procarcinogen which needs metabolic activation,at some time sufficient reactive metabolite(s) are generated to start "expression" already during exposure. However the term "expression time" is operationally defined as the time,starting at the time point at which the medium containing the carcinogen is removed(end of exposure time),and replaced by medium not containing the carcinogen up to the time point when this second medium is removed and replaced by the selective medium.This contains Ouabain which is toxic to the cells,except to those which were mutated in a gene coding for Ouabain-sensitive ATPase and have had sufficient time to replace by normal turnover the intact gene product by the defective ATPase to be able to grow in the selective medium.

SECTION II

DNA ADDUCTS

DNA LESIONS : NATURE AND GENESIS

P.A. Cerutti

Department of Carcinogenesis
Swiss Institute for Experimental Cancer Research
CH-1066 Epalinges s/Lausanne, Switzerland

SUMMARY

Most carcinogens are DNA damaging agents. They can act on DNA
directly or indirectly. Direct action means that the primary agent
or a chemical derivative of the primary agent reacts with DNA
usually resulting in the formation of a covalent adduct. Indirect
action means attack of DNA by active oxygen species which are formed
by the reaction of the primary agent with a non-DNA target. Many
carcinogens act by one or the other mechanism, others by both.

Direct action predominates for chemical carcinogens and, in
general, involves the substitution of the nucleophilic centers of
DNA with the electrophilic damaging agents. Each damaging agent
produces a characteristic spectrum of lesions. The site of
substitution and the chemical properties, size and stereochemistry
of the substituent determine the effect of the lesion on DNA and
chromatin configuration. The lesion distribution varies for different
agents and is affected by the nucleosomal and higher order chromatin
structure, e.g. bulky substituents are usually introduced in higher
concentrations into nucleosomal-linker than -core DNA.

Indirect action is mediated via active oxygen species most
importantly hydroxyl-radicals, superoxide radicals, singlet oxygen,
(hydrogen peroxide). Independent of the primary agent which elicits
the formation of active oxygen species, a similar (but not identical)
spectrum of lesions is produced. Major types of lesions formed via
indirect action are strand breaks, base damage (e.g. products of
the 5,6-dihydroxy-dihydrothymine type), apurinic- and apyrimidinic
sites and sugar damage. Indirect action can be suppressed by radical
scavengers, antioxidans and enzymes such as superoxide dismutases
and peroxidases.

Ionizing radiation may be considered as the prototype for indirect action since hydroxyl-radicals generated by water-radiolysis
are mostly responsible for the formation of DNA damage. For ultraviolet light the contribution of direct and indirect action is wavelength dependent. Indirect action is the exception for chemical DNA
damaging agents. However, these exceptions are of particular importance for cancer research. Heterocyclic-aromatic ring systems which
can form quinoid structures can partake in redox-cycles resulting
in the formation of active oxygen species. Important examples for
this class of agents are the anticancer drugs bleomycin, strepto-
nigrin, adriamycin, daunorubicin and probably certain polycyclic
aromatic hydrocarbons. Certain membrane active compounds such as
the mouse skin tumor promotors phorbol-12-myristate-13-acetate,
mezerein and teleocidin elicit a burst of superoxide radicals in
certain target cells and cause chromosomal damage via indirect
action.

These concepts are illustrated using examples from our work on
the formation and repair of chromosomal damage induced by the carcinogens aflatoxin B_1, benzo(a)pyrene and N-acetoxy-2-acetylamino-
fluorene which operate via direct action and near-ultraviolet light
and the mouse skin promotor phorbol-12-myristate-13-acetate which
operate at least in part via indirect action.

In this short overview on carcinogen induced DNA damage the
mechanisms of lesion formation via direct and indirect action are
first discussed. We will then turn to the effect which lesions may
have on local DNA conformation, the distribution of lesions relative
to the primary sequence of DNA and relative to nucleosomal and higher
order structure of chromatin. These concepts will be illustrated by
work from our laboratory on the formation and repair of bulky adducts
formed via direct action in mammalian cells by N-acetoxy-2-acetyl-
aminofluorene, benzo(a)pyrene and aflatoxin B_1 and their ultimate
metabolites. As examples for damaging agents operating via indirect
action our work on the formation and resealing of near-ultraviolet
induced DNA strand breakage in human fibroblasts will be reviewed.
Finally a short account of recent experiments on the indirect action
of the mouse skin tumor promotor TPA will be given.

Formation of DNA damage by direct and indirect action

DNA damage can be produced by direct or indirect action. Direct
action means "attack of DNA by the primary agent or a chemical
derivative of the primary agent"; indirect action: "attack of DNA
by active oxygen species which are formed by the reaction of the
primary agent with a non-DNA target" (Cerutti, 1978).

Direct action usually results in the covalent linkage of the agent to DNA and is typical for most chemical mutagens and carcinogens. Most direct agents are electrophiles or they are metabolically activated to electrophilic derivatives which then react with the nucleophilic centers of DNA and other macromolecules (Miller and Miller, 1971). For example many alkylating and arylating agents form carbonium ion intermediates. The sites of substitution on the heterocyclic bases of DNA depends on the stability of the carbonium ion, the reaction mechanism (SN_1 >< SN_2 type reaction), the space requirements, solvation and intercalation properties of the substituent etc.. Bulky substituents are usually preferentially introduced at guanine. Electrophilicity and reaction mechanism mostly determine the site of reaction of small alkylating agents which often produce a highly complex lesion spectrum since substitution occurs at nitrogen and oxygen of the pyrimidine and purine bases as well as of the phosphate groups of the backbone (Singer and Kröger, 1979). In some cases where chemically unstable adducts are formed the lesion spectrum undergoes continuous changes due to spontaneous decomposition reactions. This situation presents itself for the covalent adducts formed by the mycotoxin aflatoxin B_1 (AFB_1) (Wang and Cerutti, 1980a, 1980b). Far-ultraviolet light (far-UV < 290 nm) in the range of the absorption maximum of DNA electronically excites the heterocyclic bases and induces preferentially cyclobutane-type dimerization of neighboring pyrimidines. These reactions are a consequence of direct action since photons are interacting directly with the heterocyclic bases. Far-UV also induces photohydration of cytosin by a reaction mechanism which is not clearly established.

In contrast to direct action where each agent produces a characteristic spectrum of adducts indirect action leads to the formation of a similar family of lesions regardless of the primary agent. This is due to the fact that related active oxygen species are formed as a consequence of the reaction of the primary agent with non-DNA targets. The active oxygen species which mediate indirect action are superoxide radicals (O_2^-), singlet oxygen ($^1O_2$), hydroxyl-radicals ($^{\cdot}OH$) and hydrogen peroxide (H_2O_2). The DNA lesions which are introduced by active oxygen species are single and double strand breaks (a consequence of sugar damage), damage involving the heterocyclic bases (e.g. products of the 5,6-dihydroxy-dihydrothymine-type, 8-hydroxy-adenine etc.) and apurinic- and apyrimidinic sites. The relative amounts of these lesions are expected to vary for different indirect agents. X- and γ-rays represent the prototypes of indirect agents. In biological systems they operate to more than 90% via the formation of $^{\cdot}OH$-radicals by water radiolysis (Roots and Okada, 1972; Remsen and RotiRoti, 1977; RotiRoti and Cerutti, 1974; Johansen and Howard-Flanders, 1965). As discussed above most DNA damaging chemicals act directly

but there are exceptions. They include the anticancer drugs strepto-
nigrin, adriamycin, daunorubicin, mitomycin C (Cerutti, 1978) and
certain polycyclic aromatic hydrocarbons (Cerutti and Remsen, 1977;
Lorentzen and Ts'o, 1977). These compounds possess or are metabolically modified to quinoid structures and participate in redox-cycles
producing active oxygen species (e.g. O_2^-) (Bachur et al. 1978). The
presence of traces of transition metals may be required for the
activity of bleomycin which may produce $\cdot$OH-radicals in a Fenton-
type reaction (Lown and Sim, 1977). Since these compounds possess
high affinity to DNA they may function as site-specific producers
of active oxygen species.

Some DNA damaging agents operate both by direct and indirect
action. For example, mitomycin C in addition to its potential to
produce active oxygen forms mono-adducts and cross-links in DNA;
evidence has been presented that the polycyclic aromatic hydrocarbon
benzo(a)pyrene (Cerutti and Remsen, 1977) and 4-nitro-quinolin-N-
oxide (Ide and Cerutti, unpublished) upon metabolic activation to
quinone intermediates damage DNA via indirect action. It is well
established that both agents also form covalent adducts to guanine
adenine and cytosine (e.g. see in Roberts, 1978). Most standard
protocols for the detection and determination of chemically induced
DNA damage use radioactive damaging agents. Under these conditions
damage induced by indirect action will be unlabeled and remains
undectable. The possibility of a dual mechanism should be kept in
mind when procarcinogens can be metabolically activated to quinoid
intermediates or when the participation of transition metals is
suspected (Cerutti, 1978). Ultraviolet light also acts by both
mechanisms. As discussed above direct action is the predominant
mechanism for far-UV in the range of the absorption maximum of
DNA. In the near-UV (> 290 nm) electronic excitation still occurs
but indirect mechanisms gain in importance (Cerutti and Netrawali,
1979). Photosensitization resulting in photo-oxidation and photo-
reduction reactions may be involved. Photosensitization mostly
induces complex chain reactions in which $^1O_2$ and O_2^- participate
(Foote, 1976).

Lesions can distort the local conformation of DNA

Different types of lesions are expected to affect the conformational state of DNA to different degrees and in a characteristic
manner. Certain predictions are possible concerning the degree of
helix distortion and relaxation of superhelicity induced by different
classes of lesions. On this basis we proposed a lesion classification
which distinguished (1) monofunctional lesions causing negligible
helix distortion (2) monofunctional lesions causing minor helix
distortion and (3) lesions causing major helix distortion (Cerutti,
1975). To the first class were counted lesions with essentially

unaltered base pairing and base-stacking capacities, to the second
class lesions with only slightly altered base-pairing and base-
stacking properties, to the third class mono-functional lesions
with bulky substituents or substantially altered base pairing
properties, intercalation damage and difunctional lesions. Of
course, classifications of this type are mostly conjectural and
much biochemical and biophysical work is necessary to define the
effects of specific lesions on DNA conformation. For the case of
the guanine adducts of 2-acetylaminofluorene (AAF) and for cyclobutane-type pyrimidine dimers induced by UV (both classified as
lesions causing major helix distortion) more detailed information
has become available. In most of the work on the conformational
effects of DNA damage naked DNA was used. Extrapolation of results
obtained under these conditions to eukaryotic cells where the DNA
interactes with histone and non-histone chromosomal proteins is
not straightforward.

The ultimate carcinogen N-acetoxy-AAF preferentially reacts with
the carbon-C_8 of guanine in DNA under formation of N-(deoxyguanosin-
8-yl)-2-acetylaminofluorene or, in cells with high deacetylase
activity, of N-(deoxyguanosin-8-yl)-2-aminofluorene. In native DNA
in the usual B-conformation the introduction of this bulky substituent
is causing major helix distortion which according to an attractive
model involves the rotation of the substituted guanine residue from
the anti- to the syn-conformation. It was suggested that the aminofluorene residue is inserted into the position formerly taken up by
guanine (Fuchs, 1975; Levine et al., 1974) ("base-displacement" or
"insertion-denaturation" model). Biochemical evidence for local
distortion of the DNA helix was obtained when it was found that
single strand specific endonucleases preferentially attacked DNA
regions containing AAF substituted residues (Fuchs, 1975; Yamasaki
et al., 1977). Work with antibodies raised against AAF modified
DNA further support the notion that the AAF substituent is not
completely buried in the DNA-helix (Sage et al, 1979). In the
recently discovered Z-conformation of dG-dC sequences of DNA the
dG residues are present in syn-conformation. Z-DNA forms a left
handed, anti-parallel, narrow helix with 12 base pairs per turn.
On the basis of the "base-displacement" or "insertion-denaturation"
model discussed above it might be expected that syn-oriented dG
residues in Z-DNA are particularly reactive to AAF or that AAF-
damaged DNA might assume locally Z-conformation. Indeed, at very
high AAF substitution, double-stranded poly(dG-dC) was present in
Z-conformation. In contrast to AAF-damaged DNA the AAF damaged
regions of the polymer were remarkably resistant to digestion
with S_1-nuclease. It can be speculated that repetitive dG-dC
sequences in the genome may represent mutational hot spots to
AAF (Santella et al., 1981).

In the lesion classification mentioned above cyclobutyl-type

pyrimidine photodimers had been assigned to lesions causing major
helix distortion (Cerutti, 1975). It has been shown that the presence of dimers reduced the melting temperature of DNA (Hayes et al.,
1971), increased its reactivity to formaldehyde (Shafranovskaya et
al., 1973) and its sensitivity to single strand specific endonucleases (Legerski et al., 1977; Heflich et al., 1977). UV-irradiation also increased the sedimentation coefficient of superhelical
DNA due to a decrease in superhelical turns (Denhardt and Kato,1973).
These observations suggest local distortion and partial denaturation
of the native conformation of DNA by UV-irradiation. Recently a
highly sensitive method was developed which measures the reduction
in electrophoretic mobility of topoisomers of a small superhelical
plasmid DNA upon UV-irradiation. An unwinding angle of $-14.3 \pm$
0.2^o per dimer was determined at low doses where each DNA molecule
contained on average only one dimer. The mobility of restriction
fragments and of the RFI form of the plasmid were slightly increased, on the other hand. This latter effect was attributed to
an increase in the flexibility of DNA due to local denaturation at
dimer clusters. This method lends itself to the study of the effect
of a variety of lesions induced by chemical and physical agents on
DNA conformation (Ciarrocchi and Pedrini, in press).

The primary sequence of DNA can affect the lesion distribution

     Evidence has recently been obtained that the rate of lesion
production at a specific site in naked DNA in vitro can be affected
by the primary sequence. Using DNA restriction fragments of known
sequence the following results were obtained for 254 nm light
induced pyrimidine dimerization. The rate and level of the photo-
stationary state of dimerization was highest for sequences containing 3 (or more ?) neighboring T-residues and lowest for neighboring C-residues. Besides these effects due to the number and
chemical properties of neighboring pyrimidines, T-residues flanked
by two A-residues dimerized approximately twice as efficiently as
T-residues flanked by an A- and a G-residue (Haseltine et al., 1980).
Analogous results were obtained for highly repetitive α-sequences
irradiated in vitro and in situ in human cells although the overall
rate of reaction was diminished by approximately 50% under the
latter conditions (Lippke et al., 1981). Treatment of the DNA in
vitro with microsome activated Aflatoxin B_1 (AFB_1) results in the
formation of alkali-labile sites which probably correspond to
apurinic sites formed by spontaneous hydrolysis of the major adduct
2,3-dihydro-2-(N^7-guanyl)-3-hydroxyaflatoxin B_1. The rate of formation of alkaline-labile sites varied for different guanine residues
but no detailed analysis was carried out (D'Andrea and Haseltine,
1978). In contrast, no major differences were detected in the reactivity of the N^7-position of individual guanine residues in highly

repetitive human α-DNA in vitro and in situ towards the nitrogen
mustard methylbis(2-chloroethyl)amine. Again as for UV the overall
reactivity of DNA was approximately 50% lower in the cell (Grunberg
and Haseltine, 1980). It is concluded that the primary sequence
which determines the conformational fine structure can affect the
lesion distribution but no general rule can be given. Intracellular
chromatin structure had no major effect on the distribution of UV-
dimers or alkylation lesions induced by methylbis(2-chloroethyl)
amine. As discussed below, chromatin structure strongly affected
the distribution of bulky adducts of AFB_1, N-acetoxy-2-acetylamino-
fluorene and benzo(a)pyrene-diol-epoxide, on the other hand.

Nucleosomal structure of chromatin can affect lesion distribution

        A great deal has been learnt about the nucleosomal organization
of chromatin in eukaryotic cells and excellent reviews are available
(McGhee and Felsenfeld, 1979; Klug et al., 1980; Allan et al., 1980).
In the most basic terms the nucleosomal core consists of 3/4 turns
(145 base pairs) of superhelical DNA wound around a wedge-shaped
histone-octamer (i.e. 2 tetramers of H_{2A}, H_{2B}, H_3, H_4). This DNA is
protected from mild microccocal nuclease (MN) digestion. Twenty
additional base pairs at the entrance and exit of the DNA to the
histone octamer are partially protected to MN digestion by a single
copy of histone H_1. Two complete superhelical turns of DNA (165 b.p.)
are wrapt around the H_1-containing "chromatosomes" (Simpson, 1978).
Chromatosomes are connected by linker DNA of variable length. Human
skin fibroblasts which we have mostly used in the work described
below possess a nucleosomal repeat of 192 b.p. and therefore this
linker consists of 27 b.p. while the linker between H_1-free cores
consists of 47 b.p..
        Several laboratories have studied the role of the nucleosomal
structure of chromatin in the formation and repair of DNA damage
(see e.g. Lieberman et al., 1979; Cleaver, 1977; Bodell and Banerjee,
1979). In the context of this article I will focus on our work on
the initial distribution of bulky DNA adducts which are formed by
short treatment with the highly reactive ultimate carcinogens N-
acetoxy-2-acetylaminofluorene (AAAF) (Kaneko and Cerutti, 1980;
Cerutti et al., 1981), 7β,8α-dihydroxy-9α,10α-epoxy-7,8,9,10-tetra-
hydrobenzo(a)pyrene (BPDE I) (Feldman et al., 1980; Kaneko and
Cerutti, in press; Cerutti et al., 1981) and rat liver microsome
activated AFB_1 (Leadon et al., in press). All three carcinogens
produce a simple initial lesion spectrum in which guanine adducts
predominate. The following experimental design was used. Rapidly
growing cultures were labeled with [^{14}C]-thymidine and allowed to
reach confluency. After 2-3 days in confluency residual DNA synthesis had decreased to 2-3%. The cultures were treated with high
specific activity [^{3}H]-carcinogen for 15 to 30 min. and harvested

immediately. Nuclei were prepared and total DNA was isolated from a small aliquot and the adduct concentration (in μmoles adduct per Mol-DNA-P) determined from the ^{14}C-specific activity of the DNA and the ^{3}H-specific activity of the carcinogen. The bulk of the nuclei was mildly treated with MN and mononucleosomes were purified by sucrose gradient centrifugation. Mononucleosomal DNA was extracted and analysed by polyacrylamide gel electrophoresis which revealed major bands at 145 and 165 b.p. corresponding to core- and chromatosomal-DNA, respectively. The adduct concentrations were calculated from the ^{14}C- and ^{3}H-content of these bands. According to our protocol bona fide core- and chromatosomal DNA are being analysed in contrast to experiments using less well defined MN-resistant DNA. In our experience extensive purification of core- and chromatosomal-DNA is a prerequisite for reliable data. The adduct concentration in 47 b.p. and 27 b.p. linker DNA is calculated from the concentrations in total nuclear DNA and core- or chromato-somal-DNA, respectively. This is only justified if a random popula-tion of mononucleosomes is isolated by our procedure. While it appears unlikely that the presence of adducts induces a major change in the MN digestibility of nucleosomes it is conceivable that our preparations are enriched in mononucleosomes of higher resistance to this enzyme. Higher resistance could be a reflexion of the con-formation of a subpopulation of individual mononucleosomes or of their location in chromatin regions with a particular superstructure. At present there exists no satisfactory direct approach to measure the concentration of carcinogen DNA adducts in linker DNA in intact mammalian cells. Oligosomes can only be used under exceptional circumstances. Because of the low yields in their preparation the standard analytical procedures are not sufficiently sensitive at acceptable carcinogen concentrations and the possibility that specific nucleosome subpopulations are being isolated cannot be ignored. These limits in methodology have to be kept in mind for the evaluation of the data presented below.

All three carcinogens introduced adducts preferentially into linker DNA. For confluent human skin fibroblasts the ratio of the adduct concentrations in 47 b.p. linker-over 145 b.p. core-DNA was 4 to 5 for AAAF (Kaneko and Cerutti, 1980) and 6.3 for BPDE I (Kaneko and Cerutti, in press). The experiments with AFB_1 were carried out with mouse embryo fibroblasts 10T.1/2 which possess a 45 b.p. linker. The ratio of concentration in linker to core-DNA was 11.1 when AFB_1 was activated exogenously (for 30 min.) by rat liver microsomes and 12.7 following 4 hr activation by the cellular metabolism itself. In these experiments it was nessary to transform the chemically unstable primary adducts, AFB_1-N^7-Gua, into the more stable AFB_1-triamino-Py by short incubation of the cells at pH 9.5 immediately following AFB_1-treatment.This step is necessary because of the lengthy procedure for the isolation of highly purified

nucleosomal DNA (Leadon et al., in press). AFB_1 has also been found
to bind preferentially to linker-DNA in trout liver nucleosomes
(Bailey et al., 1980). In the case of BPDE I special attention was
given to the adduct concentration in 165 b.p. chromatosomal-DNA
relative to 145 b.p. core-DNA. Since little difference was found
it follows that the hyperreactive portion of linker DNA is reduced
to 27 b.p.. Correspondingly, the ratio of the adduct concentration
in linker over core DNA is increased to 9.2 for the shortened
"chromatosomal linker" from a value of 6.3 for the 47 b.p. "core
linker" (Kaneko and Cerutti, in press). For completeness it should
be mentioned that other carcinogens which introduce bulky substituents, e.g. benzo(a)pyrene-4,5-oxide (Feldman et al., 1980,
7-bromomethylbenzo(a)anthracene (Oleson et al., 1979) and trimethyl-
psoralene (Cech and Pardue, 1977) have been shown to damage MN
sensitive DNA (presumably mostly linker DNA) more extensively than
MN resistant DNA.

As discussed in the preceeding section cyclobutyl-type thymine
dimers cause major distortion of the native DNA conformation. However, according to our recent work using an improved chromatographic
assay comparable amounts of dimers are formed in linker and core DNA
of skin fibroblasts with 10 - 20 Jm^{-2} of 254 nm UV-light (Niggli
and Cerutti, unpublished). These results are in qualitative agreement with the work of Williams and Friedberg (1979) and Lippke et
al.(1981). In contrast, Snapka and Linn (1981) found preferential
introduction of dimers into nucleosomal cores upon 254 nm irradiation
of SV40 mini-chromosomes in vitro. This apparent discrepancy may be
due to differences in the protein complent of linker DNA. Intranuclear linker DNA is associated with a complex mixture of non-
histone proteins which may partially be lost during the preparation
of SV40 minichromosomes.

The question whether certain carcinogens may attack regulatory
regions of the genome preferentially was approached using simian
virus 40 (SV40) as a probe (Beard et al., 1981). The small DNA
viruses SV40 and polyoma represent promising systems for the study
of chromatin structure and function, since detailed information is
available about their nucleotide sequences and the expression of
their genome. For the same reasons these viruses may prove valuable
for the study of the interaction of chromatin with carcinogens.
SV40 in the infected cell is present as a minichromosome with
nucleosomal organization. In vitro studies suggest that the region
of the replication origin of SV40 may have a unique structure and
may be free of nucleosomes (Saragosti et al., 1980; Yakobovits et
al., 1980). We infected monkey kidney cells BSC-B with SV40 and
treated them in the late phase of the lytic cycle, during viral
DNA replication, with tritiated AAAF. SV40 was extracted and
digested with the restriction endonucleases Hae III and Kpn I. The
restriction fragments were separated by agarose gel electrophoresis

and the adduct concentrations determined in each fragment. It was
found that the origin region of SV40, i.e. the restriction fragment
Hae III Flb/Kpn I, was hypermodified by a factor of 1.5 to 2
relative to the rest of the SV40 genome. No hypermodification of
the same fragment was observed when free SV40 DNA was reacted with
AAAF in vitro (Beard et al., 1981). From our results it appears
likely that SV40 DNA in situ possesses a stretch of DNA in the
origin region which is nucleosome free and more reactive to the
carcinogen, therefore. The region of the SV40 chromosome which
reacts preferentially with AAAF contains regulatory sequences
controlling the origin of replication of DNA (Danna and Nathans,
1972), T-antigen binding sites (Tjian, 1978) and likely promoters
for late transcription (Ghosh et al.,1978; Handa et al., 1981).
SV40 uses cellular enzymes for its replication (Tooze, 1980), and
SV40 chromatin probably resembles certain regions of cellular
chromatin in structure (Shelton et al., 1978). Therefore, regulatory
sequences of some cellular genes may likewise be particularly
susceptible to modification by AAAF and similar carcinogens (Beard
et al., 1981).

The effect of the nucleosomal distribution of carcinogen
adducts on their excisability and persistence is only shortly
summarized (but see in Cerutti, in press). In confluent and growing
human fibroblasts AAF-adducts were removed preferentially from
linker DNA resulting in the relative enrichment of lesions in core-
DNA. Even at low toxicity (> 80% survival of colony forming ability
and under conditions where excision repair was not saturated)
approximately 50% of the initial adducts persisted in the DNA after
24 hr incubation (Kaneko and Cerutti, 1980). Similar results were
obtained for BPDE I (Kaneko and Cerutti, in press). It follows that
nucleosomal linker DNA was both preferentially damaged and repaired
by these carcinogens. The adducts which persist in the DNA over
longer periods are predominantly, but not exclusively, located in
core-DNA and may not be amenable to excision because of constraints
in nucleosomal- and higher-order chromatin structure.

Indirect action of near-ultraviolet light

While direct action predominates in the far-UV below 290 nm
indirect action represents the major mechanism in the long wavelength UV above 320 nm where DNA absorption has become very low.
In the intermediate region of the near-UV between 290 - 320 nm
both mechanisms operate at the same time. This can be demonstrated
by comparing the action spectrum for the formation of thymine
photodimers (TT, characteristic for direct action) to those for
single-strand breakage (SS-breaks, characteristic for indirect
action) and the formation of monomeric, ring-saturated thymine
derivatives of the 5,6-dihydroxy-dihydrothymine type (t_{sat},

characteristic for indirect action). The ratio of the lesion concentrations TT/SS for 12.5 Jm^{-2} light at 254 nm was 5.7 x 10^3 and for 2.25 KJm^{-2} at 313 nm 8.9 in the DNA of human skin fibroblasts. It follows that the predominance of photodimerization has decreased by a factor of 640 in going from 254 to 313 nm. The same trend was observed for the ratio TT/t_{sat} which decreased from 21 at 265 nm to 1.3 at 313 nm (Cerutti and Netrawali, 1979).

There is no reliable data on the removal of t_{sat} in mammalian cells following near-UV irradiation. However, experiments with high doses of aerobic γ-rays which induce a similar spectrum of lesions suggest very rapid excision (Mattern et al., 1975). Because of the high sensitivity of the alkaline elution procedure it was possible to determine the kinetics of the rejoining of near-UV induced SS-breaks at a physiological dose of 2.25 KJm^{-2} of 313 nm light in human skin fibroblasts, on the other hand. In Xeroderma pigmentosum fibroblasts of complementation group A the kinetics of rejoining of radiation-induced SS-breaks could be measured without interference from enzymatic breaks resulting from the excision repair of pyrimidine photodimers. More than 90% of the initial breaks were rejoined within 30 min post-treatment incubation (Cerutti and Netrawali, 1979).

In Bloom Syndrome (BS) excessive amounts of DNA-damage may be induced by near-UV and agents operating via indirect action, in general. BS is an autosomal recessive disease with increased cancer incidence, growth abnormalities, immunodeficiency and sensitivity of the facial skin to solar radiation. Lymphocytes and fibroblasts of BS-patients possess increased frequencies of spontaneous chromosomal aberrations and sister chromatid exchanges (SCE) (German, 1972). We found that near-UV at 313 nm at $37^{O}C$ induced abnormally high numbers of SS-breaks in 6 of 8 BS fibroblast strains tested (Hirschi et al., 1981). Furthermore, a majority of BS strains were hypersensitive to the lethal action of near-UV at 313 nm (Zbinden and Cerutti, 1981) as well as of mitomycin C and 4-nitroquinolin-N-oxide (i.e. chemical agents operating partially via indirect action) (Zbinden and Cerutti, unpublished). We speculate that BS-cells possess increased stationary concentrations of active oxygen species either due to overproduction or deficient detoxification. This notion is supported by the discovery of a clastogenic factor (CF, i.e. a component breaking chromosomes) in the culture medium of BS-fibroblasts which could be inhibited by the addition of superoxide dismutase (SOD) (Emerit and Cerutti, 1981a; Cerutti, in press). BS may supply a valuable experimental system for the study of the biological effects of excessive damage induced via indirect action. For completeness it should be added that near-UV also induced excessive SS-breakage in Xeroderma pigmentosum variants by an unknown mechanism (Netrawali and Cerutti, 1979).

Indirect action of the tumor promotor phorbol-12-myristate-13-acetate

As discussed above indirect action is characteristic for physical damaging agents and direct action for chemicals. However, chemicals which possess or are metabolically transformed to quinoid structures and certain reducing agents in the presence of transition metals(Fenton-type reagents) form exceptions. A third class of cell-membrane active chemicals may lead to the formation of active oxygen species via the induction of a respiratory burst and it might be expected that some of them may damage DNA via indirect action. We were particularly interested in the tumor promotors phorbol-12-myristate-13-acetate (PMA), mezerein and teleocidin for which it has been shown that they interact with the cell-membrane and elicite a burst of superoxide radicals in bovine and human polymorphonuclear leukocytes and possibly other types of cells (Goldstein at al., 1979; Mueller et al., 1980; De Chatelet et al., 1976). It has been suggested that the intermediate formation of active oxygen may be a necessary but insufficient step in tumor promotion. Most investigators agree that PMA does not form covalent adducts with DNA, that it is non-mutagenic and that it is at best a weak inducer of SCE (Slaga et al.,eds, 1978; Diamond et al., 1980; Kinsella and Radman, 1978; Thompson et al., 1980; Nagasawa and Little, 1979; Loveday and Latt, 1979). These negative properties by no means excluded the possibility that PMA could be a potent clastogen via indirect action. It should be remembered that ionizing radiation which may be considered as the prototype of indirect agents is known to be a strong clastogen but a weak mutagen.

Our prediction turned out to be correct. When we tested PMA on phytohemagglutinin stimulated, normal human lymphocytes, we found that it induced chromosomal aberrations with high efficiency while it was only a weak inducer of SCE. 10 ng/ml PMA induced 33.9 ± 13.9 (mean ± S.D.) aberrations relative to 7.2 ± 8.6 aberrations per 100 mitosis in untreated controls; the same concentration of PMA induced only 7.7 ± 3.4 SCE relative to 5.2 ± 2.2 SCE per mitosis for untreated controls. The structurally related weak promotor 4-0-methyl-PMA possessed only marginal clastogenicity and the non-promotor phorbol was inactive. Care was taken in our experiments to use solvents and media with a low content in radical scavengers. The observation that the addition of superoxide dismutase (50 μg/ml) strongly inhibited the clastogenic activity of PMA supports our notion that PMA induces chromosomal damage via indirect action (Emerit and Cerutti,1981b). However, the possibility that superoxide dismutase may decrease PMA binding to the cell surface is also being considered. It is not known whether PMA is only clastogenic in white blood cells which respond with a strong respiratory burst

to a variety of stimuli. However, recent results with mouse epidermal
cells suggest that the clastogenicity of PMA may be a more general
phenomenon (Dzarlieva et al., 1980). We are presently studying the
mechanism of the clastogenic action of PMA and have found that a
CF is produced with properties which are similar to those of the
CF isolated from the culture medium of BS-fibroblasts.

ACKNOWLEDGEMENT

This work was supported by grants 3'627.80 of the Swiss
National Science Foundation and a grant from the Swiss Association
of Cigarette Manufacturers.

REFERENCES

Allan, J., Hartman, P.G., Crane-Robinson, C., and Aviles, F.X.,
        1980, The structure of histone H_1 and its location in
        chromatin, Nature 288:675.
Bachur, N.R., Gordon, S.L., and Gee, M.V., 1978, A general mechanism
        for microsomal activation of quinone anticancer agents to
        free radicals, Cancer Res. 38:1745.
Bailey, G.S., Nixon, J.E., Hendricks, J.D., Sinnhuber, R.O., and
        Van Holde, K.E., 1980, Carcinogen aflatoxin B_1 is located
        preferentially in internucleosomal deoxyribonucleic acid
        following exposure in vivo in rainbow trout, Biochem. 19:
        5836.
Beard, P., Kaneko, M., and Cerutti, P., 1981, N-acetoxy-acetylamino-
        fluorene reacts preferentially with a control region of
        intracellular SV40 chromosome, Nature 291:84.
Bodell, W., and Banerjee, M., 1979, The influence of chromatin
        structure on the distribution of DNA repair synthesis
        studied by nuclease digestion, Nucl. Acid. Res. 6:359.
Cech, T., and Pardue, M., 1977, Cross-linking of DNA with trimethyl-
        psoralen is a probe for chromatin structure, Cell 11:631.
Cerutti, P., 1975, Repairable damage in DNA: Overview, in: "Molecular
        mechanisms for repair of DNA", P.C. Hanawalt and R.B. Setlow,
        eds., Plenum Publishing Corp, New York.
Cerutti, P., and Remsen, J., 1977, Formation and repair of DNA
        damage induced by oxygen radical species in human cells,
        in: "DNA Repair Processes", W. Nichols and D. Murphy, eds.,
        Symposia Specialists, Miami.
Cerutti, P., 1978, Repairable damage in DNA, in: "DNA Repair
        Mechanisms", P. Hanawalt, E. Friedberg and C. Fox, eds.,
        Academic Press, New York.
Cerutti, P., and Netrawali, M., 1979, Formation and repair of DNA
        damage induced by indirect action of ultraviolet light in
        normal and Xeroderma pigmentosum skin fibroblasts, in:

Proceedings of VIth Int. Congr. of Radiat. Res. Tokyo,
Toppan Printing Co., Ltd., Tokyo.

Cerutti, P., Kaneko, M., and Beard, P., 1982, Chromosome Damage
and Repair, in: NATO-ASI series Vol. 40, pp.49-61, E. Seeberg
and K. Kleppe, eds., Plenum Press, New York.

Cerutti, P., in press, Persistence of carcinogen-DNA adducts in
cultured mammalian cells, in: "Mechanisms in chemical
carcinogenesis", C. Harris and P. Cerutti, eds., Academic
Press, New York.

Cerutti, P., in press, Abnormal oxygen metabolism in Bloom Syndrome,
in: "DNA-Repair, Chromosome Alterations and Chromatin
Structure", A. Natarajan, H. Altman and G. Obe, eds.
Elsevier North Holland Biomedical Press.

Ciarrocchi, G., and Pedrini, A., in press, Determination of
pyrimidine dimer unwinding angle by measurement of DNA
electrophoretic mobility, J. Mol. Biol.

Cleaver, J., 1977, Nucleosome structure controls rates of excision
repair in DNA of human cell, Nature 270:451.

D'Andrea, A., and Haseltine, W.A., 1978, Modification of DNA by
aflatoxin B_1 creates alkali-labile lesions in DNA at
positions of guanine and adenine, Proc. Natl. Acad. Sci. US
75:4120.

Danna, K., and Nathans, D., 1972, Bidirectional replication of
simian virus 40 DNA, Proc. Natl. Acad. Sci. 69:3097.

De Chatelet, L., Shirley, P., and Johnston, R., 1976, Blood 47:
545.

Denhardt, D., and Kato, A., 1973, Comparison of the effect of ultraviolet radiation and ethidium bromide intercalation on the
conformation of superhelical ØX174 replicative form DNA,
J. Mol. Biol. 77:479.

Diamond, L., O'Brien, G., and Baird, W., 1980, Tumor promotors and
mechanism of tumor promotion, Avd. Canc. Res. 32:1.

Dzarlieva, R., Breitkreuz, D., Schütz, S., and Fusenig, N., 1980,
Effect of phorbol esters on differentiation, sister chromatid
exchange and structural chromosomal aberrations in keratinizing mouse epidermal cell lines, in: "Cocarcinogenesis
and Biological Effects of Tumor Promotors", Abstr. 115,
Castle Elman, West Germany.

Emerit, I., and Cerutti, P., 1981a, Clastogenic activity from
Bloom's Syndrome fibroblast cultures, Proc. Natl. Acad.
Sci. USA, 78:1868.

Emerit, I., and Cerutti, P., 1981b, Tumor promotor phorbol-12-
myristate-13-acetate induces chromosomal damage via indirect action, Nature 293:144.

Feldman, G., Remsen, J., Wang, T.V., and Cerutti, P., 1980,
Formation and excision of covalent deoxyribonucleic acid
adducts of benzo(a)pyrene 4,5-epoxide and benzo(a)pyrene-

diol epoxide I in human lung cells A549, Biochem. 19:1095.

Foote, C.F., 1976, Photosensitized oxidation and singlet oxygen: consequences in biological systems, in: "Free Radicals in Biology" Vol.2, W.A. Pryor, ed., Academic Press, New York.

Fuchs, R., 1975, In vitro recognition of carcinogen-induced local denaturation sites in native DNA by S_1 endonuclease from Aspergillus oryzae, Nature 257:151.

German, J., 1972, Genes which increase chromosomal instability in somatic cells and predispose to cancer, in: "Medical Genetics", Vol.8, A. Steinberg and A. Bearn, eds., Grune & Stratton, New York.

Ghosh, P., Reddy, V., Swinscoe, J., Lebowitz, P., and Weissman, S., 1978, Heterogeneity and 5'-terminal structures of the late RNAs of simian virus 40, J. Mol. Biol. 126:813.

Goldstein, B., Witz, G., Amoruso, M., and Troll, W., 1979, Protease inhibitors antagonize the activation of polymorphonuclear leukocyte oxygen consumption, Biochem. Biophys. Res. Commun. 88:854.

Grunberg, S., and Haseltine, W.A., 1980, Use of an indicator sequence of human DNA to study DNA damage by methylbis (2-chloroethyl) amine, Proc. Natl. Acad. Sci. 77:6546.

Handa, H., Kaufman, R., Manley, J., Gefter, M., and Sharp, P., 1981, Transcription of simian virus 40 DNA in the HeLa whole cell extract, J. Biol. Chem. 256:478.

Haseltine, W.A., Gordon, L.K., Lindan, C.P., Grafstrom, R.H., Shaper, N.L., and Grossman, L., 1980, Cleavage of pyrimidine dimers in specific DNA sequences by a pyrimidine dimer DNA-glycosylase of M. luteus, Nature 285:634.

Hayes, F.N., Williams, D.L., Ratliff, R.L., Varghese, A., and Rupert, C.S., 1971, J. Am. Chem. Soc. 93:4940.

Heflich, R., Dorney, D., Maher, V., and McCormick, 1977, Reactive derivatives of benzo(a)pyrene and 7,12-dimethylbenz(a)-anthracene cause S_1 nuclease sensitive sites in DNA and "UV-like" repair, Biochem. Biophys. Res. Commun., 77:634.

Hirschi, M., Netrawali, M., Remsen, J., and Cerutti, P., 1981, Formation of DNA single-strand breaks by near-ultraviolet and γ-rays in normal and Bloom's syndrome skin fibroblasts, Cancer Res. 41:2003.

Johansen, I., and Howard-Flanders, P., 1965, Macromolecular repair and free radical scavenging in the protection of bacteria against X-rays, Radiat. Res., 24:184.

Kaneko, M., and Cerutti, P., 1980, Excision of N-acetoxy-2-acetyl-aminofluorene-induced DNA adducts from chromatin fractions of human fibroblasts, Cancer Res. 40:4313.

Kaneko, M., and Cerutti, P., in press, Excision of benzo(a)pyrene diol epoxide I adducts from nucleosomal DNA of confluent normal human fibroblasts, Chem. Biol. Interactions.

Kinsella, A.R., and Radman, M., 1978, Tumor promoter induces sister chromatid exchanges: relevance to mechanisms of carcinogenesis, Proc. Natl. Acad. Sci. USA 75:6149.

Klug, A., Rhodes, D., Smith, J., Finch, J.T., and Thomas, J.O., 1980, A low resolution structure for the histone core of the nucleosome, Nature 287:509.

Leadon, S., Amstad, P., and Cerutti, P., in press, Repair and expression of aflatoxin B_1-induced DNA damage, in: "Proceedings of NATO Advanced Study Institute on "The use of human cells for the assessment of risk for physical and chemical agents", Plenum Press, New York.

Legerski, R., Gray, H., and Robberson, D., 1977, A sensitive endonuclease probe for lesions in deoxyribonucleic acid helix structure produced by carcinogenic or mutagenic agents, J. Biol. Chem. 252:8740.

Levine, A., Rink, L., Weinstein, I., and Grunberger, D., 1974, Effect of N-2-acetylaminofluorene modification on the conformation of nucleic acids, Cancer Res., 34:319.

Lieberman, M., Smerdon, M., Tlsty, T., and Oleson, F., 1979, The role of chromatin structure in DNA repair in human cells damaged with chemical carcinogens and ultraviolet irradiation, in: "Environmental Carcinogenesis, Occurrence, Risk evaluation and Mechanisms", P. Emmolot and E. Kriek), Elsevier/North-Holland, Amsterdam.

Lippke, J.A., Gordon, L.K., Brash, D.E., and Haseltine, W.A., 1981, Distribution of UV light-induced damage in a defined sequence of human DNA: detection of alkaline-sensitive lesions at pyrimidine nucleoside-cytidine sequences, Proc. Natl. Acad. Sci. US 78:3388.

Lorentzen, R., and Ts'o, P., 1977, Benzo(a)pyrenedione/benzo(a)pyrenediol oxidation-reduction couples and the generation of reactive reduced molecular oxygen, Biochemistry 16:1467.

Loveday, K.S., and Latt, S.A., 1979, The effect of a tumor promoter, 12-0-tetradecanoyl-phorbol-13-acetate (TPA) on sister-chromatid exchange formation in cultured Chinese hamster cells, Mutat. Res. 67:343.

Lown, J.W., and Sim, S.K., 1977, The mechanism of the bleomycin-induced cleavage of DNA, Biochem. Biophys. Res. Commun. 77:1150.

Mattern, M.R., Hariharan, P.V., and Cerutti, P.A., 1975, Selective excision of gamma ray damaged thymine from the DNA of cultured mammalian cells, Biochim. Biophys. Acta 395:48.

McGhee, J., and Felsenfeld, G., 1979, Reaction of nucleosome DNA with dimethyl sulfate, Proc. Natl. Acad. Sci. 76:2133.

Miller, J.A., and Miller, E.C., 1971, Chemical Carcinogenesis: mechanisms and approaches to its control, J. Natl. Cancer Inst. 47:V.

Mueller, G., Wertz, P., Kwong, C., Anderson, K., and Wrighton, J., 1980, Dissection of the early molecular events in the activation of lymphocytes by 12-0-tetradecanoylphorbol-13-acetate, in: "Carcinogenesis: Fundamental Mechanisms and Environmental Effects", B. Pullman, P. Ts'o and H. Gelboin, eds, pp 319, D. Reidel Publ. Co. Holland.

Nagasawa, H., and Little, J.B., 1979, Effect of tumor promoters, protease inhibitors and repair processes on X-ray-induced sister chromatid exchanges in mouse cells, Proc. Natl. Acad. Sci. USA 76:1943.

Netrawali, M.S., and Cerutti, P., 1979, Increased near-ultraviolet induced DNA fragmentation in Xeroderma pigmentosum variants, Biochem. Biophys. Res. Commun. 87:802.

Oleson, F., Mitchell, B., Dipple, A., and Lieberman, M., 1979, Distribution of DNA damage in chromatin and its relation to repair in human cells treated with 7-bromomethylbenzo(a)-anthracene, Nucl. Acid Res. 7:1343.

Remsen, J., and RotiRoti, J., 1977, Formation of 5,6-dihydroxy-dihydrothymine-type products in DNA by hydroxyl radicals, Int. J. Radiat. Biol. 32:191.

Roberts, J.J., 1978, Repair of DNA by cytotoxic, mutagenic and carcinogenic chemicals, Advances in Radiat. Biol. 7:212.

Roots, R., and Okada, S., 1972, Protection of DNA molecules of cultured mammalian cells from radiation induced single-strand scission by various alcohols and SH compounds, Int. J. Radiat. Biol. 21:329.

RotiRoti, J., and Cerutti, P., 1974, Gamma-ray induced thymine damage in mammalian cells, Int. J. Radiat. Biol. 25:413.

Sage, E., Fuchs, R.P., and Leng, M., 1979, Reactivity of the anti-bodies to DNA modified by the carcinogen N-acetoxy-N-acetyl-2-aminofluorene, Biochemistry 18:1328.

Santella, R., Grunberger, D., Weinstein, I., and Rich, A., 1981, Induction of the Z conformation in poly(dG-dC) poly (dG-dC) by binding of N-2-acetylaminofluorene to guanine residues, Proc. Natl. Acad. Sci. US 78:1451.

Saragosti, S., Moyne, G., and Yaniv, M., 1980, Absence of nucleosomes in a fraction of SV40 chromatin between the origin of replication and the region coding for late leader RNA, Cell 20:65.

Shafranovskaya, N., Trifonov, E., Lazurkin, Yu., and Frank-Kamenetshii, M., 1973, Clustering of thymine dimers in ultraviolet irradiated DNA and the long-range transfer of electronic excitation along the molecule, Nature New Biol. 241:58.

Shelton, E., Wassarman, P., and DePamphilis, M., 1978, Structure of simian virus 40 chromosomes in nuclei from infected monkey cells, J. Mol. Biol. 125:491.

Simpson, R.T., 1978, Structure of the chromatosome, a chromatin
          particle containing 160 base pairs of DNA and all the
          histones, Biochem. 17:5524.
Singer, B., and Kröger, M., 1979, Participation of modified nucleo-
          sides in translation and transcription, in: "Progress in
          Nucleic Acid Research and Molecular Biology", Vol. 23,
          pp. 151-191, W.E. Cohn, ed., Academic Press, New York.
Slaga, T., Sivak, A., and Boutewell, R., eds., 1978, in:"Carcino-
          genesis", Vol. 2, Raven Press, New York.
Snapka, R., and Linn, St., 1981, Efficiency of formation of pyrimi-
          dine dimers in SV40 chromatin in vitro, Biochemistry 20:68.
Thompson, L., Baker, R., Carrano, A., and Brookman, K., 1980,
          Failure of the phorbol 12-0-tetradecanoylphorbol-13-acetate
          to enhance sister chromatid exchange, mitotic segregation,
          or expression of mutations in chinese hamster cells,
          Cancer Res. 40:3245.
Tjian, R., 1978, The binding site on SV40 DNA for a T antigen-
          related protein, Cell 13:165.
Tooze, J., ed., 1980, "DNA Tumor Viruses", Cold Spring Harbor
          Laboratory, New York.
Wang, T.V., and Cerutti, P.A., 1980a, Effect of formation and removal
          of aflatoxin B_1: DNA adducts in 10T1/2 mouse embryo fibro-
          blasts on cell viability, Cancer Res. 40:2904.
Wang, T.V., and Cerutti, P.A., 1980b, Spontaneous reaction of afla-
          toxin B_1-modified DNA in vitro, Biochemistry 19:1692.
Williams, J., and Friedberg, E., 1979, DNA excision repair in
          chromatin after ultraviolet irradiation of human fibro-
          blasts in culture, Biochemistry 18:3965.
Yakobovits, E., Bratosin, S., and Aloni, Y., 1980, A nucleosome-
          free region in SV40 minichromosomes, Nature 285:263.
Yamasaki, H., Pulkrabek, P., Grunberger, D., and Weinstein, I.,
          1977, Differential excision from DNA of the C-8 and N^2-
          guanosine adducts of N-acetyl-2-aminofluorene by single
          strand-specific endonucleases, Cancer Res. 37:3756.
Zbinden, I., and Cerutti, P., 1981, Near-ultraviolet sensitivity
          of skin fibroblasts of patients with Bloom's syndrome,
          Biochem. Biophysical Res. Commun. 98:579.

DNA ALKALINE ELUTION: PHYSICAL BASIS OF THE ELUTION PROCESS AND VALIDATION OF THIS METHOD AS A SCREENING PROCEDURE TO IDENTIFY CHEMICAL CARCINOGENS

Claudio Nicolini**, Marco Cavanna*,Annalisa Maura*, Albiana Pino*, Luigi Robbiano*, Felice Biassoni*, Rossella Ricci*, A. Belmont*, S. Zietz*, and Giovanni Brambilla*.

*National Research Councyl, Italy, and Division of Biophysics of Temple University, Philadelphia, Pa. USA**; Institute of Pharmacology, School of Medicine University of Genoa, Italy**

INTRODUCTION

The alkaline elution technique, developed by Kohn and coworkers (Kohn and Ewig, 1973; Kohn et al., 1976; Kohn, 1979), provides a sensitive measurement of DNA single-strand size distribution in mammalian cells and represents an advanced alternative to the technique of alkaline sucrose gradient sedimentation. Alkaline elution of DNA from cell lysates allows size measurement of DNA single strands longer than the sizes that can be measured by sedimentation in alkaline sucrose gradients. The elution technique requires relatively simple and not expensive apparatuses, and is less time-consuming in comparison with the latter. Moreover, it gives more repeatable results and is more suitable to assess DNA damage from various tissues following *in vivo* exposure to DNA interacting agents. In the last few years, this technique has been widely applied by different groups of researchers to the study of various DNA lesions induced by several physical or chemical agents (ranging from carcinogens to antineoplastic agents), and a large series of results have been

collected. The aims of this review are: to discuss the physical basis that governs DNA elution, to summarize the possible application
of this method, to revise the use of alkaline elution and its reliability in the assessment of DNA fragmentation in various organs of
mice and rats following *in vivo* exposure to chemical agents, and to
evaluate critically its role as a screening procedure for carcinogenic compounds.

PHYSICAL BASIS OF THE ALKALINE ELUTION PROCESS

The alkaline elution technique that utilizes membrane filters
to discriminate DNA single-strand sizes from mammalian cells, in
the typical procedure consists of the following steps. 1) Cells (or
nuclei) are isolated and brought into suspension, looking out not
to introduce (specially when cells are obtained from tissues) into
DNA any *technical* fragmentation. 2) Cells are collected and washed
on the filter. 3) Cell lysis is accomplished on the filter by adding a lysis solution at high ionic strength, containing NaCl, EDTA
and an anionic detergent (pH 10), with spontaneous dripping. This
step removes almost all of the non-DNA material of the cells (protein, RNA, lipid). 4) The lysate on the filter is then washed with
EDTA solution (pH 10). The previous steps do not denature DNA, so
that DNA still exists on the filter as double-stranded helices. 5)
The filter is then eluted with an alkaline solution (pH approx. 12.1)
which is pumped slowly through with a peristaltic pump, while fractions containing single stranded DNA are regularly collected. 6) DNA
is dosed in the eluted fractions, in the filter, and in the filter
holder to determine the kinetics of DNA release.

By working with L1210 mouse leukemia cells grown in suspension
Kohn et al. (1976) showed that for DNA to be eluted, the base-paired
structure requires to be disrupted, which occurs owing to the high
pH of eluting solution. Only if the cells are much damaged or heav-
ily exposed to X ray, a fraction of DNA will be eluted in neutral
solution as double stranded molecules (Bradley and Kohn, 1979). During alkaline elution, the elution rate is governed by the properties
of DNA itself, being dependent on average single-strand size. Always
according to Kohn et al. (1976), the elution kinetics is not affected
by the attachment of DNA to a non-DNA cell component that sticks to
the filter, since its characteristic pattern can be demonstrated to
be not at variance after nearly all non-DNA material of the cell has
been removed from the filter (e.g. by further incubation of the lysates before elution step with proteolytic enzyme and strong detergent). In addition, the elution rate is independent of the number
of cells deposited onto the standard filter (25 mm in diameter) in
the range of 0.1 to 2×10^6 cells. Moreover, the retention on the
filter of DNA was shown to be substantially independent either of
the composition of the filter membrane or of its pore size, since
qualitatively similar results were obtained using filters composed

of various materials and with different pore size (from 1 to 5 µm).
The retention of DNA on the filter as depending on the large size
of the strands is confirmed by the observations that the elution is
highly sensitive to shearing, and that visible light can interfere
with the assay by producing single-strand breaks in DNA both in alkali and in intact cells. The transition pH for DNA elution was found
to depend on the nature of the cation in the eluting solution, occurring at pH 11.3 - 11.7 with the organic tetrapropylammonium cation and at pH 11.9 - 12.5 with sodium cation. Above the transition
pH for DNA elution, the kinetics of elution of DNA from mammalian
cells, exposed to low doses of X ray, was found to consist of two
phases. In the initial phase of elution, DNA exhibits alkaline elution curves which accurately fit first-order kinetics, as indicated
by a linear plot of log of fraction of DNA retained on the filter
versus elution time (i.e. versus eluted volume). In this phase the
elution rate is inversely dependent on the size of DNA strands resulting from strand breakage elicited by X ray. In the later phase
the rate is accelerated due to a slow alkali-catalyzed hydrolysis
of phosphodiester bonds; in addition, it becomes dependent on pH.

Calibration relative to the effect of X ray showed that the
range of DNA single strand lengths which can be discriminated by
elution above the transition pH is $5 \times 10^8 - 10^{10}$ daltons (Kohn et
al., 1976).

Assuming that DNA of uniform length elutes according to first-
-order kinetics,

$$DNA_{eluted} = \left[DNA\right]_0 \times \left\{1 - e^{-v(l)t}\right\}$$

the equation for elution of a distribution of DNA strands of different length will be:

$$\left[DNA\right]_{eluted}^{total} = \int_0^\infty l \, dn \, (l) \left[1 - e^{-v(l)t}\right] \qquad (1)$$

where: $dn \, (l)$ = DNA of length l to $l + dl$; $v(l)$ = elution rate;
t = elution time.

It is known that $n(l)$ for a distribution created by random
breaks is:

$$n(l) = \frac{NT}{l_1^2} e^{-l/l_1}$$

where l_1 = average strand length, and (NT) = total number of DNA
units = $\sum_l^\infty n(l)l$. If we begin with a distribution as above (control), and then introduce an additional probability (per nucleotide)
of breakage p', we have:

$$n(l) = NT \left[e^{-l(p' + 1/l_1)}\right] (p' + 1/l_1)^2 \qquad (2)$$

In order to solve equation (1), the problem is to find elution rate, v(l), as function of l. It seemed that the best course was to come up with v(l) from first principles. In this respect a hypothesis has already been published (Kohn et al., 1976) on the assumption that, since the contour length of each DNA strand is large relative to the size of filter pores, the elution would occur when one pore achieves *dominance* over the other pores which are covered by the same molecule. However, it seemed to us that the important parameter is not the contour length but rather the radius (r) of the random coil that the DNA strand will find itself in. For a coil in which there is no angle restriction for rotation of adjoining links, assuming a *random walk* type model, the radius distribution is given by:

$$P(r) = (\frac{1}{2\pi\alpha^2})^{3/2} \; e^{-r^2/2\alpha^2} \quad . \qquad (3)$$

where $\alpha^2 = <r^2> = B \; \nu^2$

B being the number of nucleotides for the given strand, and ν the length between successive nucleotides. For a DNA strand of 10^7 nucleotides, assuming a length of 3.4 Å (ν) for each nucleotide, we obtain a DNA *ball* radius of $\cong 1.1 \times 10^{-6}$ m.

On these bases, Nicolini et al. (1981a) have developed a new analytical model which takes into consideration both all the physicochemical properties of *in situ* DNA strand (length and flexibility//superpacking) and the geometric and hydrodynamic configuration of the elution apparatus (flow and filter conditions). This model is based on the following assumption.

1) About a filter pore there is a radius, A, for which any DNA strand lying within it elutes with a characteristic rate, independently of strand length. This radius is physically close in size to the actual pore size, but may be slingthly larger.

2) The average elution rate, v(l), is not length independent, as the probability of being positioned within the radius A is not the same for DNA strands of different length. This probability to first order can be taken as proportional to the area of the circle of radius A - r, where r is the radius of the *ball* conformation of the DNA strand. Thus,

$$v(l) \propto (R - r)^2 = K(A - r)^2$$

where K is a constant depending on the flow conditions. Considering that the ball radius r is function of both chain flexibility/superpaking and length, elution rate will increase for a DNA with similar length and higher flexibility/superpacking, or for a DNA with similar flexibility/superpacking but smaller length.

3) The radius of the *ball* formed by a DNA strand will be defined in terms of the standard deviation, σ, of the *random walk chain* model. For a completely flexible chain, $\sigma^2 = l\mu^2$, where l = number of links and μ = length of each link. For a preliminary test of this model, r (strand) was set equal to σ, but a better fit was attained with $r = c\sigma$, where c is a constant related to chain flexibility, which may change in DNA from different cells. Changes in the constant c should reflect changes in the viscoelastic properties of DNA, which indeed are clearly changing during carcinogenesis and cell proliferation (Nicolini et al., 1981b).

Thus, from the above considerations and equations 1-3 we have for the DNA eluted as function of time,

$$\left[DNA\right]_{el} (t) = \int_0^{A^2/\mu^2c^2} \left(\frac{1}{l_l^2}\right) e^{-l/l_l} \left(1-e^{-K(A-c\mu\sqrt{l})^2t}\right) dl \qquad (4)$$

Note that for DNA of radius greater than or equal to A, the elution rate is zero, hence the integration limit, $l = A^2/\mu^2c^2$ (for which

$r = c \sqrt{A^2/\mu^2c^2} \cdot \mu = A$).

To evaluate the fraction of eluted DNA versus time, we solve then the integral in equation (4) (see Appendix in Nicolini et al., 1981a), yielding:

$$\left[DNA\right]_{el} (t) = \left[1-(1+P_1^2)\exp(-P_1^2)\right] -2\exp\left(\frac{-P_2 P_1^2 t}{P_2 t+P_1^2}\right) \int_0^t f(\omega,\alpha,\beta) \, d\omega \qquad (5)$$

where:
$$P_1 = \frac{1}{c\sqrt{l_l}} (A/\mu) \quad ; \quad P_2 = KA^2$$

$$\alpha = \frac{P_2}{P_1} (t + 1); \quad \beta = \frac{P_2}{P_1} t$$

$$f(\omega,\alpha,\beta) = \omega^3\exp\left[-\alpha(\omega-\beta/\alpha)^2\right]$$

In order to probe the capability of this model to quantitatively explain and predict experimental observations, several simulations have been performed to search for the optimal combination of previously defined DNA chain parameters which best fit the experimental data. Initially (Fig.1) our attention has been addressed to typical alkaline elution profiles such as those previously obtained (Cavanna et al., 1980) with liver DNA from untreated control mice and from

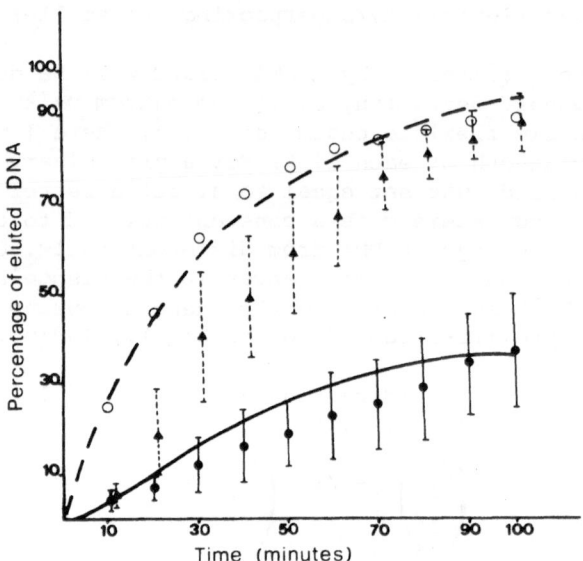

Fig. 1 Experimental time-dependence of eluted DNA from control liv-
         er (●) and DGA-treated liver cells, with (○) and without
         (▲) 30 minutes incubation in alkaline solution. The contin-
         uous (———) and dashed (----) lines refers to the theoretical
         time dependence obtained from a best fitting of the data (con-
         trol ● and treated ▲ respectively) with the model described
         in the text. Vertical bars indicate S.D.

mice treated with 1000 mg/kg of N-diazoacetylglycine amide (DGA).
The theorical time-dependence of eluted DNA, as shown in Fig. 1, was
computed from equation (5) by best fitting the experimental data obtained with a 5 μm pore size filter, eluted at the rate of 0.2 ml/
/min for a total of 20 ml, which gives a constant

$$K = 3.2 \times 10^{-12} \left(\frac{\text{fraction eluted DNA}}{\text{min} \times \text{area}} \right).$$

     For the control mice, the optimization was carried out search-
ing simultaneously for the values of two independent dimensionless
parameters, $P_1 = \dfrac{A}{c \mu \sqrt{l_1}}$ and $P_2 = KA^2$, which yielded the minimum χ^2,
where A (*equivalent* pore size), l_1 (average strand molecular weight),
K (flow rate per unit area), and c (DNA flexibility and superpacking).
They were respectively: 1.8 (P_1) and 0.0182 (P_2), with a $\chi^2 = 2 \times 10^{-3}$.

Assuming known the value of K, which depends from the experimental flow conditions and is approximately equal to 3.2×10^{-12} fraction of total DNA, per minute and Angstrom square, we then compute the effective pore size $A = \sqrt{\dfrac{P_2}{K}} = 5.6 \times 10^4$ Angstrom, which is sligthly larger than actual pore size as expected on theorical grounds. From A and P_1 we obtain $c\sqrt{l_1} = \dfrac{A}{\mu P_1} = 9.1 \times 10^3$, i.e. for a perfectly flexible chain (c=1) an average molecular weight l_1 equal to 8.2×10^7 links or 2.7×10^{10} daltons (considering that on link is equal to 330 daltons).

Considering that the flow and filter conditions were kept constant when the DNA-damaging effect of DGA was explored, we then mantained P_2 constant (i.e., the same value of 0.0182 of the above controls) and best fitted ($\chi^2 = 2 \times 10^{-2}$) the elution profiles of the 1000 mg/kg DGA dosage to find the value of P_1 (16.5) and then, for c=1, that of l_1 of DGA-altered DNA strand (3.3×10^8 daltons). Interestingly, the DNA average molecular weight theoretically computed before and after DGA administration is in good agreement with values obtained by independent determination by calibrated alkaline sucrose gradients (respectively $\simeq 1.5 \times 10^9$ and 2.0×10^8 daltons in hepatocyte preparations).

The quality of the fit 'for the *treated* data set was, however, improved when also P_2 was optimized and not kept constant (0.0182), yielding a better fit ($\chi^2 = 10^{-3}$) for $P_2 = 0.064$ and $P_1 = 3.8$. This implies a different value of A (13×10^4 Angstrom) possibly related to the fact that a DNA strand of quite shorter length and different flexibility may actually *see* a larger *effective* pore size. The theoretical average DNA length after DGA treatment would then become 3.3×10^{10} daltons, i.e. quite larger than the one actually measured with alkaline sucrose gradients. Both theoretical values have been computed for a perfectly flexible chain (c=1); to yield values identical to the experimentally determined length (l_1^E), the overall chain flexibility ($c = \dfrac{A}{\mu P_1 \sqrt{l_1^E / 330}}$) has to be equal to 4 and to 12 for control and DGA-treated DNA respectively, suggesting a dramatic increase in chain rigidity. It is conforting to note that the DNA chain elasticity/flexibility and superpacking dramatically decreases of similar magnitude after interaction with chemical carcinogens (Nicolini et al., 1981b).

In the theoretical profile, but not in the experimental one (see Fig. 1) the concavity is upward at the early times, in a wide distribution of randomly-broken DNA the smaller fragments should indeed elute faster than the larger ones, yielding a downward concavity in the broken DNA elution profiles (in the intact DNA, as for controls, unwinding may play a role in the elution rate). Incidentally at the later times the concavity is also upward suggesting the appearance with time of new single-strand breaks, progressively generated by alkali-labile sites. In the first 50 minutes the predicted values are significantly larger than the experimental ones obtained in standard washing solution (pH 10.4 and $\chi^2 = 2 \times 10^{-2}$), but where exactly those obtained after a 30 minutes incubation in alkaline eluting solution (pH 12.3, and $\chi^2 = 10^{-14}$), when most alkali-labile sites induced by DGA had sufficient time for conversion to single-strand breaks. Our model then proved to be quite accurate even in predicting the *true* elution sequence of DNA strands of given length, since the apparent discrepancies at early times are the result of inherent experimental pitfalls (Cavanna et al., 1980). The theoretical profiles is indeed obtained by best fitting over the entire range, where the size (and consequent distribution) of the overall single-strand breaks are properly estimated.

Our simulation therefore has shown that the elution profiles for constant flow (K) and filter (A) conditions depend, not only upon the DNA molecular weight, but also upon a parameter (c) critically related to chain flexibility and supercoiling. This dependency, expected from our model, has been confirmed to be quite relevant to the elution rate by the following experiment. As shown in Fig. 2, intact nuclei from untreated control rats, lysed with 2 M NaCl, 0.2% Sarcosyl, 20 mM Na_2EDTA, pH 10.0 (i.e. below the transition value) for different length of time (ranging from 30 min to 48 hr) exhibited drastically different elution profiles in standard alkaline conditions (pH 12.3). On the contrary, they yielded a constant low fraction of DNA eluted from the filter for identical lysing times and neutral (pH 7.5) eluting conditions.

Parallel studies performed on the same samples determining DNA molecular weight by sedimentation in alkaline sucrose gradients confirm that, indeed, with the DNA molecular weight remaining similar (1.2×10^9 daltons after 0.5 hr of lysis; 1.1×10^9 daltons after 24-48 hr of lysis), as expected during lysis at pH equal to 10.0 in the presence of EDTA and high ionic strength, the visco-elastic properties and higher order superpacking (Nicolini et al.,1981b) of the DNA chain do change with lysis time, increasing up to 48 hr its elasticity, viscosity and uncoiling toward a B-form double stranded DNA. The predictions of our model, with l_1 (average strand length) K and A remaining constant, are compatible with all above observations, yielding a constant value of effective pore size of 5.6×10^4 Angstrom (as expected from the actual pore size) and progressively lower values for the parameter c with the increasing elution

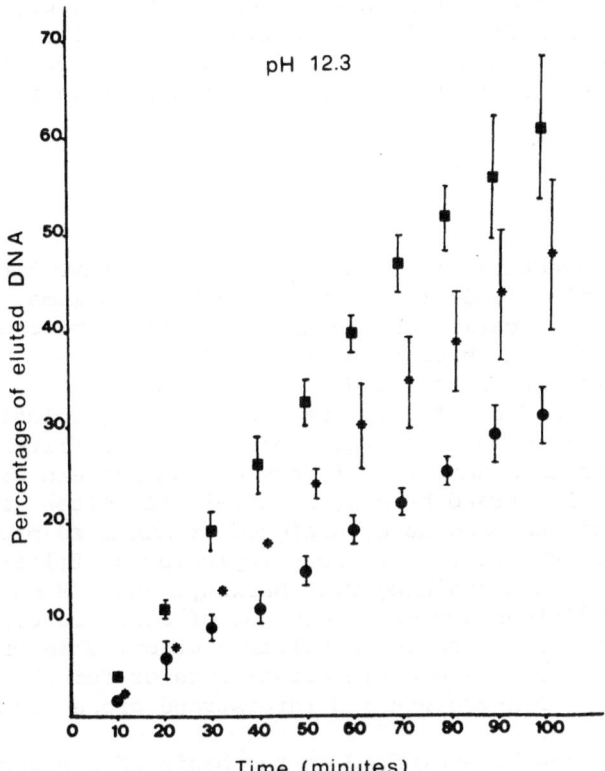

Fig. 2 Elution profiles of DNA from untreated rat liver cell nuclei
after incubation in lysing solution (pH 10) for different
periods of time: ● 30 min, ✳ 24 hr, ■ 48 hr. Subsequent elution was carried out at pH 12.3. The data are the average
of 4 independent experiments; vertical bars indicated S.E..

rate, which suggests an increase in chain flexibility and/or a decrease in radius ball size (as found for nuclear DNA in similar experimental conditions) (Nicolini et al., 1981b).

In conclusion, the described physico-chemical model is capable
indeed to yield quantitative explanation, from first principles, of
the elution data available in the literature, yielding a quantitative
estimate of DNA molecular weight (at least its upper limit obtainable in the hypothesis of a perfectly flexible chain) both within
and outside the range of calibrated alkaline sucrose gradients, and
most important of DNA chain elasticity and supercoiling, critical parameters highly associated with DNA length. The modifications of these
two latter parameters during mutation and carcinogenesis, which have

been so far largely underestimated and can be independently monitored by complex viscosimetric assays (Chase and Shafer, 1979; Shafer
and Chase, 1980; Parodi et al., 1981a; Nicolini et al., 1981b), have
been shown to occur dependently or independently of changes in DNA
length and are then co-factors in determining elution rates of native giant DNA.

TYPES OF ASSAYS

Two basic procedures of DNA alkaline elution have been developed by Kohn et al. (1980) in order to reach the maximal sensitivity
and to allow quantification of the damage. A first procedure, designed to minimize protein absorption, is based on the use: a) of polycarbonate filters, b) of sodium dodecylsulfate in both lysing and
eluting solution, and c) of proteinase-K in lysing solution. In this
way, less than 0.1% of cell protein remains on the filter. This procedure is used to eliminate the effects of DNA-protein cross-links
in assays of single-strand breaks, alkali-labile sites or interstrand
cross-links. A second procedure, designed to maximize protein absorption, is based on the use: a) of polyvinylchloride filters, and b)
of a lysing solution containing 0.2% Sarkosyl and 2 M NaCl. In these
experimental conditions approximately 20% of cell protein remains absorbed to the filter during the alkaline elution. This procedure is
used for the assay of DNA protein cross-links or for the study of the
combined effect of DNA-protein and interstrand cross-links.

Cross-links can be evaluated on the basis of a reduction in the
elution rate. In the case of interstrand cross-links the elution rate
is reduced bacause of an effective increase in strand length and probably also because of the obstacle to the unwinding process. The absorption of protein to the filter reduces the elution rate when DNA-
-protein cross-links are present. To evaluate the effect of cross-
-links on DNA elution rate, the cells are exposed prior to elution
assay to an appropriate dose of X ray in order to introduce a given
frequency of single-strand breaks. A detailed description of the procedures for the assay and the quantitation of total, interstrand and
DNA-protein cross-links, as well as for the assay of strand breaks
and cross-links mixtures has been published by Kohn et al. (1980).
The application of these procedures to the study of the mechanism
of action of some alkylating agents, platinum compounds, and chemical carcinogens was the object of several papers (e.g.: Ross et al.,
1978; Thomas et al., 1978; Ewig and Kohn, 1978; Fornace and Little,
1979; Laurent et al., 1981).

Double-strand breaks can be detected by measuring the rate of
DNA elution through the filter under neutral conditions (Bradley and
Kohn, 1979). A number of variables were found to be important in order to optimize the sensitivity of this procedure to the X ray effect. By the use of a stringent deproteinization, polycarbonate

straight-through pore filters, eluting solution at pH 9.6, and a
total cell number less than $0.5x10^{-6}$, the assay has been shown to be
capable of detecting the number of double-strand breaks induced by
as little as 1000 rad of X-ray.

DNA DAMAGE *IN VIVO*/ALKALINE ELUTION ASSAY AS A SHORT-
-TERM TEST FOR PREDICTING CARCINOGENIC POTENTIAL OF
CHEMICAL AGENTS

The use of alkaline elution for the screening of chemical carcinogens has been initially proposed by Swenberg et al. (1976). Dose-
dependence of DNA damage was evaluated in V79 cultured cells either
in the absence or in the presence of liver microsomal activation
systems. The results of 71 chemicals (Swenberg, 1979) indicate that
alkaline elution appears to correctly identify carcinogens from non-
carcinogens 85-90% of the time. Other data (Cavanna et al., 1977;
Cerutti et al., 1978) confirm the satisfactory correlation between
positive results in the *in vitro* alkaline elution assay and carcinogenicity. However, the use of cultured cells presents at least a
substantial limitation (Langenbach et al., 1978; Bigger et al., 1980),
that is the lack of proper metabolic activation, since the usual S-9
activating systems from liver of induced or noninduced rats do not
reproduce exactly the metabolic capacity of liver *in vivo*. Moreover,
the metabolic activation of the procarcinogens to ultimate carcinogens could take place in organs other than the liver, or be performed by the intestinal bacterial flora. This limitation may be circum-
vented by evaluating the ability of a chemical to cause DNA damage
in vivo. With this aim, the alkaline elution technique has been adapted by Petzold and Swenberg (1978) and by Parodi et al. (1978) to
detect DNA fragmentation induced in various tissues of rats and mice
by treatment with a chemical agent.

The DNA damage *in vivo*/alkaline elution assay has been put to
practical use in our laboratory for more than three years. The results that have been accumulated in this period allow to determine
its reliability both in terms of repeatability and of sensitivity.
The standard procedure followed, already published (Brambilla et al.
1978; Cavanna et al., 1980), briefly is as now to be given. Tissues
to be tested for DNA damage are dissected and processed in order to
obtain cells or nuclei in suspension with as little as possible sub-
cellular debris and a minimum of DNA damage. Aliquots of $0.5-1x10^{6}$
cells and/or nuclei are deposited on a Millipore mixed esters of
cellulose filter (25 mm diameter; 5 μm pore size). The cells are
washed on the filter with cold Merchant's solution (0.14 M NaCl, 1.47
mM KH_2PO_4, 2.7 mM KCl, 8.1 mM Na_2HPO_4, 0.53 mM Na_2EDTA; pH 7.4), and
lysed with 0.2% sodium lauroyl sarcosinate, 2 M NaCl, 0.02 M Na_2EDTA,
pH 10. After an additional wash with 0.02 M Na_2EDTA, pH 10, single-
-stranded DNA eluted from the filter in the dark by controlled flow
of a solution of 0.02 M Na_2EDTA, 0.06 M tetraethylammonium hydroxide,

pH 12.3. The flow rate was usually 0.13 ml/min. The content of DNA
in the 13 ml of eluate and that remaining on the filter is determined as previously described (Cavanna et al., 1980) by a modification
of the microfluorometric technique of Kissane and Robins (1958). In
these experimental conditions the recovery of applied DNA is 80% or
greater. DNA damage (single-strand breaks and alkali-labile sites)
induced by a chemical agent is evaluated as increase over controls
in the percentage of eluted DNA (or as increase over controls of DNA
elution rate, K (ml^{-1})).

Since the variability of results in mainly dependent on differences in tissue handling for obtaining cells or nuclei in suspension,
and such differences are operating in single samples even if run in
the same day, it is important to be able to check a positive result
either against a large spectrum of controls data or against data
obtained with breaks-inducing agents of known potency. Figures 3,4
and 5 show some elution data obtained in our laboratory in the last
12 months. By comparing (Figures 3 and 4) the distributions of the
percentage of eluted DNA from different tissues of control mice, it
is evident that the variability of results is greater for those organs (thymus, bone marrow, stomach and colon mucosa) presenting more
difficulty in obtaining a suspension of cells without any *technical*
damage. For these organs a larger set of data will be required to
reach a statistical significance for the same average increase in
the percentage of eluted DNA induced by a chemical agent. Figures 3
and 5 show the variability in the percentage of DNA eluted from the
liver of mice and rats treated with N-nitrosodimethylamine. Dose-
-dependence of DNA fragmentation elicited in rat by i.p. treatment
with this procarcinogen, in the low dose range, is clearly evident
from histograms of Fig. 5.

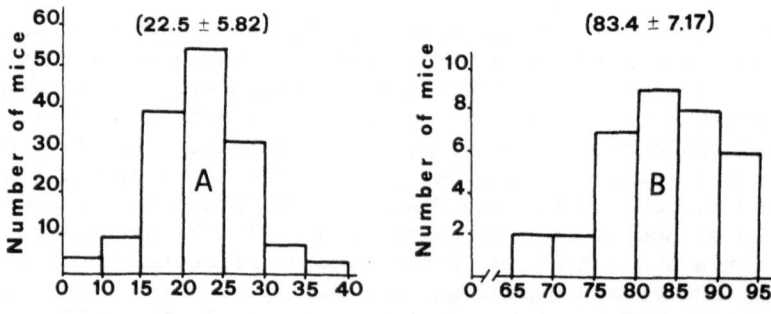

% of eluted **DNA** in each mouse

Fig. 3   Distribution of the values of DNA eluted from livers of:
A) 148 control mice; B) 34 mice given i.p. 37 mg/kg of
N-nitrosodimethylamine 4 hr before killing. In brackets,
mean ± S.D.

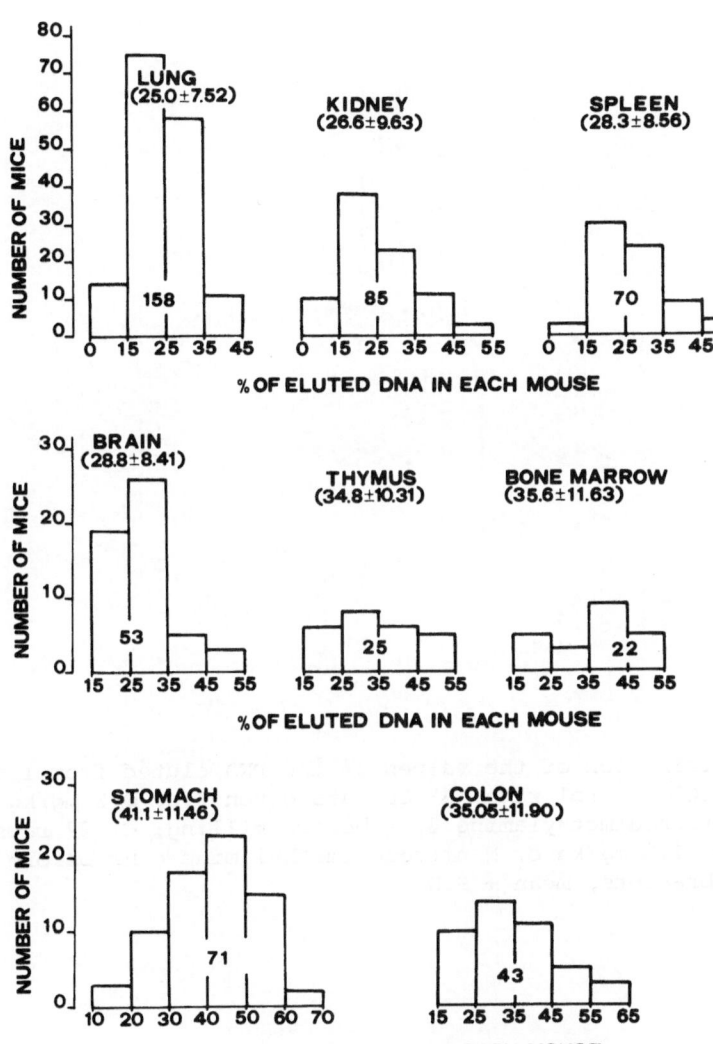

Fig. 4   Distribution of the values of DNA eluted from various organs of control mice. Data in brackets are the mean ± S.D.;
inside the histograms the number of mice for each organ.

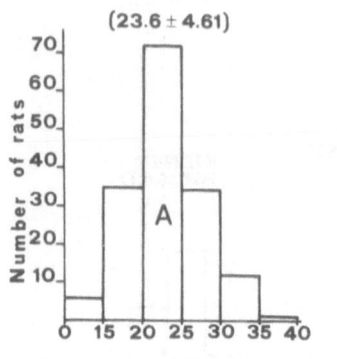

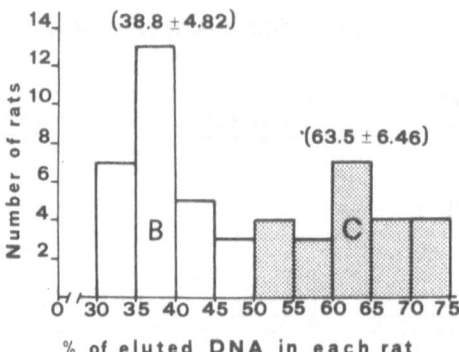

Fig. 5   Distribution of the values of the DNA eluted from livers of:
         A) 160 control rats; B) 28 rats given i.p. 0.6 mg/kg of N-
         -nitrosodimethylamine 4 hr before killing; C) 22 rats given
         i.p. 1.2 mg/kg of N-nitrosodimethylamine 4 hr before killing.
         In brackets, mean ± S.D.

        It is evident that DNA damage *in vivo*/alkaline elution assay
accounts for host mediation of the compound and thereby affords several other advantages over *in vitro* systems, beyond that of assuring
a *normal* metabolic behaviour. These advantages can be summarized as
follows. a) The assay accounts for the role of physiological factors
which include the route of administration, the rate of absorption,
the type of distribution, and the rate of elimination. b) It permits,
allowing multiple tissue analysis, the assessment of tissue specific
level of risk for genotoxic damage. A satisfactory correlation was

indeed found to exist between target organs for tumor formation and
tissues showing increased elution after treatment with procarcinogens (Petzold and Swenberg, 1978; Cavanna et al., 1979). c) Since
the acute LD50's are usually known, it is easy to choose doses to
be tested. d) It can provide information otherwise unobtainable,
as the formation of DNA damaging agents in the gastric environment
from the reaction of nitrite with amino-group carrying compounds
(Parodi et al., 1980), or in the gut from activating reactions
carried out by bacterial flora (Cavanna et al., 1979).

    Because of such advantages, the capability of inducing DNA dam-
age *in vivo* seems to be more suitable than *in vitro* tests to evaluate the potential carcinogenic activity of chemical agents. As a
consequence, an examination of whether there is a quantitative correlation between the carcinogenic potency in experimental animals
and the potency in inducing DNA fragmentation is of some interest.
Starting with the work of Damjanov et al. (1973) on the induction by
methylating agents of single-strand breaks in rat liver DNA, several
carcinogens have been shown to cause a dose-dependent DNA fragmentation in various organs of rats and/or mice. Unfortunately, in most
cases DNA-damage was evaluated by sedimentation velocity in alkaline
sucrose gradients and results, usually published as sedimentation
profiles,do not allow a quantitative estimate of the degree of DNA
fragmentation. On the contrary, DNA elution rate, which in first
approximation may be considered proportional to the number of single-
-strand breaks (Kohn et al., 1976), provides a quantitative datum
which can be utilized to calculate DNA-damaging potency. Consequently, the following analysis of the correlation between DNA-damaging
and carcinogenic potency is based only on results obtained *in vivo*
by the use of the alkaline elution technique. DNA-damaging potency
was calculated from the ratio:

$$\frac{(K_t - K_c)}{mol/kg}$$

where $(K_t - K_c)$ is the average elution rate over controls, being
K_t the average elution rate of DNA from treated animals and K_c the
average elution rate of DNA from control animals. K was obtained
from the following formula

$$K = \ln \frac{1}{(\text{fraction of DNA retained on filter})} \times \frac{1}{V}$$

where V in the elution volume in ml.

    Data obtained in the last few years by testing the ability of
41 known carcinogens of inducing DNA fragmentation in various organs of mice and rats are listed,in terms of DNA-damaging potency,
in Table 1. When a compound was tested for various routes of admin-

istration and/or at various doses, and/or in independent experiments, the values given in Table 1 are the potency range. If the DNA-damaging activity of the compound was measured in various organs, the potency is that observed in the most affected organ, and other organs showing DNA damage are listed in order of decreasing effect. Tissues which are the target of carcinogenic activity are indicated by an asterisk. Unfortunately a precise evaluation of DNA damaging activity sometimes was not possible, since published data provide for both dose and % of eluted DNA only the range; in these cases the interpolated values are given in brackets. Furthermore, no indication was often given of the statistical significance of the results.

The carcinogenic potency was computed from literature data usually obtained from IARC Monographs on the Evaluation of Carcinogenic Risk of Chemicals to Man (1972-81) and from Survey of Compounds which have been Tested for Carcinogenic Activity (1972-73), by utilizing, when necessary, more complete information from original papers. This carcinogenic potency was calculated according to the suggestion of Ames (1979), as TD50 (tumor dose 50), which is the daily dose rate required to decrease by half the probability of an animal remaining tumor-free at the end of a standard lifetime (taken as 104 weeks for rats and mice). The calculation of this index, which takes into account spontaneous tumor incidence in control animals, was performed according to the formula

$$TD50 = \frac{(\ln 2)\,dt^3}{\ln\left(\dfrac{P_c}{P_e}\right)}$$

where d is the experimental dose in mmol/kg/day averaged over experiment time, t is the experiment time/standard life time, and P_c and P_e are the probabilities of being tumor-free at the end of the experiment in the control group and in the experimental group respectively. Data reported in Table 1 indicate the range of TD50 computed from the experiments considered.

On the whole, data of Table 1 suggest that the variability in DNA-damaging potencies obtained from independent experiments is usually smaller than the variability in TD50. To set an example of the variability of DNA damaging potency, Table 2 lists the values obtained from experiments performed in different strains of rats and mice treated i.p. or p.o. with various doses of N-nitrosodimethylamine. It must be pointed out that a general greater variability of TD50 could be expected, since carcinogenesis is a multistep process of which DNA damage could be the initial step.

Concerning the qualitative relationship between the ability of a chemical to cause tumor growth and that to induce DNA fragmentation,

Table 1. Summary of DNA damage induced *in vivo* by chemical agents[a]

Chemical	Animal species	DNA-damaging potency $\frac{K_t-K_c}{mol/kg}$	Ref.	Carcinogenic potency (TD50 mmol/kg)
Alkylating Agents				
Methyl methane-sulfonate	rat	St:84-131;br,* si,ki,lu,th,li	1	NC
	mouse	Li:12-94;ki,lu*	2,3,4	2.02-50.65
Ethyl methane-sulfonate	rat	Th:(16);li,ki*	1	0.59-2.69
β-Propiolactone	rat	Li:(5-13);st,si*	1	13.43
Cyclophosphamide	rat	Bm:*(44-700)	1	NC
Azaserine	rat	Li:(74-370);ki	1	0.009
N-Diazoacetyl-glycine amide	mouse	Th:11-30;ki,li,* sp,bm,lu*	5	0.11-0.68
N-Nitroso Compounds				
N-Nitrosodimethyl-amine	rat	Li:*174-778;lu,ki,* th	1,6,7	0.16-0.78
	mouse	Li:*207-1256;lu,* ki*	3,8	0.16-11.34
N-Nitrosodiethyl-amine	rat	Li:*30-273;si,ki,*	1,6	NC
	mouse	Li:*20-42	3	0.02-0.80
N-Nitrosodi-n-propylamine	rat	Li:*15-64	6	0.63-1.12
N-Nitrosodi-n-butylamine	rat	Li:*17-21	6	NC
N-Nitroso-pyrrolidine	rat	Li:*6-22	6	9.20-13.21

(Table 1 continued)

Table 1.

Chemical	Animal species	DNA-damaging potency $\dfrac{K_t-K_c}{mol/kg}$	Ref.	Carcinogenic potency (TD50 mmol/kg)
N-Nitroso-morpholine	mouse	Li:32-40 *	3	10.22-58.6
N-Nitroso-N-methylurea	rat	Ki:(231);mg,br*, th,li	1,6	NC
	mouse	Ki:103-116;br, sp,li	8	0.07-1.19
N-Nitroso-N-ethylurea	rat	Mg:(68-137);lu, br,li,ki *	1	0.9-3.73
N-Methyl-N'-nitro-N-nitroso-guanidine	rat	Si:15-24;st,li *	1	0.52-44.79
N-nitrosohexa-methylenimine	rat	Li: 0 *	1	NC
Streptozotocin	rat	Ki:(97-194);li *	1	0.04-0.15
Hydrazo-,Azo-,Azoxycompounds				
1,2-Dimethyl-hydrazine	rat	Si:(55-277);li*, ki *	1	0.08
	mouse	Li:26-76;lu,ki, st,cm *	9,10	0.17-4.5
1,1-Dimethy-hydrazine	mouse	Lu:1-3;li *	9	85-300
Hydrazine	mouse	Lu:2-7;li *	9	3.3-131
Carbamyl-hydrazine	mouse	Lu:0.3-3[ns];li *	9	2523-6934
Phenylhydrazine	mouse	Li:13-63;lu *	9	71.96

(Table 1 continued)

Table 1.

Chemical	Animal species	DNA-damaging potency $\frac{K_t-K_c}{mol/kg}$	Ref.	Carcinogenic potency (TD50 mmol/kg)
1-Carbamyl-2-phenylhydrazine	mouse	$\overset{*}{L}u:2-3^{ns};li$	9	1562-2405
Phenelzine	mouse	$\overset{*}{L}u:6-11;li$	9	409-1351
Isoniazid	mouse	$Li:5-10;\overset{*}{l}u$	9	11.5-85.2
Iproniazid	mouse	$Li:0.3-0.4^{ns};\overset{*}{l}u$	9	183
Hydralazine	mouse	$\overset{*}{L}u:3-26;li$	9	830-1240
Procarbazine	mouse	$Li:4-41;\overset{*}{l}u,bm,$ ki,sp,th	9,11	0.03-0.25
Azoxymethane	rat	$\overset{*}{L}i:(72-195);\overset{*}{s}i$	1	0.03
Cycasin	rat	$\overset{*}{L}i:145;\overset{*}{s}i,\overset{*}{k}i$	12	0.005-0.12
	mouse	$\overset{*}{L}i:60$	12	0.17
Various Compounds				
2-Acetylamino-fluorene	rat	$\overset{*}{L}i:(110-275)$	1	0.01-17.83
N-Hydroxy-2-acetylamino-fluorene	rat	$\overset{*}{L}i:(74-147)$	1	0.41
4-Dimethylamino-azobenzene	mouse	$\overset{*}{L}i:7$	3	2.06-243
Benzidine	rat	$\overset{*}{L}i:(13)$	1	NC
7,12-Dimethyl-benz(a)anthracene	rat	$St:(76-201);\overset{*}{m}g,lu$	1	0.002-0.06
Benzo(a)pyrene	rat	$Li:841^{ns}$	13	0.63
	mouse	$Li:0.8^{ns}$	13	0.05-0.18

(Table 1 continued)

Table 1.

Chemical	Animal species	DNA-damaging potency $\dfrac{K_t - K_c}{mol/kg}$	Ref.	Carcinogenic potency (TD50 mmol/kg)
Aflatoxin B$_1$	rat	Ki:(11425-22850); *li,th	1	0.0008-0.002
4-Nitroquinoline--1-oxide	rat	*Lu:23-75;br,ki,li	1	NC
Ethylcarbamate	rat	*Br:2-46;ki	1	0.02-30.45
Chloroform	rat	*Li: 0	1	NC
Nickel carbonate	rat	Ki:40-249	14	0.007-0.39

[a]Legends of the body of Table 1 are as follows.

- For DNA-damaging potency and carcinogenic potency, see text pp.15-16.

- st= stomach mucosa; br= brain; si= small intestine; ki= kidney; lu= lung; th= thymus; li= liver; sp= spleen; bm= bone marrow; mg= mammary gland; cm= colon mucosa; *= organ susceptible to tumor formation.

- NC= not calculated because of lack of sufficient data in reported animal species.

- ns= increase in DNA elution rate not significantly different from controls (p>0.05).

References: 1) Petzold and Swenberg, 1978. 2) Eastman and Bresnick, 1978. 3) Schwarz et al., 1979. 4) Unpublished data. 5) Cavanna et al., 1980. 6) Brambilla et al., 1981a. 7) Parodi et al., 1980. 8) Parodi et al., 1978. 9) Parodi et al., 1981b. 10) Brambilla et al., 1978. 11) Brambilla et al., 1981b. 12) Cavanna et al., 1979. 13) Parodi et al., 1981c. 14) Ciccarelli et al., 1981.

Table 2. Distribution of some DNA-damaging potency values obtained
         from independent experiments performed on liver from rats
         and mice treated with single doses of N-nitrosodimethyl-
         amine.

Animal species	Dose (mg/kg)	DNA-damaging potency	Reference
Rat (♂♂,♀♀) (Upj:TUC(SD)spf) (i.p.)	0.4 1.0 3.0 10.0	778 568 726 433	Petzold and Swenberg,1978
Rat (♂♂) (Sprague-Dawley) (p.o.)	5.2 26.0	471 451	Brambilla et al.,1981a
Rat (♂♂) (Sprague-Dawley) (i.p.)	10.0 20.0 40.0	267 196 174	Parodi et al., 1980
Mouse (♀♀) (BALB/c) (i.p.)	2.3 9.4 18.7 37.5	1256 560 405 207	Parodi et al., 1978
Mouse (♂♂,♀♀) (NMRI) (i.p.)	1 5 10	1004 489 474	Schwarz et al., 1979

as determined by increase of DNA elution rate over controls, the data of Table 1 show that such relationship is positive for 35 of the
41 (85%) tested carcinogens, being negative in the alkaline elution
test six known carcinogenic chemicals (nitrosohexamethylenimine,
carbamylhydrazine, 1-carbamyl-2-phenylhydrazine, iproniazid, benzo(a)-
pyrene and chloroform).

On a quantitative basis, the data of Table 1 point out that the
DNA-damaging potency of the 35 carcinogens found positive in the alkaline elution varies over an approximately 20,000-fold range, being
maximal for aflatoxin B1 and minimal for some hydrazine derivatives.
For the 35 carcinogens of which Table 1 lists carcinogenic potency,
this value varies over an approximately 8.5×10^6-fold range, being,
as above, maximal for aflatoxin B1 and minimal for carbamylhydrazine.

        Concerning the usefulness of examining the quantitative correl-
ation existing between DNA-damaging potency and carcinogenic potency, this analysis may be open to discussion because of several reasons. In first place,while tumor growth is the final result of a
multistep process, DNA damage is only a first consequence of the DNA-
-carcinogen interaction. In second place, the increase in DNA elution
rate provides only a measure of DNA fragmentation without giving any
information about the nature of alkylation or arylation sites, which
have been demonstrated to be differently correlated with tumor induction (Lawley, 1980). Moreover, when interstrand (and/or DNA-protein) crosslinks and single-strand breaks occur simultaneously the
apparent alkaline elution rate is an understimate of single-strand
break frequency. Notwithstanding, from the practical point of view
of the use of DNA damage *in vivo*/alkaline elution assay as a short-
-term test for detecting chemical carcinogens, it may be.of some
interest to know the degree of quantitative correlation existing
between DNA-damaging potency an carcinogenic potency, either for all
compounds so far tested or for selected chemical families.

        A preliminary approach to the analysis of this correlation is
given in Table 3, where the regression of log DNA-damaging potency
as linear function of log carcinogenic potency is computed according
to three different criteria. In the first case, for each compound
two couples of data were considered whenever possible; they consisted
respectively of the inferior limits and of the superior limits of the
ranges of carcinogenic potency and DNA-damaging potency. This relationship is identified in Table 3 as *high-low potency regression*.
In the second case, only the higher limits of each of the two ranges
were taken to form the couples of data (*high potency regression* of
Table 3). In the third case, the geometric means of the limits of
each range were computed for the regression (*mean potency regression*
of the Table 3). It must be pointed out that in the computation the
reciprocal value of TD50 was used. The first type of regression
showed significant correlations between DNA-damaging and carcinogenic potencies either for all compounds examined or for the five subsets of selected chemical families. However, the good correlations
observed throughout could be due to the increased number of couples,
since each compound furnished two couples of values with some degree
of internal correlation. The second and third types of regression
gave positive correlation coefficients for every group considered,
with significant statistical values for all of the compounds grouped
together, for hydrazine derivatives and for the group of miscellan-
eous compounds listed as *various* in Table 1. Alkylating agents and
N-nitroso compounds did not reach statistical significance showing,
however, threshold values. As regards N-nitroso compounds, this result is substantially in agreement with that reported in a previous
paper (Brambilla et al., 1981a) where only six N-nitroso compounds
were considered and carcinogenic potency was computed according to
a different formula.

Table 3. Statistical analysis of the correlation between DNA-dam-
          aging potency and carcinogenic potency, by plotting for
          linear regression their log values [a].

Type of regression		Correlation coefficient	Statistical significance (one-sided)
High-low potency regression[b]			
All compounds	(67)	r = 0.71	p<0.0005
Alkylating agents	(10)	r = 0.75	p<0.010
Nitroso compounds	(20)	r = 0.50	p<0.025
Hydrazine derivatives	(23)	r = 0.74	p<0.0005
Various	(14)	r = 0.79	p<0.0005
High potency regression[c]			
All compounds	(34)	r = 0.67	p<0.0005
Alkylating agents	(5)	r = 0.70	0.05<p<0.10
Nitroso compounds	(10)	r = 0.43	0.10<p<0.15
Hydrazine derivatives	(12)	r = 0.69	p<0.010
Various	(7)	r = 0.78	p<0.025
Mean potency regression[d]			
All compounds	(34)	r = 0.73	p<0.0005
Alkylating agents	(5)	r = 0.78	0.05<p<0.10
Nitroso compounds	(10)	r = 0.45	0.10<p<0.15
Hydrazine derivatives	(12)	r = 0.78	p<0.005
Various	(7)	r = 0.85	p<0.010

a) The couples of data are the carcinogenic and the DNA-damaging potencies computed for each compound in the same species, as shown
   in Table 1. The number of the couples of data is reported in brackets.
b) Regression based on both the extreme values of the 2 potency ranges
   shown in Table 1.
c) Regression based on the higher potency value in each of the 2 potency ranges shown in Table 1.
d) Regression based on the geometric means of the estreme values of
   the 2 potency ranges shown in Table 1

     These results, although so far limited in number, seem to sug-
gest that DNA fragmentation, as evaluated *in vivo* by the alkaline
elution assay, correlates satisfactorily both qualitatively and quantitatively with tumorigenic activity and may be considered ,as a consequence, a useful endpoint for a rapid prescreening of oncogenic

potential of chemical agents. It is evident that a more extensive evaluation is needed in order to establish which ones among the several chemical families of carcinogenic agents are better identified with this assay. This prerequisite is further underlined by the existence in this book itself of another chapter by Parodi et al. (of which we had knowledge only after having prepared this chapter) dealing more extensively with the correlations existing, not only between carcinogenic potency and DNA-damaging potency, but also among carcinogenic potency and other biological effects.

ACKNOWLEDGEMENTS

This work was supported by CNR grants 80.01485.96 (Finalized Project *Control of Neoplastic Growth*) and 79.02360.65. Claudio Nicolini was supported by a Research and Study Leave Award from Temple University and by the National Research Council, Italy.

REFERENCES

Ames, B.N.,1979,Identifying environmental chemicals causing mutations and cancer, *Science*, 204: 587-593.

Bigger, C.A.H., Tomaszewski, I.E., Dipple, A., and Lake, R.S., 1980, Limitations of metabolic activation systems used with *in vitro* tests for carcinogens, *Science*, 209: 503-505.

Bradley, M.O., and Kohn, K.W., 1979, X-ray induced DNA double strand break production and repair in mammalian cells as measured by neutral filter elution, *Nucleic Acid. Res.*, 7: 793-804.

Brambilla, G., Cavanna, M., Parodi, S., Sciabà, L., Pino, A., and Robbiano, L., 1978, DNA damage in liver, colon, stomach, lung and kidney of BALB/c mice treated with 1,2-dimethylhydrazine, *Int. J. Cancer*, 22: 174-180.

Brambilla, G., Cavanna, M., Parodi, A., and Robbiano, L., 1981a, Quantitative correlation among DNA damaging potency of six N-nitroso compounds and their potency in inducing tumor growth and bacterial mutations, *Carcinogenesis*, 2: 425-429.

Brambilla, G., Cavanna, M., Pino, A., and Robbiano, L., 1981b, DNA damage and repair in mouse tissues following procarbazine administration. *Pharmacol. Res. Commun.*, 13: 213-222.

Cavanna, M., Parodi, S., Sciabà, L., Maura, A., Carlo, P., Cajelli, E., and Brambilla, G., 1977, DNA damage and repair by alkaline elution in N-diazoacetylglycine amide-treated cells, *Toxicol. Letters*, 1: 115-120.

Cavanna, M., Parodi, S., Taningher, M., Bolognesi, C., Sciabà, L., and Brambilla, G., 1979, DNA fragmentation in some organs of rats and mice treated with cycasin,*Br. J. Cancer*, 39: 383-390.

Cavanna, M., Parodi, S., Robbiano, L., Pino, A., Sciabà, L., and Brambilla, G., 1980, Alkaline elution assay as a potentially useful method for assessing DNA damage induced *in vivo* by diazoalkanes, *Gann*, 71: 251-259.

Cerutti, P.A., Sessions, F., Hariharan, P.V., and Lusby, A., 1978,
    Repair of DNA damage induced by benzo(a)pyrene diol-epoxides
    I and II in human alveolar tumor cells, *Cancer Res.*, 38: 2118-
    2122.
Chase, E.S., and Shafer, R.H., 1979, Viscoelastic behaviour of mam-
    malian DNA, *Biophys. J.*, 28: 93-106.
Ciccarelli, R.B., Hampton, T.H., and Jennette, K.W., 1981, Nickel
    carbonate induces DNA-protein cross links and DNA strand breaks
    in rat kidney, *Cancer Lett.*, 12: 349-354.
Damjanov, I., Cox, R., Sarma, D.S.R., and Farber, E., 1973, Patterns
    of damage and repair of liver DNA induced by carcinogenic methyl-
    ating agents *in vivo*, *Cancer Res.*, 33: 2122-2128.
Eastman, A., and Bresnick, E., 1978, A technique for the measurement
    of breakage and repair of DNA alkylated *in vivo*, *Chem. Biol.
    Interact.*, 23: 369-377.
Ewig, R.A.G., and Kohn, K.W., 1978, DNA-protein cross-linking and
    DNA interstrand cross-linking by haloethylnitrosoureas in L1210
    cells, *Cancer Res.*, 38: 3197-3203.
Fornace, A.J., Jr., and Little, J.B., 1979, DNA-protein cross-linking
    by chemical carcinogens in mammalian cells, *Cancer Res.*, 39:
    704-710.
International Agency for Research on Cancer, 1972-1981, in: *IARC
    Monographs on the Evaluation of the Carcinogenic Risk of Chem-
    icals to Humans*, vols., 1-26, IARC, Lyon.
Kissane, J.M., and Robins, E., 1958, The fluorometric measurement of
    deoxyribonucleic acid in animal tissue with special reference
    to the central nervous system, *J. Biol. Chem.*, 233: 184-188.
Kohn, K.W., 1979, DNA as a target in cancer chemotherapy: measure-
    ment of macromolecular DNA damage produced in mammalian cells
    by anticancer agents and carcinogens, *Methods in Cancer Res-
    earch*, 16: 291-345.
Kohn, K.W., and Ewig, R.A.G., 1973, Alkaline elution analysis, a new
    approach to the study of DNA single-strand interruption in cells,
    Cancer Res., 33: 1849-1853.
Kohn, K.W., Erickson, L.C., Ewig., R.A.G., and Friedman, C.A., 1976,
    Fractionation of DNA from mammalian cells by alkaline elution,
    Biochemistry, 15: 4629-4637.
Kohn, K.W., Ewig, R.A.G., Erickson, L.C., and Zwelling, L.A., 1980,
    Measurement of strand breaks and crosslinks in DNA by alkaline
    elution, in: *DNA Repair a Laboratory Manual of Research Proce-
    dures*. Friedberg and Hanawalt (eds.) Marcel Dekker, N.Y.
Langenbach, R., Freed, H.J., Raveh, D., and Huberman, E., 1978.
    Cell specificity in metabolic activation of aflatoxin B_1 and
    benzo(a)pyrene to mutagens for mammalian cells, *Nature*, 276:
    277-279.
Laurent, G., Erickson, L.C., Sharkey, N.A., and Kohn, K.W., 1981,
    DNA cross-linking and cytotoxicity induced by cis-diammine-
    dichloroplatinum(II) in human normal and tumor cell lines,
    Cancer Res., 41: 3347-3351.
Lawley, P.D., 1980, DNA as a target of alkylating carcinogens, *Br.
    Med. Bull.*, 36: 19-24.

Nicolini, C., Belmont, A., Zietz, S., Maura, A., Pino, A., Robbiano, L., and Brambilla, G., 1981a, Physico-chemical model for DNA alkaline elution: new experimental evidence and differential role of DNA length, chain flexibility and superpacking, sub-*J. Theor. Biol.*, In Press.

Nicolini, C., Carlo, P., Martelli, A., Finollo, R., Bignone, F.A., and Brambilla, G., 1981b, Viscoelastic propertier of native DNA from intact nuclei of mammalian cells, submitted for publication to J. Mol. Biol..

Parodi, S., Taningher,M.,Santi,L.,Cavanna, M., Sciabà, L., Maura, A., and Brambilla, G., 1978, A practical procedure for testing DNA damage *in vivo* proposed for a prescreening of chemical carcinogens, *Mutat. Res.*, 54: 39-46.

Parodi, S., Taningher, M., Pala, M., Brambilla, G., and Cavanna, M., 1980, Detection by alkaline elution of rat liver DNA damage induced by simultaneous subacute administration of nitrite and aminopyrine, *J. Toxicol. Environ. Health*, 6: 167-174.

Parodi, S., Carlo, P., Martelli, A., Taningher, M., Finollo, R., Pala, M., and Giaretti, W., 1981a, A circular channel crucible oscillating viscometer: detection of DNA damage induced *in vivo* by exceedingly small doses of dimethylnitrosamine, *J. Mol. Biol.*, 147: 501-521.

Parodi, S., De Flora, S., Cavanna, M., Pino, A., Robbiano, L., Bennicelli, C., and Brambilla, G., 1981b, DNA-damaging activity *in vivo* and bacterial mutagenicity of sixteen hydrazine derivatives as related quantitatively to their carcinogenicity, *Cancer Res.*, 41: 1469-1482.

Parodi, S., Taningher, M., Pala, M., Santi, L., 1981c, Alkaline DNA fragmentation *in vivo*: borderline or negative results obtained respectively with 7,12-dimethylbenz(a)anthracene and benz(a) pyrene, *Tumori*, 67: 87-93.

Petzold, G.L., and Swenberg, J.A., 1978, Detection of DNA damage induced *in vivo* following exposure of rats to carcinogens, *Cancer Res.*, 38: 1589-1598,

Ross, W.E., Ewig, R.A.G., and Kohn, K.W., 1978, Differences between melphalan and nitrogen mustard in the formation and removal of DNA cross-links, *Cancer Res.*, 38: 1502-1506.

Schwarz, M., Hummel, J., Appel, K.E., Rickart, R., Kunz, W., 1979, DNA damage induced *in vivo* evaluated with a nonradioactive alkaline elution technique, *Cancer Lett.*, 6: 221-226.

Shafer, R.G., Chase, E.C., 1980, DNA damage in rat (L cells treated with nitrogen mustard and 1,3-bis(2-chloroethyl)-1-nitrosourea assayed by viscoelastometry and S_1 nuclease, *Cancer Res.*, 90: 3186-3193.

Survey of Compounds which have been Tested for Carcinogenic Activity, 1972-73, USPHS Publication no. 149, Washington, D.C.

Swenberg, J.A., 1979, The value of *in vitro* and *in vivo* alkaline elution assays for predicting the carcinogenic potential of chemicals, in: *Short Term Tests for Prescreening of Potential carcinogens*, Santi, L., and Parodi, S. (Eds.), Istituto Scientif-

ico per lo Studio e la Cura dei Tumori, Genova, pp. 20-30.
Swenberg, J.A., Petzold, G.L., and Harback, P.R., 1976, *In vitro*
    DNA damage/alkaline elution assay for predicting carcinogenic
    potential, *Biochem. Biophys. Res. Commun.*, 72: 732-738.
Thomas, C.B., Osieka, R., and Kohn, K.W., 1978, DNA cross-linking by
    in vivo treatment with 1-(2-chloroethyl)-3-(4-methylcyclohexyl)-
    -1-nitrosourea of sensitive and resistant human colon carcinoma
    xenografts in nude mice, *Cancer Res.*, 38: 2448-2454.

DNA FRAGMENTATION: ITS PREDICTIVITY AS

A SHORT TERM TEST

Silvio Parodi, Maurizio Taningher and Leonardo Santi

Istituto Scientifico per lo Studio e la Cura dei Tumori
and Department of Oncology, University of Genoa
I-16132 Genoa, Italy

INTRODUCTION

In order to assess the carcinogenic risk it is important not only to know qualitatively if a chemical is a carcinogen, but also to have an idea of its carcinogenic potency. Unfortunately, the epidemiological data almost never allow for a correlation between tumour frequency and dose of a carcinogen. Perhaps the only exception is the carcinogenic effect of ionizing radiations. Because of this general deficiency in the epidemiological data, it is impossible to know if carcinogenic potencies in humans and carcinogenic potencies in small rodents are quantitatively correlated. A quantitative correspondence of scales could exist, even if obviously the latency time of tumours is much longer in humans than in small rodents. Qualitatively, all the compounds found to be carcinogenic in humans were also found to be carcinogenic in small rodents, except for the arsenic derivatives[37]. On this basis, and on the generic biological basis that carcinogenicity in small rodents is the closest thing to carcinogenicity in humans, carcinogenicity data in small rodents are considered the most relevant for human risk assessment, especially when epidemiological data are not available. For these reasons, the results obtained in the short term tests are always compared with carcinogenicity in small rodents.

On a qualitative basis, three parameters are usually taken into consideration: sensitivity, specificity and accuracy. Sensitivity is the ratio between number of positives in the short term test considered and the number of carcinogens examined. Specificity is

the ratio between number of negative results in the short term test
and number of non carcinogens examined. Accuracy is the ratio between number of correct responses in the short term test and number
of compounds examined. This qualitative approach has the advantage
that it avoids the complex problems related to a quantitative evaluation of carcinogenicity in small rodents, but it has the disadvantage that it gives no information whatsoever about the carcinogenic
potency, and two chemicals could differ even one million fold in
terms of carcinogenic potency. Moreover, if the short term test and
the carcinogenicity assay differ significantly in the threshold of
sensitivity, all the compounds falling between the two thresholds
of sensitivity will be positive in one test and negative in the other. For these reasons it is interesting to have an idea of the quantitative correlation existing between a given short term test and
carcinogenic potency.

To our knowledge the studies examining quantitative correlations are few in the literature. Coombs et al.[38] evaluated the mutagenicity in the Ames' test and the carcinogenicity (skin painting)
of 54 polycyclic aromatic compounds. All the 37 carcinogens were
found to be mutagens. Of the 16 non carcinogens 7 appeared to be mutagens. However, from a quantitative point of view, a very poor quantitative correlation seemed to exist between carcinogenic and mutagenic potency. In an other study on the predictivity of the Ames'
test, Meselson and Russell[39] found a good quantitative correlation
between mutagenic potency and oncogenic potency for a selected group
of ten heterogeneous compounds (discarding some nitrosamines).Bartsch
et al.[40], examining only five polycyclic aromatic hydrocarbons found
a poor quantitative correlation (r = 0.26) between oncogenic potency
and mutagenic potency in the Ames' test; on the contrary the five
corresponding bay region dihydrodiols showed a better correlation.
Glatt et al.[41] examined an homogenous series of 43 polycyclic aromatic hydrocarbons with heteroatoms. The appearance of sarcomas in
situ after subcutaneous injection was evaluated, and compared with
the mutagenicity in the Ames' test. We want to underline that the
Ames' test uses a rat liver microsomal fraction as an enzymatic activating system, while in vivo metabolic activation occurred in subcutaneous tissue. 17/18 carcinogens were found to be mutagens and
13/25 non carcinogens were also found to be mutagens. No quantitative correlation was found between mutagenic and oncogenic potency;
mutagenic potency of non carcinogens was similar to mutagenic potency
of carcinogens. Bartsch et al.[42], studying the quantitative corre-

lation between oncogenic potency and mutagenic potency in the Ames'
test, did not find the test to be predictive for seven alkylating
agents. Clive et al.[43] studying the mutagenicity in mammalian cells,
with the metabolic help of a rat liver microsomal fraction, examined
the quantitative predictivity of a short term test using a mouse lymphoma cell line (L5178Y/TK$^{+/-}$); 25 heterogeneous compounds were studied and a good quantitative correlation was found between oncogenic
and mutagenic potencies.

From what we have mentioned, it appears that there is not much
information about the quantitative relationships existing between
potency in a given short term test and carcinogenic potency.

In this report we will examine mainly the quantitative relation—
ship existing between DNA damage (evaluated with the alkaline elution technique in rat cells in vivo) and carcinogenicity. As a reference point two other short term tests will be considered: the autoradiographic repair (unscheduled DNA synthesis) in liver cells in
vitro, and the Ames' test. An other reference parameter that we considered important was the number of adducts formed with rat and mouse
liver DNA in vivo. If a short term test has some specific correlation
with carcinogenicity, this correlation should be clearly better
than the correlation existing between acute toxic potency and carcinogenicity. For this reason, as a kind of negative reference point,
the degree of predictivity of the parameter acute toxicity was also
examined.

From a theoretical point of view the evaluation of alkaline DNA
fragmentation in rat liver in vivo has both advantages and disadvantages. The main advantage is that in this short term test the metabolic activation is the natural one existing in vivo in the liver,
considered the most important organ for metabolic transformations.
A second important advantage is that the test is very rapid and practical. For instance it is much more rapid than mutagenicity in mammalian cells, transformation in vitro, and even SCE induction. The
main disadvantage is represented by the fact that the number of alkaline breaks does not correctly reflect the number of adducts and
even less the intrinsic mutagenic potency of a given adduct. Another
disadvantage, that is common to all short term tests, except perhaps
transformation in vitro, is that only initiation processes are
monitored by the test, and not processes related to promotion or epigenetic causes. The balance of advantages and disadvantages cannot
be known a priori, and only experimental investigation will tell us
the degree of quantitative predictivity of this test.

METHODS FOR CALCULATING THE DIFFERENT POTENCIES

Oncogenic potency was expressed with an Oncogenic Potency Index (OPI). Potency in inducing DNA fragmentation was expressed with a DNA Fragmentation Index (DFI). Mutagenic potency in the Ames' test was expressed with a Mutagenic Potency Index (MPI). Potency in inducing DNA adducts was expressed with a Covalent Binding Index (CBI). Potency in inducing autoradiographic repair was expressed with an Unscheduled DNA synthesis Index (UDI). Finally, toxic potency was expressed with a Lethal Dose Index (LDI).

Common conditions and criteria selected for estimation of DFI, CBI and LDI

   a) Only adult mice and rats studies.
   b) Only oral and parenteral routes (exotic routes excluded).
   c) For DFI and CBI studies, only data referred to liver DNA
      were considered.
   d) Only acute treatments (most often a single administration)
      followed by sacrifice within a few days were considered.
   e) For DFI and CBI, when more than one dosage was available in
      the same work, the highest potency value, usually from lower
      dosages, was selected, considering that the highest dosage
      usually tends to saturate the metabolic activation systems.
   f) When more than one DFI, CBI or LDI value was found from
      different studies, only the first five available were con-
      sidered. The arithmetic mean of the different values was
      used for correlation studies.

Normalization of data from DNA damage in vivo/alkaline elution

a)   The number of groups utilizing the in vivo alkaline elution
     assay is relatively small (Bolognesi et al.[26], Brambilla et al.
     [24,28,29], Parodi et al.[19,20,22,25,27], Petzold and Swenberg[21],
     Schwarz et al.[23]). The procedures adopted are rather homogeneous,
     and essentially referred to the basic publication of Kohn et al.
     [44]. However, in order to normalize the data of different authors
     some criteria had to be assumed.
b)   From an analysis of the data taken from Kohn and our own stud-
     ies, it appears that the fraction of eluted DNA depends only in-
     directly on the elution time, but it depends primarily on the
     elution flow (ml of eluting-solution passing through a cm^2 of the
     filter).
c)   The number of breaks is proportional not to the percentage of
     eluted DNA, but to the elution rates, as a first approximation
     (Kohn et al.[44]). According to the above points a), b) and c) we

transformed all the data of different authors in terms of:

$$K = \frac{-\ln Q_v}{V} \qquad\qquad (\underline{1})$$

where Q_v is the fraction of DNA remaining on the filter and V is the eluted volume in ml for filters of constant diameter (2.5 cm).

d)   In order to consider a result significantly different from control values, it was required not only that the difference be statistically significant (p<.05, preferably according to a non parametric Mann-Whitney test, or according the Student's t test), but also that K_t (elution rate for treated animals) $\geqslant 1.5$ K_c (elution rate for control animals). Most often these two criteria coincide, but the second condition protects against hidden bias that could reach statistical significance for relatively large samples (Parodi et al.[20])

e)   The relationship: $-\ln Q_v = f(V)$ draws away significantly from linearity; as a consequence, whenever possible, K was calculated for the same, or a similar, total volume ($\sim$13 ml).

f)   The DNA fragmentation index was calculated by the following equation:

$$DFI = \frac{K_t - K_c}{\text{dosage in millimoles/kg}} \times 1000 \qquad (\underline{2})$$

where K_t is the elution rate constant per unit volume for treated samples and K_c the same for control samples.

g)   For most authors a reference standard for alkaline elution rate constants was not available. However, an idea of the variability of the elution rate constant against differences at present difficult to normalize, (such as flow velocity, eluant composition, filter type, pore size between 2 and 5 μm in diameter, and other possible minor differences), can be given by a comparison of data obtained from Kohn et al.[44] and ourselves[45] after standard X ray dosages. The data reported in Fig.2 of the work of Kohn et al.[44] (average pumping speed = 0.045 ml/min and filter area of $\sim$4.9 cm^2), were normalized in terms of elution rate constant per unit volume as K = 0.18 per Krad. From Fig.2 of our data (Brambilla et al.[45]) we obtained a K = 0.09 per Krad, which is a ratio of two to one. This order of difference seems completely compatible with the purpose of our present correlation study.

Computation of MPI in the Ames' test

MPI was defined according to McCann et al.[30] as follows:

$$MPI = \frac{\text{Histidine revertants over controls per plate}}{\text{nanomole of chemical per plate}} \qquad (\underline{3}).$$

The MPI that we utilized for our comparison was obtained from data reported by: De Flora[33], Kawachi et al.[31], McCann et al.[30], Painter and Howard[32], Parodi et al.[19,20].

Computation of CBI

CBI was defined by Lutz as follows:

$$CBI = \frac{\text{micromole chemical bound per mole nucleotides}}{\text{millimole chemical administered/kg}} \quad (\underline{4})$$

The CBI data that we utilized for our comparison was taken directly from the data reported by Lutz[34] in his Tables 13-20 of a recent study, without any further elaboration. We considered already adequate for our comparison the criteria adopted by Lutz. CBI values for benzidine and chloroform, and additional values for ethylnitrosourea, 2-naphthylamine, 1,2-dimethylhydrazine and carbon tetrachloride were kindly given to us directly from Dr. W.K. Lutz (personal communication).

Computation of UDI

The data on autoradigraphic repair were obtained from report No.7 of an IARC publication on screening assay for carcinogens[35]. In this report the grain per nucleus and dose were given for 46 different compounds assayed in the hepatocyte primary culture (DNA repair assay). In this single homogeneous work we could find 22 compounds that had also been tested for carcinogenic potency. The compounds belonged to eight different classes of chemicals, as reported in Table 3 of the above report. Calculation of potency in the assay was straightforward, we used the following formula:

$$UDI = \frac{\text{grain/nucleus}}{\text{dose in millimoles}} \quad (\underline{5})$$

where UDI is the index of unscheduled DNA synthesis.

Computation of LDI

The lethal dose index was evaluated as the reciprocal of the lethal dose 50 in moles per kg:

$$LDI = (LD_{50} \text{ in moles/kg})^{-1} \quad (\underline{6}).$$

The utilized LD_{50} were as reported in literature[18]. Additional LD_{50} values were obtained from our own studies[19,20].

Evaluation of oncogenic potency (OPI)

The data on long term assays of carcinogenicity were obtained from studies quoted in the Survey of Compounds which have been test-

ed for carcinogenic activity, vol. 1972–73 and vol. 1978[1,2], and in
the IARC Monographs on the evaluation of carcinogenic risk to humans[3].
Data were obtained also from Medline, Toxline and Cancerline of the
Blaise Data Bank (British Library Automated Information Service,
London).

Establishing well defined conditions for normalization of the
different types of data and determination of the set to be submitted
to statistical analysis appeared to be a difficult task, for which
only compromise solutions were possible. The conditions adopted for
defining the set of data were the following:

a) Only adult mice and rats studies.

b) Only oral and parenteral routes (exotic routes excluded).

c) Tumours in the inoculum site excluded.

d) Pathological examination level required: level 2 or 3, according
   to the Survey classification.

e) We utilized experiments where the following minimum information
   was available: control data; tumour bearing animals data; duration
   of experiment or average time at tumour diagnosis.

f) Method of calculation of oncogenic potency index (OPI) according to Meselson and Russell[39]:

   $$OPI = - \ln (1 - I) / D\ t^n \qquad\qquad (\underline{7})$$

   where I is the cumulative single-risk incidence of tumours; t the
   time of exposure (time unit = 2 years); D the dose (in milli-
   moles/kg/day) equivalent to the total dose divided for a two year
   exposure; n was empirically set equal to 1, because no improvement of predictivity could be observed with higher exponents. Values of I were calculated exactly according to methods C, and sometimes D, as indicated by the above authors. When more than one study
   was found, only the first five available were considered. The arith-
   metic mean of different OPI values was utilized. We adopted the
   simplest computation because it was difficult to find a rationale
   for a different type of mean.

g) Requirements for accepting positive results:
   - only experiments lasting longer than 5 months were considered
   - the dose giving the highest potency was selected
   - the most responsive strain or species were selected
   - at least 5 tumour bearing animals in excess of controls
   - $p < .05$ according to the χ^2 test.

h) Requirements for accepting negative results:
   - only experiments lasting longer than 12 months were considered
   - the dose given had important chronic toxic effects
   - no other positive experiments existed at higher dosages in the
     same study

- at the end of the experiment more than 20 treated animals and 20 controls survived, (with substantially the same tumour frequency).

Problems related to the dose-response relationship

In order for the potencies in the different tests to be more significant, each response should be obtained from a point on an increasing (and possibly quasi linear) dose-response curve. For the majority of the mutagenicity data, obtained from the study of McCann et al.[30] and our own studies[19,20], the revertants per plate are single points from an increasing dose-response curve. The OPI, DFI and CBI data corresponds to single values. Usually for each experiment two-three different dosage schedules were available, the most active dosage was utilized. The UDI values[35] were obtained from studies spaced 10 fold. As a consequence the active dose could already be in a plateau region of the dose-response curve and the actual maximum potency could be 3-5 times higher, but probably no more than that. We are aware that the lack of sufficient dose-response data, especially for OPI, DFI and CBI values, could cause an apparent (probably moderate) reduction in the level of correlation found between different couples of parameters.

RESULTS AND DISCUSSION

Internal consistence of carcinogenicity data

Normalization of potencies of carcinogenicity data is a serious problem. As it clearly appears from the previous section (Evaluation of oncogenic potency (OPI)), the calculation of these potencies requires compromise solutions. We will not repeat what was already mentioned in the previous section. We want only to underline one point. Calculating the potencies from the animals with at least one tumour, gives the same weight to all different types of tumours. This is a serious compromise. However, it is absolutely impossible to find enough data for a single type of tumour, except for special classes of compounds (for instance: hydrazine derivatives and lung adenomas). Considering all these problems, in order to test if the carcinogenicity data have some degree of internal consistence, we made the following type of comparison. For 44 compounds more than one OPI value was available. We randomly generated two subsets of 44 single data. We examined the correlation existing between these two subsets. We found an $r = 0.73$, p (that $r = 0$) $\ll .001$. The equation of the regression line between (Log OPI_1) and (Log OPI_2) was $y = 0.50 + 0.70 x$.

Log OPI spaced between -1.5 and 5. In the central part of the regression line (Log OPI = 2) the belt zone including 90% of the values spanned in the following range: 2 $\pm$ 2.07. On an arithmetical scale, this is equivalent to a range $\frac{1}{117}$ - 117 X, for an interval of potencies more than a million times. The above correlation coefficient and the above amplitude of the belt zone can be considered as the upper limit of correlation possible between carcinogenicity and any short term test, at least for our approach to normalization of carcinogenic potencies. The reason is that no short term test can be considered closer to carcinogenicity than carcinogenicity itself. In any way, the above result gives an idea of the degree of "noise" that affects our investigation.

Correlation studies amongst OPI, DFI, MPI, LDI, CBI and UDI

In Table 1 and 2 is listed a series of 65 compounds, belonging to different chemical classes. For almost all of these compounds we could find simultaneously data concerning oncogenic potency (OPI), DNA fragmentation in liver in vivo (DFI), mutagenic potency in the Ames' test (MPI) and acute toxicity (LDI), (see Table 1). For a fraction of these compounds we could also find DNA adducts in liver in vivo (CBI) and/or unscheduled DNA synthesis in liver cells in vitro (UDI), (see Table 2).

Table 3 is divided in five parts (A, B, C, D, E). Table 3-A) compares the predictivity of DFI, MPI and LDI for the same 50 compounds. DFI and MPI have practically the same degree of predictivity and this predictivity is clearly statistically significant. This predictivity is also apparently better than the predictivity of LDI. However, this is only a trend; the difference ($r_{MPI} - r_{LDI}$) is not significant, even for a $p < .1$.

Table 3-B) compares the predictivity of DFI and CBI for the same 28 compounds. CBI is apparently more predictive, however the difference ($r_{CBI} - r_{DFI}$) is not significant, even for a $p < .1$.

Table 3-C) compares the predictivity of DFI and UDI for the same 16 compounds. There is clearly no significant difference among the two.

Table 3-D) compares the predictivity of CBI and MPI for the same 33 compounds. There is no significant difference amongst the two parameters in terms of predictivity.

Table 3-E) compares the predictivity of CBI and UDI for the same 19 compounds. There is a trend in favour of CBI, but the difference between ($r_{CBI} - r_{UDI}$) is not significant, even for a $p < .1$.

In conclusion, we sustain that DFI and MPI, for which the largest

Table 1. Different potencies of the compounds examined[a]

No.	Chemical	OPI	S,R	Ref.	LDI	S,R	Ref.	DFI	S,R	Ref.	MPI	Ref.
Nitrosocompounds												
1)	Dimethylnitrosamine	408	m,ip	(1)	2850	r,po	(18)	373	r,ip	(21)	.02	(30)
		3330	m,ip	"	2060	r,ip	"	341	r,ip	(22)	.022	(31)
		720	m,po	"	1650	r,sc	"	527	m,ip	(23)	.017	(32)
		2190	r,ip	"				471	r,po	(24)	.014	(33)
		120	m,po	"								
2)	Diethylnitrosamine	1420	m,po	"	473	r,ip	"	214	r,ip	(21)	.01	(30)
		185	m,ip	"				42.4	m,ip	(23)		
		871	r,iv	"				162	r,po	(24)		
		1640	m,ip	"								
		517	m,ip	(2)								
3)	Di-n-propyl-nitrosamine	294	r,sc	(3)	271	r,po	"	63.5	r,po	(24)	.08	(30)
					189	m,sc	"					
4)	Di-n-butyl-nitrosamine	17.3	m,sc	(3)	132	r,po	"	20.8	r,po	(24)	.15	(30)
		17.0	m,sc	"	132	r,sc	"				.317	(31)
		3.26	m,iv	"								
5)	Methylnitrosourea	3980	r,iv	(1)	573	r,po	"	43.3	r,$^{ip}_{iv}$	(21)	4.4	(30)
		4580	m,ip	(2)	937	r,ip	"	103	m,ip	(25)	1.65	(31)
		1580	r,iv	(3)	955	r,iv	"	42.3	r,po	(24)		
		655	r,iv	"	716	m,ip	"					
6)	Ethylnitrosourea	666	r,ip	(1)	390	r,po	"	18.8	r,$^{ip}_{iv}$	(21)	1.1	(30)
		283	m,ip	"	488	r,sc	"					
		652	m,ip	(2)	488	r,iv	"					

No.	Chemical	OPI	S,R	Ref.	LDI	S,R	Ref.	DFI	S,R	Ref.	MPI	Ref.
7)	N-Methyl-N'-nitro-	69.5	r,po	(1)	368	r,po	(18)	14.1	r,po	(21)	1380	(30)
	-N-nitrosoguanidine	322	r,po	(2)	350	r,sc	"				1100	(32)
		119	r,po	(3)								
8)	Nitrosohexa-	10400	m,sc	(1)	382	r,po	"	ns	r,ip/po	(21)	--	
	methyleneimine	242	r,po	(4)								
9)	Nitrosomorpholine	150	r,po	(1)	411	r,po	"	40.6	m,ip	(23)	.06	(30)
		35.0	r,po	(2)	411	r,ip	"					
		29.1	r,po	(3)	683	r,sc	"					
		315	r,po	(3)	1190	r,iv	"					
10)	Nitrosopyrrolidine	3.43	r,po	(1)	111	r,po	"	22.2	r,po	(24)	.02	(30)
		33.0	r,po	(3)								
11)	Nitrosopiperidine	97.2	r,po	(1)	571	r,po	"	--			.01	(30)
		26.7	m,ip	"	1140	r,sc	"					
					1900	r,iv	"					
12)	Streptozotocin	2060	r,iv	(3)	1920	r,iv	"	126	r,iv	(21)	1950	(30)
		2150	r,iv	"	1000	m,po	"					
Aromatic amines and amides, aminoazodyes												
13)	1-Naphthylamine	1.15	m,po	(3)	184	r,po	"	11.6	r,ip	(19)	.42	(30)
		ns	m,sc	"	231	r,ip	(19)	49.6	m,ip	(26)	.501	(31)
											1.23	(19)
											.71	(33)
14)	2-Naphthylamine	3.88	m,po	(3)	197	r,po	(18)	34.7	m,ip	(27)	8.5	(30)
		ns	r,po	"	716	m,ip	"	50.5	r,ip	(19)	8.31	(31)
		.367	m,sc	"				87.8	m,ip	(26)	26.3	(19)
		4.50	m,sc	(5)								

(Continued)

Table 1.   (continued)

No.	Chemical	OPI	S,R	Ref.	LDI	S,R	Ref.	DFI	S,R	Ref.	MPI	Ref.
15)	Aniline	ns	r,po	(3)	212	r,po	(18)	8.37	r,ip	(27)	ns	(30)
		.0752	r,po	(6)	222	r,ip	"	13.5	r,ip	(19)	ns	(19)
					201	m,po	"				ns	(33)
					189	m,ip	"					
16)	2,4-Diaminotoluene	17.2	r,po	(3)	831	r,ip	(19)	13.0	r,ip	(19)	.43	(30)
		5.98	r,po	(7)							.075	(19)
17)	2,4-Diaminoanisole	.0338	r,po	(8)	300	r,po	(18)	54.7	r,ip	(19)	36.1	(19)
		6.84	r,po	(9)	2760	r,ip	(19)					
18)	Benzidine	12.2	m,sc	(3)	596	r,po	(18)	12.2	r,ip/sc	(21)	1.4	(30)
		.725	m,sc	"	861	m,po	(18)	65.1	m,ip	(27)	1.2	(32)
		23.5	r,sc	"	366	r,ip	(19)	51.1	r,ip	(19)	.358	(19)
		4680	r,po	(10)				229	m,ip	(26)		
19)	4,4'-Oxydianiline	7.11	m,po	(3)	276	r,po	(18)	16.3	r,ip	(19)	1.29	(19)
		7.12	r,sc	(11)	549	r,ip	"					
		9.43	r,po	(12)	292	m,po	"					
					668	m,ip	"					
20)	4,4'-Methylene-dianiline	ns	r,po	(3)	571	r,po	"	140	r,ip	(19)	1.89	(19)
		5.54	r,sc	"	991	r,sc	"					
					2680	m,ip	"					
21)	4-Biphenylamine	32.5	m,po	"	338	r,po	"	--			31	(30)
											6.77	(31)
22)	2',3-Dimethyl-4-biphenylamine	27.1	r,sc	(1)	--			--			75	(30)
		424	r,sc	(2)								
23)	Auramine O	2.46	m,po	(3)	2380	r,ip	(19)	561	r,ip	(19)	.003	(19)
		2.85	r,po	(3)	671	m,po	(18)					

No.	Chemical	OPI	S,R	Ref.	LDI	S,R	Ref.	DFI	S,R	Ref.	MPI	Ref.
24)	Rhodamine B	ns	r,po	(13)	5320	r,ip	(19)	ns	r,ip	(19)	.101	(31)
		1.69	m,po	(3)							ns	(19)
		ns	r,po	(14)e								
25)	2-Acetylamino-fluorene	228	r,po	(1)	219	m,po	(18)	153	r,ip	(21)	108	(30)
		138	r,po	"	172	r,ip	(19)	ns	m,po ip	(23)	13.8	(31)
		4280	r,ip	"				ns	r,ip	(19,27)	22.6	(19)
		227	r,po	"								
		195	r,po	"								
26)	N-Hydroxy-2--acetylamino-fluorene	2950	r,ip	"	4600	r,ip	(18)	95.7	r,ip	(21)	--	
		395	r,po	"								
		52	r,po	"								
27)	p-Aminoazobenzene	.222	r,po	(3)	687	r,ip	(19)	32.0	r,ip	(19)	.29	(30)
		ns	r,po	"							.473	(31)
											.347	(19)
28)	o-Aminoazotoluene	320	m,po	(1)	131	r,ip	(19)	ns	r,ip	(19)	15	(30)
		40.8	m,sc	(3)							5.86	(31)
		54.4	m,ip	"							11.6	(19)
29)	4-Dimethylamino-azobenzene	4.27	r,po	(1)	1130	r,po	(18)	ns	m,po ip	(23)	.12	(30)
		127	r,po	"	451	r,ip	"	16.6	r,ip	(19)	.080	(19)
		15.6	r,po	"	751	m,po	"				.11	(33)
		19.3	r,po	(2)	980	m,ip	"					
		36.4	m,po	(3)b								
30)	3'-Methyl-4-dimethyl-aminoazobenzene	290	r,po	(1)c	--			ns	r,ip	(19)	.34	(30)
		759	r,po	"							4.31	(31)
											ns	(19)

(Continued)

Table 1. (continued)

No.	Chemical	OPI	S,R	Ref.	LDI	S,R	Ref.	DFI	S,R	Ref.	MPI	Ref.
31)	Ponceau MX	ns 1.97 .644 .104	m,po r,po m,po m,po	(3) " " "	240 480	m,ip r,ip	(18) (19)	ns	r,ip	(19)	.0690	(19)
	Hydrazine derivatives											
32)	Hydrazine	2.85	m,po	(15,20)	321 422 197	m,ip r,ip m,ip	(20) (18) "	6.4	m,ip	(20)	.00440	(20)
33)	1,1-Dimethylhydrazine	4.79	m,po	"	589 481 5010	r,ip m,ip m,sc	" " "	ns	m,ip	(20)	.000881	(20)
34)	1,2-Dimethylhydrazine	44.9	m,po	"	601 273 1400	r,po r,sc m,ip	" " (20)	75.5 36.7 653	m,ip r,sc m,sc	(20) (21) (28)	ns .00884	(30) (20)
35)	Carbamylhydrazine	.258	m,po	"	536 434 427 610 715	r,ip r,sc r,po m,ip m,sc	(18) " " " "	ns	m,ip	(20)	.000179	(20)
36)	Phenylhydrazine	3.82	m,po	"	636 575	m,ip r,po	(20) (18)	34.3	m,ip	(20)	.0163	(20)
37)	1-Carbamyl-2-phenyl-hydrazine	.228	m,po	"	2750 764	r,ip m,ip	" (20)	ns	m,ip	(20)	ns	(20)
38)	Phenelzin	.821	m,po	"	1120 1500	r,po m,po	(18) "	ns	m,ip	(20)	.0823	(20)

No.	Chemical	OPI	S,R	Ref.	LDI	S,R	Ref.	DFI	S,R	Ref.	MPI	Ref.
39)	Procarbazine	995	m,po	(15,20)	1410	m,ip	(18)	40.6	m,ip	(20)	ns	(30)
					1870	m,sc	"					
					1490	m,iv	"					
40)	Isoniazid	.579	m,po	"	322	m,ip	(20)	ns	m,ip	(20)	.000509	(20)
					328	r,po	(18)				.000137	(31)
					211	r,po	"				.000158	(20)
					417	r,sc	"					
					863	m,ip	"					
					857	m,sc	"					
					921	m,iv	"					
41)	Iproniazid	1.69	m,po	"	491	r,po	"	ns	m,ip	"	ns	(20)
					333	r,sc	"					
					263	m,po	"					
					280	m,ip	"					
					239	m,sc	"					
42)	Hydralazine	.118	m,po	"	2370	m,ip	"	ns	m,ip	(20)	.0499	(20)
	Other compounds											
43)	Methylmethanesulphonate	.829	m,po	(3)	881	r,sc	"	91.8	r,ip	(21)	.63	(30)
		ns	m,ip	"	630	r,iv	"	93.9	m,ip	(23)	.67	(32)
		ns	m,ip	"				38.8	m,ip	(27)	1.5	(33)
44)	Ethylmethanesulphonate	ns	m,ip	(1)	--			14.9	r,ip	(21)	.16	(30)
		274	r,ip	"							.15	(32)
		34.8	m,ip	(2)								
		1250	m,ip	(3)								
		33.4	r,ip	"								

(Continued)

Table 1. (continued)

No.	Chemical	OPI	S,R	Ref.	LDI	S,R	Ref.	DFI	S,R	Ref.	MPI	Ref.
45)	β-Propiolactone	20.7	r,po	(3)[d]	209	m,iv	(18)	8.58	r^{ip}_{po}	(21)	4.1	(30)
											7.21	(31)
											1.2	(33)
											.23	(32)
46)	Myleran	ns	m,ip	(3)	13700	r,ip	(18)	--				
		ns	m,iv	"	1230	m,po	"					
47)	Nitrogen mustard	909	m,sc	"	78000	r,ip	"	--			1.3	(30)
		3610	m,sc	"	142000	r,iv	"					
		146	m,ip	"	60000	m,sc	"					
		8970	m,iv	"								
		6390	r,iv	"								
48)	Cyclophosphamide	132	r,iv	(1)	2970	r,po	"	ns	r,ip	(21)	1.4	(30)
		91.9	m,sc	"	6980	r,ip	"				1.2	(32)
		45.2	m,sc	"	1740	r,iv	"					
		127	m,sc	(3)	2040	m,po	"					
					1020	m,iv	"					
49)	Chloroform	1.00	m,po	(3)	149	r,po	"	ns	r,po	(21)	--	
					107	m,po	"					
					71.5	m,ip	"					
					170	m,sc	"					
50)	Carbon tetrachloride	.471	r,sc	(1)	54.9	r,po	"	ns	m,po	(23)	ns	(30)
		ns	r,sc	"	103	r,ip	"				ns	(33)
		ns	r,po	"	12.0	m,po	"					
		ns	m,ip	(2)	39.9	m,ip	"					
		.362	m,po	(3)								

No.	Chemical	OPI	S,R	Ref.	LDI	S,R	Ref.	DFI	S,R	Ref.	MPI	Ref.
51)	1,2-Dibromoethane	36.8	r,po	(3)	1740	r,po	(18)	--			.06	(30)
					854	m,ip	"					
52)	Azaserine	933	r,ip	"	1020	r,po	"	145	r,ip	(21)	12000	(30)
					1730	r,ip	"					
					1150	m,po	"					
					1730	m,ip	"					
53)	Azoxymethane	1250	r,sc	(2)	2740	r,sc	"	144	r,sc	(21)	--	(30)
54)	Methylazoxy-methanol acetate	10300	r,iv	(1)	13200	m,iv	"	400	m,ip	(29)	.021	(31)
		368	r,ip	(16)								
55)	Cycasin	231	m,po	(1)	934	r,po	"	296	r,po	(29)	ns	(30)
		56.1	r,po	(3)	505	m,po	"					
56)	3-Methylcholanthrene	364	m,po	(1)	--			--			58	(30)
		62.7	r,po	"								
57)	Benz(a)anthracene	ns	r,iv	(3)	--			--			11	(30)
											12	(33)
58)	7,12-Dimethyl-benz(a)anthracene	73400	r,iv	(1)	784	r,po	"	ns	r,po	(21)	19	(30)
		8710	m,sc	"	4750	r,iv	"	ns	m,ip	(27)	11.3	(31)
		4300	r,po	"	754	m,po	"					
		6700	r,po	"								
		20900	r,po	"								
59)	Benzo(a)pyrene	ns	r,ip	"	5050	r,sc	"	ns	m,ip	(27)	121	(30)
		372	r,po	"							42.9	(31)
		144	m,po	(3)[c]							110	(32)
		3860	r,ip	"							185	(33)
		178	m,ip	(17)								

(Continued)

Table 1.   (continued)

No.	Chemical	OPI	S,R	Ref.	LDI	S,R	Ref.	DFI	S,R	Ref.	MPI	Ref.
60)	Aflatoxin B$_1$	2510	r,po	(1)	44600	r,po	(18)	14900	r,ip	(21)	7060	(30)
		59300	r,po	"	52000	r,ip	"				7600	(32)
		612	r,po	"	34700	m,po	"				1950	(33)
		43700	r,po	(2)	32900	m,ip	"					
		23100	r,po	(3)								
61)	Aflatoxin B$_2$	223	r,ip	(3)[f]	--			--			2.1	(30)
62)	Aflatoxin G$_1$	8920	r,po	(3)	8210000	r,po	"	--			116	(30)
63)	Urethane	.344	m,po	(1)	59.4	r,ip	"	ns	r,ip	(21)	ns	(30)
		ns	m,po	"	63.7	r,im	"	ns	m,ip	(27)		
		.177	m,po	"	33.0	m,po	"					
		ns	m,ip	"	40.0	m,sc	"					
		5720	m,ip	(2)								
64)	Diethylstilbestrol	6380	m,po	(3)	7890	r,ip	"	--			ns	(30)
		1950	m,po	"	4000	m,ip	"					
		1650	r,po	"								
65)	Phenobarbital	1.77	m,po	"	1430	r,po	"	ns	m,po	(23)	ns	(30)
		7.95	m,po	"	1160	r,sc	"					
		1.67	m,po	"	1110	r,iv	"					
		1.52	r,po	"	1380	m,po	"					
					929	m,ip	"					

[a]The abbreviations used are: OPI, oncogenic potency index; LDI, lethal dose index; DFI, DNA fragmentation index; MPI, mutagenic potency index; S, species; R, route; r, rat; m, mouse; po, oral; ip,

intraperitoneal; iv, intravenous; im, intramuscular; sc, subcutaneous; ns, not significant.
b,cDuration of experiment 120 days and 140 days respectively.
d3/5 tumour bearing animals.
e0/18 tumour bearing animals; minimum duration of experiment = 307 days.
f3/9 tumour bearing animals.

Table 2. Different potencies of the compounds examined[a]

No. Chemical	CBI	S,R	UDI
Nitrosocompounds			
1) Dimethylnitrosamine	5900	r,ip	3.96
	7100	r,ip	
	516	r,ip	
	8050	r,ip	
	1800	r,ip	
2) Diethylnitrosamine	104	r,po	3.77
	42	r,ip	
	125	r,po	
	430	r,ip	
5) Methylnitrosourea	400	r,po iv	--
	640	r,ip	
	490	r,iv	
	500	m,ip	
6) Ethylnitrosourea	9	r,iv	--
	377	r,iv	
7) N-Methyl-N'-nitro- -N-nitrosoguanidine	1000	r,po	176
8) Nitrosohexamethylene- imine	126	r,po	--
	104	r,po	
9) Nitrosomorpholine	44	r,po	4.11
10) Nitrosopyrrolidine	176	r,po	3.32
11) Nitrosopiperidine	118	r,po	--
Aromatic amines and amides, aminoazodyes			
14) 2-Naphthylamine	.53	m,ip	--
	2.7	r,ip	
15) Aniline	3.7	r,ip	.100
18) Benzidine	180	r,ip	2780
21) 4-Biphenylamine	--		71800
22) 2',3-Dimethyl-4- -biphenylamine	--		5410
25) 2-Acetylaminofluorene	83	r,ip	42.4
	77	r,ip	
	245	r,ip	
	59	r,ip	
	73	r,ip	
26) N-Hydroxy-2-acetyl- aminofluorene	225	r,ip	--
	287	r,ip	
	290	r,ip	

No.	Chemical	CBI	S,R	UDI
		949	r,iv	
		182	r,ip	
27)	p-Aminoazobenzene	2.4	r,ip	251
28)	o-Aminoazotoluene	59	m,po	--
		230	m,ip	
29)	4-Dimethylamino-	6.5	r,ip	125
	azobenzene	10	r,ip	
		4.5	r,ip	
		7.1	r,po	
		5.8	r,ip	
30)	3'-Methyl-4-dimethyl-	66	r,ip	221
	aminoazobenzene			
Hydrazine derivatives				
34)	1,2-Dimethylhydrazine	1730	r,sc	--
		1570	r,$^{ip}_{sc}$	
		4260	r,sc	
Other compounds				
43)	Methylmethanesulphonate	556	r,iv	233
		272	r,ip	
		360	r,iv	
44)	Ethylmethanesulphonate	62	r,ip	--
46)	Myleran	21	m,ip	--
47)	Nitrogen mustard	83	r,ip	--
48)	Cyclophosphamide	62	r,ip	--
49)	Chloroform	7.3	m,ip	--
50)	Carbon tetrachloride	51	m,ip	--
		ns	m,ip	
51)	1,2-Dibromoethane	180	r,ip	--
54)	Methylazoxymethanol acetate	4400	r,iv	1.75
56)	3-Methylcholanthrene	ns	r,ip	112
		5.6	m,po	
57)	Benz(a)anthracene	--		ns
58)	7,12-Dimethylbenz(a)	4	r,po	37.8
	anthracene	37	r,iv	
		20	r,ip	
		28	r,ip	

(Continued)

Table 2.   (continued)

No.	Chemical	CBI	S,R	UDI
59)	Benzo(a)pyrene	7	m,po	190
		14	m,po	
		20	r,ip	
		19	r,iv	
		6	r,ip	
60)	Aflatoxin B_1	17000	r,ip	350
		24000	r,ip	
		10500	r,ip	
		10300	r,po	
		250	m,po	
61)	Aflatoxin B_2	560	r,ip	168
62)	Aflatoxin G_1	680	r,ip	1970
63)	Urethane	35	m,ip	--
		29	m,ip	
		23	m,ip	
		25	m,ip	
		90	m,ip	
64)	Diethylstilbestrol	.4	r,po	--
		.6	r,sc	

[a]The abbreviations used are: CBI, covalent binding index;
UDI, unscheduled DNA synthesis index; S, species; R ,
route; r, rat; m, mouse; po, oral; ip, intraperitoneal;
iv, intravenous; sc, subcutaneous; ns, not significant.
CBI values were obtained from Reference (34). The CBI
values for Benzidine and Chloroform and additional values for Ethylnitrosourea, 2-Naphthylamine, 1,2-Dimethyl-
hydrazine and Carbon tetrachloride were kindly given to
us directly from Dr. W.K. Lutz.
All the UDI values were obtained from Reference (35).

Table 3. Correlations between paired parameters

Pair of parameters	N. of compounds	Correlation coefficient r	Probability that r = 0
A) (Log OPI) = f(Log DFI)	50	0.42	p < .005
(Log OPI) = f(Log MPI)	50	0.45	p < .005
(Log OPI) = f(Log LDI)	48	0.23	.1 < p < .2
B) (Log OPI) = f(Log DFI)	28	0.26	.1 < p < .2
(Log OPI) = f(Log CBI)	28	0.56	p < .005
C) (Log OPI) = f(Log DFI)	16	0.29	.2 < p < .4
(Log OPI) = f(Log UDI)	16	0.21	.2 < p < .4
D) (Log OPI) = f(Log CBI)	33	0.40	p < .025
(Log OPI) = f(Log MPI)	33	0.34	.05 < p < .10
E) (Log OPI) = f(Log CBI)	19	0.52	p < .025
(Log OPI) = f(Log UDI)	19	0.27	.2 < p < .4

set was available, are definitely predictive, more or less at the same degree. In addition to this fact, we can perhaps say that we have two trends, which however are not statistically demonstrated. The first trend is that perhaps LDI is less predictive than DFI and MPI. The second trend is that because CBI compared favourably with all the other three short term tests, perhaps it could be slightly more predictive.

In Table 4 we have examined the predictivity of some short term tests for special classes of chemical compounds. This subdivision generates subsets of 10-15 compounds. A lot of caution must be exerted before accepting that 10-15 compounds can be considered representative of a chemical class. However, even with this reservation in mind, it seemed interesting to explore if trends of higher or lower predictivity exist for a specific short term test, with respect to a specific chemical class of compounds. For instance, the difference in predictivity of CBI for aromatic amines and aminoazodyes with respect to nitrosocompounds is at least slightly significant (p < .1).

Considering LDI, it appears clearly significant (p < .02) the difference between nitrosocompounds and hydrazine derivatives. Toxicity correlates much better with carcinogenicity of nitrosocompounds than with carcinogenicity of hydrazine derivatives.

Considering MPI, this parameter appears to be more predictive

Table 4. Correlations between paired parameters
for specific classes of chemicals

Chemical class	N. of compounds	Correlation coefficient r	Probability that r = 0
(Log OPI) = f(Log CBI)			
Nitrosocompounds	10	0.31[a]	.2 < p < .4
Aromatic amines and amides, aminoazodyes	9	0.88[a]	p < .005
(Log OPI) = f(Log LDI)			
Nitrosocompounds	13	0.54[a,b]	p < .05
Aromatic amines and amides, aminoazodyes	17	0.067[a]	p > .5
Hydrazine derivatives	11	−0.51[b]	.1 < p < .2
(Log OPI) = f(Log DFI)			
Aromatic amines and amides, aminoazodyes	17	0.053[b]	p > .5
Hydrazine derivatives	11	0.75[b]	p < .01
(Log OPI) = f(Log MPI)			
Aromatic amines and amides, aminoazodyes	18	0.61[b]	p < .01
Hydrazine derivatives	11	−0.19[b]	p > .5

[a,b]In each section the r values with the same index are significantly different with a p < .1 or a p < .05 for index a and b
respectively (according to Ref.36, p.185-186).

for aromatic amines and aminoazodyes than for hydrazine derivatives
(p < .05). Conversely, DFI appears to be significantly more predictive
for hydrazine derivatives than for aromatic amines and aminoazodyes`
(p < .05).

In conclusion, we have identified four cases, corresponding to
the four sections of Table 4, for which CBI, LDI, DFI and MPI have
degrees of predictivity significantly different for different classes of chemical compounds. We strongly suspect that this could be
a general trend, and that in the future we will be able to identify
the most suitable short term test for a given class of chemical compounds. Obviously, in order to arrive at this stage, we need
larger sets of chemical compounds.

Statistical considerations on the possible gains in predictivity
obtainable from a multivariate linear regression analysis

In this section we make reference to a previous work[27]. The
mathematical part of that work was developed by one of the coauthors:
Dr. P. Boero. We examined the multiple linear regression described
by the equation:

$$Y_R = a + \beta_2 X_2 + \beta_3 X_3 \qquad (\underline{8})$$

where Y_R is (Log OPI), X_2 is (Log MPI) and X_3 is (Log DFI). (For this
statistical analysis and for the symbols used we made reference to
Chapter XIII of the book of Snedecor and Cochran[36]).

It seemed interesting to have an idea of the dependence (in our
type of situation) of the multiple correlation on different simple-
correlation coefficients. To explore the variation of the multiple
correlation r_{123} for different values of r_{12}, r_{13} and r_{23}, we plotted
the four graphs reported in Figure 1 (Panel a, b, c, d) with the aid
of a convenient programme, run on a HP85 Hewlett-Packard microcomput-
er. (The index 1 refers to OPI, the index 2 refers to MPI and the index 3 refers to DFI):

Panel a, where $r_{13}=.32$; $r_{12}=.345$; .445; .545; .645; .745.
Panel b, where $r_{13}=.42$; $r_{12}=.345$; .445; .545; .645; .745.
Panel c, where $r_{13}=.52$; $r_{12}=.345$; .445; .545; .645; .745.
Panel d, where $r_{13}=.62$; $r_{12}=.345$; .445; .545; .645; .745.

In each graph a family of curves was plotted, corresponding to
$r_{123}= f(r_{23})$, for increasing values of r_{12}, from bottom to top.

$r^2_{123} =f(r_{12},r_{13},r_{23})$ is described by the equation:

$$r^2_{123} = r_{12} \cdot \frac{r_{12} - r_{13} \cdot r_{23}}{1 - r^2_{23}} + r_{13} \cdot \frac{r_{13} - r_{12} \cdot r_{23}}{1 - r^2_{23}} \qquad (\underline{9})$$

From our family of curves the following facts are shown:
r_{123} decreases (for constant values of r_{12} and r_{13}) when r_{23} increases. At worst, however, r_{123} can only become equal to the better simple correlation between r_{12} and r_{13}. Moreover, the size of the improvement of r_{123} is rather resistant to increases of r_{23}.

In the case of our MPI and DFI correlations, the predictivity
of the two associated tests increases from an r_{12} of .45 or an r_{13}
of .42 respectively, to an r_{123} of .54. This increase is shown in
Figure 1, panel b. The degree of increment of r_{123} is inversely dependent on the correlation between MPI and DFI. In our case the correlation between the above two parameters was $r_{23} =.32$.

This increase of the multiple correlation above the higher value
of the simple correlations shows that a battery of tests represents

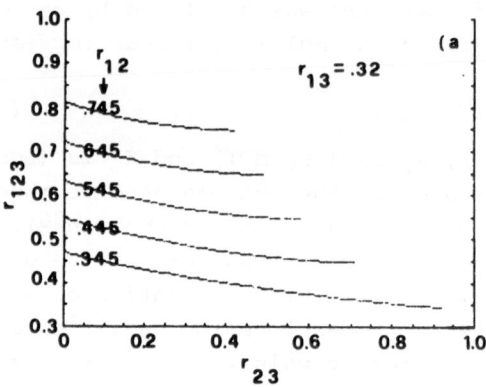

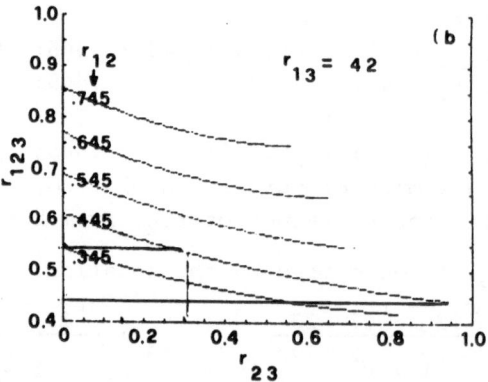

Figure 1 (Panel a-b).   Analysis of the dependence of multiple
correlation on simple correlations for three parameters. In pan-
els a and b the analysis of a trivariate correlation is presented. r_{123} (the dependent variable) and r_{23} are represented as
continuous variables, r_{13} is represented in four decimal steps
(from .32 to .62), r_{12} is represented in five decimal steps
(from .35 to .75). In panel b is also represented the gain of
the multiple correlation r_{123} for (Log OPI) = f(Log DFI,Log MPI)
in respect to the two simple correlations r_{12} , r_{13}.

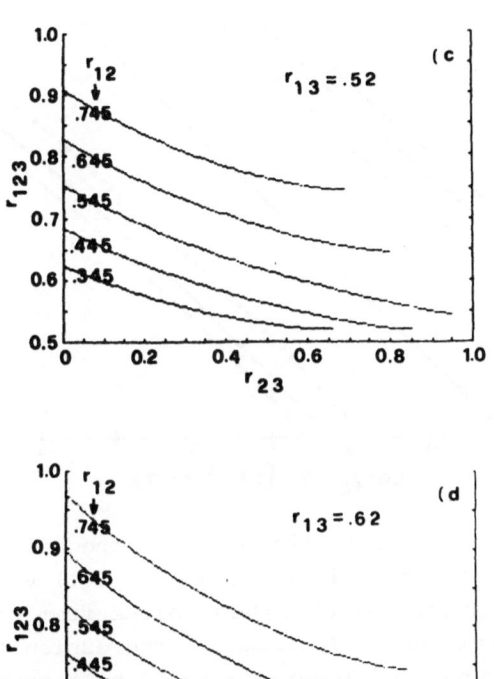

Figure 1   (Panel c-d).   Analysis of the dependence of multiple
correlation on simple correlations for three parameters. In pan-
els c and d the analysis of a trivariate correlation is presented. r_{123} (the dependent variable) and r_{23} are represented as
continuous variables, r_{13} is represented in four decimal steps
(from .32 to .62), r_{12} is represented in five decimal steps
(from .35 to .75).

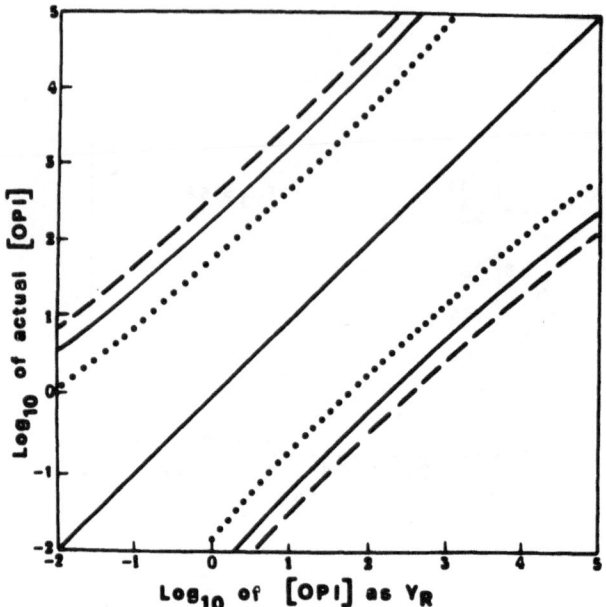

Figure 2.   Progressive shrinking of the belt zones including 90% of actual individual (Log OPI) values, as
function of predicted (Log OPI) values from single and
multiple parameters.   (―――――): regression line;
(– – – –): upper and lower limits of belt zone for (Log DFI);
(―――――): belt zone for (Log DFI, Log MPI); (•••••):
limit of internal consistency of (Log OPI) versus (Log OPI)
data.

an improvement over each single test, not only from a qualitative,
but also from a quantitative point of view. Moreover, the gain is
larger if the two short term tests measure components both related
to carcinogenicity, but rather independent one from the other. This
fact is not immediately obvious from a qualitative point of view.

    If Y_R is the value predicted from the regression equations, it
is equally true both for a simple and for a multiple regression that
r of Y versus Y_R is always equal to the r intercurring between Y and
X_2 or Y and X_2, X_3 respectively. This being the case, we can examine
the shrinking of the belt zone including 90% of the Y values, for

$Y = f(Y_R)$ obtained from the simple regressions: (Log OPI) =f(Log DFI);
(Log OPI) = f (Log MPI) and, finally, from the multiple regression:
(Log OPI) = f (Log DFI, Log MPI). The results obtained are shown in
Figure 2. Utilizing for prediction of OPI only DFI values, 90% of
actual OPI values will fall in a belt zone approximately 1/275 - 275 X.
Utilizing MPI only, 90% of actual OPI values will fall in a belt zone
approximately 1/250 - 250 X. Utilizing both MPI and DFI values, 90%
of actual OPI values will fall in a belt zone approximately 1/200 -
200 X. For a comparison, the belt zone related to the internal consistency of (Log OPI) versus (Log OPI) data was roughly 1/100-100X.

We can ask ourselves what is the practical significance, in
terms of predictivity, of this order of amplitude of the belt zones.
Looking at Figure 2, if a compound was weak both for MPI and DFI, it
will be in 90% of the cases weak or at most medium in terms of OPI,
and vice versa, if a compound was potent both for MPI and DFI, it
will be in 90% of the cases potent or at least medium in terms of
OPI.

CONCLUSIONS

     In our opinion, the main conclusions of this study are the fol-
lowing.
1)   An investigation on the quantitative predictivity of short term
      tests, as an alternative to the qualitative approach, can be im-
      portant for risk assessment. Moreover, it is by itself a valid
      independent way of probing the value of these tests, both alone
      and in combination.
2)   There are problems in evaluating carcinogenic potencies in rats
      and mice, and in order to normalize the data compromise solutions
      have to be accepted.
3)   The internal consistency of the carcinogenicity data gave an
      $r = .73$, with a 90% belt zone roughly around 1/100 - 100 X. This
      could be considered the upper limit of quantitative predictivity
      of any short term test.
4)   The quantitative predictivities of both MPI and DFI were sta-
      tistically significant and of the same level ($r = .45$ and $r = .42$
      respectively).
5)   The use of MPI and DFI in a battery brings the correlation
      coefficient to .54, with a 90% belt zone 1/200 - 200 X, that is
      only two times larger than the belt zone for the internal consis-
      tency of carcinogenicity data.
6)   Different short term tests have very different predictivities

for different classes of chemical compounds. Perhaps, in the future, we will be able to indicate the test most appropriate for a given class of chemical compounds.

7)   CBI and UDI should be examined more adequately. Very important tests, like mutagenicity in mammalian cells, transformation <u>in vitro</u> and SCE induction in bone marrow cells were not examined in this investigation.

ACKNOWLEDGEMENTS

We are grateful to Dr. P. Boero (Dept. of Mathematics, University of Genoa) for the helpful discussions concerning statistical problems and computer drawing of Fig. 1.

We are also grateful to Dr. W.K. Lutz (Institute of Toxicology, Swiss Federal Institute of Technology and University of Zurich) for the personal communication of some CBI data.

This work was supported by the Consiglio Nazionale delle Ricerche (Progetto Finalizzato "Controllo della Crescita Neoplastica"; Contracts No. 80.01608.96 and No. 80.01650.96).

REFERENCES

1.   National Cancer Institute, "Survey of compounds which have been tested for carcinogenic activity," Government Printing Office, Washington D.C. (1972-73).

2.   ibidem (1978).

3.   International Agency for Research on Cancer, "Monographs on the evaluation of carcinogenic risk of chemicals to humans," vols.1-24, IARC, Lyon (1972-80).

4.   C. M. Goodall, W. Lijinsky and L. Tomatis, Tumorigenicity of N-nitrosohexamethyleneimine, Cancer Res., 28: 1217-1220 (1968).

5.   G. M. Bonser, D. B. Clayson, J. W. Jull and L. N. Pirah, The carcinogenic activity of 2-naphthylamine, Br. J. Cancer, 10: 533-538 (1956).

6.   National Cancer Institute, Bioassay of aniline hydrochloride for possible carcinogenicity, Natl. Cancer Inst. Carcinog. Tech. Rep. Ser., 130:1-55 (1978).

7.   R. H. Cardy, Carcinogenicity and chronic toxicity of 2,4-toluenediamine in F344 rats, J. Natl. Cancer Inst., 62:1107-1114 (1979).

8.   J. M. Ward, S. F. Stinson, J. F. Hardisty, B. Y. Cockrell and D. W. Hayden, Neoplasms and pigmentation of thyroid glands

in F344 rats exposed to 2,4-diaminoanisole sulfate, a hair
dye component, J. Natl. Cancer Inst., 62:1067-1073 (1979).

9. R. P. Evarts and C. A. Brown, 2,4-Diaminoanisole sulfate: early
effect on thyroid gland morphology and late effect on gland-
ular tissue of Fisher 344 rats, J. Natl. Cancer Inst., 65:197-
204 (1980).

10. D. P. Griswold Jr., A. E. Casey, E. K. Weisburger and J. H.
Weisburger, The carcinogenicity of multiple intragastric doses
of aromatic and heterocyclic nitro or amino derivatives in
young female Sprague-Dawley rats, Cancer Res., 28:924-933
(1968).

11. D. Steinhoff, Cancerogene Wirkung von 4,4'-Diamino-diphenyläther
bei Ratten, Naturwissenschaften, 64:394 (1977).

12. National Cancer Institute, National Institutes of Health, National Toxicology Program, "Bioassay of 4,4'-oxydianiline for
possible carcinogenicity," U.S. Department of Health and Human Services, DHHS Publication No. (NIH) 80-1761.

13. H. Zeller, H. Birnstel, K. O. Freisberg, P. Kirsch and K. H.
Hempel, Chronic toxicity of auramine, Naturwissenschaften,
60:523-524 (1973).

14. M. Umeda, Experimental study of xanthene dyes as carcinogenic
agents, Gann, 47:51-78 (1956).

15. B. Toth, Sinthetic and naturally occurring hydrazines as possible
cancer causative agents, Cancer Res., 35:3693-3697 (1975).

16. G. L. Laqueur and H. Matsumoto, Neoplasms in female Fisher rats
following intraperitoneal injection of methylazoxymethanol,
J. Natl. Cancer Inst., 37:217-225 (1966).

17. S. D. Vesselinovitch, A. P. Kyriazis, N. Mihailovich and K. V.
N. Rao, Conditions modifying development of tumours in mice
at various sites by benzo(a)pyrene, Cancer Res., 35:2948-
2953 (1975).

18. National Institute for Occupational Safety and Health, "Registry
of toxic effects of chemical substances," R. J. Lewis (Ed.),
U.S. Government Printing Office, Washington D.C. (1978).

19. S. Parodi, M. Taningher, P. Russo, M. Pala, M. Tamaro and C.
Monti-Bragadin, DNA-damaging activity in vivo and bacterial
mutagenicity of sixteen aromatic amines and azo-derivatives,
as related quantitatively to their carcinogenicity, Carcinogenesis, in press.

20. S. Parodi, S. De Flora, M. Cavanna, A. Pino, L. Robbiano, C.
Bennicelli and G. Brambilla, DNA-damaging activity in vivo
and bacterial mutagenicity of sixteen hydrazine derivatives
as related quantitatively to their carcinogenicity, Cancer

Res., 41:1469-1482 (1981).

21. G. L. Petzold and J. A. Swenberg, Detection of DNA damage indu-
    ced in vivo following exposure of rats to carcinogens,
    Cancer Res., 38:1589-1594 (1978).

22. S. Parodi, M. Taningher, M. Pala, G. Brambilla and M. Cavanna,
    Detection by alkaline elution of rat liver DNA damage induced
    by simultaneous subacute administration of nitrite and amino-
    pyrine, J. Toxicol. Environm. Health, 6:167-174 (1980).

23. M. Schawarz, J. Hummel, K. E. Appel, R. Rickart and W. Kunz,
    DNA damage induced in vivo evaluated with a non-radioactive
    alkaline elution technique, Cancer Letters, 6:221-226 (1979).

24. G. Brambilla, M. Cavanna, A. Pino and L. Robbiano, Quantitative
    correlation among DNA damaging potency of six N-nitroso-
    compounds and their potency in inducing tumor growth and bac-
    terial mutations, Carcinogenesis, 2:425-429 (1981).

25. S. Parodi, M. Taningher, L. Santi, M. Cavanna, L. Sciabà, A.
    Maura and G. Brambilla, A practical procedure for testing
    DNA damage in vivo, proposed for a pre-screening of chemical
    carcinogens, Mutation Res., 54:39-46 (1978).

26. C. Bolognesi, C. F. Cesarone and L. Santi, Evaluation of DNA
    damage by alkaline elution technique after in vivo treatment
    with aromatic amines, Carcinogenesis, 2:265-268 (1981).

27. S. Parodi, M. Taningher, P. Boero and L. Santi, Quantitative
    correlations amongst alkaline DNA fragmentation, DNA covalent
    binding, mutagenicity in the Ames' test and carcinogenicity,
    for twenty-one different compounds, Mutation Res., in press.

28. G. Brambilla, M. Cavanna, S. Parodi, L. Sciabà, A. Pino and L.
    Robbiano, DNA damage in liver, colon, stomach, lung and
    kidney of BALB/c mice treated with 1,2-dimethylhydrazine,
    Int. J. Cancer, 22:174-180 (1978).

29. M. Cavanna, S. Parodi, M. Taningher, C. Bolognesi, L. Sciabà
    and G. Brambilla, DNA fragmentation in some organs of rats
    and mice treated with cycasin, Br. J. Cancer, 39:383-390
    (1979).

30. J. McCann, E. Choi, E. Yamasaki and B. N. Ames, Detection of
    carcinogens as mutagens in the Salmonella/microsome test:
    Assay of 300 chemicals, Proc. Natl. Acad. Sci. USA, 72:5135-
    5139 (1975).

31. T. Kawachi, T. Komatsu, T. Kada, M. Ishidate, M. Sasaki, T.
    Sugiyama and Y. Tazima, Results of recent studies on the
    relevance of various short-term screening tests in Japan,
    in: "The predictive value of short-term screening test in
    carcinogenicity evaluation," G. M. Williams, R. Kroes, H. W.

Waaijers and K. W. van de Poll (Eds.), Elsevier, Amsterdam, pp.253-257 (1980).

32. R. Painter and R. Howard, A comparison of the HeLa DNA synthesis inhibition test and the Ames' test for screening of mutagenic carcinogens, Mutation Res., 54:113-115 (1978).

33. S. De Flora, Study of 106 organic and inorganic compounds in the Salmonella/microsome test, Carcinogenesis, 2:283-298 (1981).

34. W. K. Lutz, In vivo covalent binding of organic chemicals to DNA as a quantitative indicator in the process of chemical carcinogenesis, Mutation Res., 65:289-356 (1979).

35. G. M. Williams, C. Bordet, P. A. Cerutti, R. P. Fuchs, J. Laval, S.-H. Lu, S. Parodi, A.E. Pegg and M.F. Rajewsky, DNA damage and repair in mammalian cells, in: "Long-term and short-term screening assays for carcinogens: a critical appraisal," IARC Monographs on the evaluation of the carcinogenic risk of chemicals to humans, Supplement 2, International Agency for Research on Cancer, Lyon, pp.201-226 (1980).

36. G. W. Snedecor and W. G. Cochran, "Statistical methods," The Iowa State University Press, Ames (1967).

37. L. Tomatis, C. Agthe, H. Bartsch, J. Huff, R. Montesano, R. Saracci, E. Walker and J. Wilbourn, Evaluation of the carcinogenicity of chemicals: A review of the Monograph Program of the International Agency for Research on Cancer, Cancer Res., 38:877-885 (1978).

38. M. M. Coombs, C. Dixon and A. M. Kissonerghis, Evaluation of the mutagenicity of compounds of known carcinogenicity belonging to the benzo(a)anthracene, chrysene, and cyclopenta(a)-phenanthrene series, using Ames test, Cancer Res., 36:4525-4529 (1976).

39. M. Meselson and K. Russell, Comparison of carcinogenic and mutagenic potency, in: "Origins of Human Cancer," H. H. Hiatt, J. D. Watson and J. A. Winsten (Eds.), Cold Spring Harbor Laboratory, Book C, pp.1473-1481 (1977).

40. H. Bartsch, C. Malaveille, B. Tierney, P. L. Grover and P. Sims, The association of bacterial mutagenicity of hydrocarbon-derived "bay-region" dihydrodiols with the Iball indices for carcinogenicity and with the extents of DNA-binding on mouse skin of the parent hydrocarbons, Chem-Biol. Interact., 26:185-196 (1979).

41. H. R. Glatt, H. Schwind, F. Zajdela, A. Croisy, P. C. Jacquignon and F. Oesch, Mutagenicity of 43 structurally related heterocyclic compounds and its relationship to their carcinogenicity, Mutation Res., 66:307-328 (1979).

42. H. Bartsch, C. Malaveille, A.-M. Camus, G. Martel-Planche, G.
     Brun, A. Hautefeuille, N. Sabadie, A. Barbin, T. Kuroki, C.
     Drevon, C. Piccoli and R. Montesano, Validation and compara-
     tive studies on 180 chemicals with S. typhimurium strains
     and V79 chinese hamster cells in the presence of various met-
     abolizing systems, Mutation Res., 76:1-50 (1980).

43. D. Clive, K. O. Johnson, J. F. S. Spector, A. G. Batson and M.
     M. M. Brown, Validation and characterization of the L5178Y/
     TK$^{+/-}$ mouse lymphoma mutagen assay system, Mutation Res.,
     59:61-108 (1979).

44. K. W. Kohn, L. C. Erickson, R. A. G. Ewig and C. A. Friedman,
     Fractination of DNA from mammalian cells by alkaline elution,
     Biochemistry, 15:4629-4637 (1976).

45. G. Brambilla, M. Cavanna, P. Carlo, R. Finollo, L. Sciabã, S.
     Parodi and C. Bolognesi, DNA damage and repair induced by
     diazoacetyl derivatives of amino acids with different mecha-
     nism of cytotoxicity. Correlations with mutagenicity and
     carcinogenicity, J. Cancer Res. Clin. Oncol., 94: 383-390
     (1979).

MEASUREMENT OF VISCOUS AND ELASTIC COMPONENTS OF NATIVE DNA FIBER

FOLLOWING CARCINOGEN ADMINISTRATION

Claudio Nicolini and Giuseppe Accornero

National Research Council, Italy and Institute of
Pharmacology, Medical School, University of Genova, Italy
Temple University, Department of Biophysics-physiology
Philadelphia, USA

The problem of determining the physical properties of giant DNA molecules in native conditions from intact mammalian nuclei (or cells) remains one of the most challenging and intriguing, especially considering their critical dependence on cell proliferation and transformation: DNA length (1), structure (2), and intrinsic viscosity (3) have been shown to be critically related to early events occurring during chemical carcinogenesis. Progressively lower amounts of "putative" single DNA strand breaks are detectable by alkaline sucrose gradients (1), alkaline elution (4), and viscometry (3), but numerous questions concerning the role of higher order structure (dealt with in a separate communication (5)) or the relative contribution of elastic and viscous components on the latter more sensitive viscoelastic measurements remain unanswered. Mammalian DNA molecules "in situ" have a pronounced tendency to associate to form gelled networks of nucleofilament fibers (2) with high elastic modulus and intrinsic viscosity which lend themselves to quantitative measurements (6,7).

We describe here a simple "Couette" elastoviscometer with a horizontal buoyant inner cylinder capable of discriminating between viscosity and molecules, either damaged or undamaged. The design is similar to both the low-shear-rate viscometer built by Zimm and Crothers (6) to study DNA solutions and to the elastometer of Carr et al.(7) built to study fibrinogen.

We believe that with the prototype here described we have satisfied several practical criteria for a technique which may have routine laboratory applications: the instrument (a) is versatile, being capable of discriminating in a single experiment between two critical independent physical parameters (viscosity and elasticity); (b) is inexpensive and easy to build and use; (c) requires an extremely smooth quantity of nuclear DNA; (d) yields highly reproducible and significant measurements with very little time and effort.

ELASTOVISCOMETER APPARATUS

Figure 1 shows the new simple elastoviscometer, consisting of an outer and an inner cylinder, separated by a narrow space filled with the liquid sample. The inner cylinder is hollow, and enough sample suspension is added to make it just buoyant in the horizontal position. A torque is then applied to the outer cylinder, either manually or with a stepping mechanism, to yield a rotation through a fixed angle (Fig. 2). Depending on the viscosity of the liquid sample, the inner cylinder will also rotate through an angle Θ_I, equal or larger, depending on its inertia, ultil it comes to a stop. The position reached by the inner cylinder with respect to the outer cylinder can be measured as a function of time by means of markers placed on both cylinders.

Whenever solutions of giant DNA molecules with long retardation times possess elastic properties, the direction of rotation of the inner cylinder after the driving torque is suddenly removed is reversed with a recoil angle (Θ_R) measured as a function of time with respect to the point of inversion.

On the other hand, if the inner cylinder is suspended in lysing solution or in a medium without any elastic recovery (such as 20% glycerol), its rotational velocity simply decays exponentially to zero due to frictional forces once the torque is removed. With a DNA solution, however, the direction of motion is reversed as a result of forces exerted on it as the DNA chains relax back exponentially to the equilibrium configuration. Figure 3 summarized the typical time dependence of the rotation angle (with respect to the unperturbed position) of the buoyant inner cylinder when the outer cylinder is rotated 90° and the inner space is filled with an intact DNA suspension from rat liver nuclei, with its solvent alone (lysing solution), or with 20% glycerol solution.

A calibration of the instrument is carried out with glycerol at different concentrations of known intrinsic viscosity (and no elastic component). Figure 4 shows a plot of the equilibrium inertia angle (Θ_I) for glycerol at 0%, 10%, 20%, 50%, and 100% concentration versus the known intrinsic viscosity expressed in centipoises. These samples do not display any recoil as would be expected from their lack of elasticity. For a range of 1 to 5 cp a strict linear correlation appears evident; for larger viscosity this correlation disappears progressively up to 100% glycerol, where

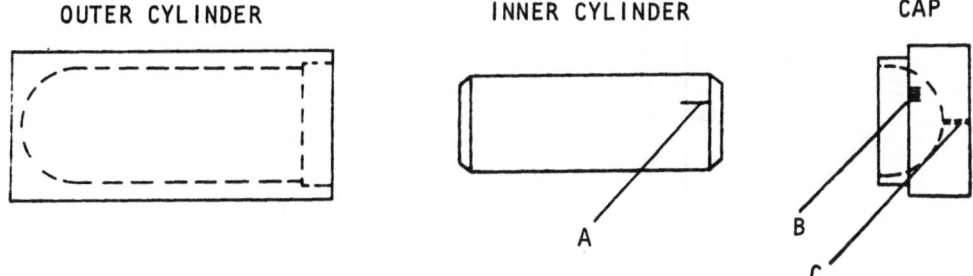

Fig. 1 Schematic diagram of the elastoviscometer: A marker of
        the inner cylinder, B markers (placed every 5 degrees)
        of the outer cylinder, C hole to complete the filling
        of the elastoviscometer.

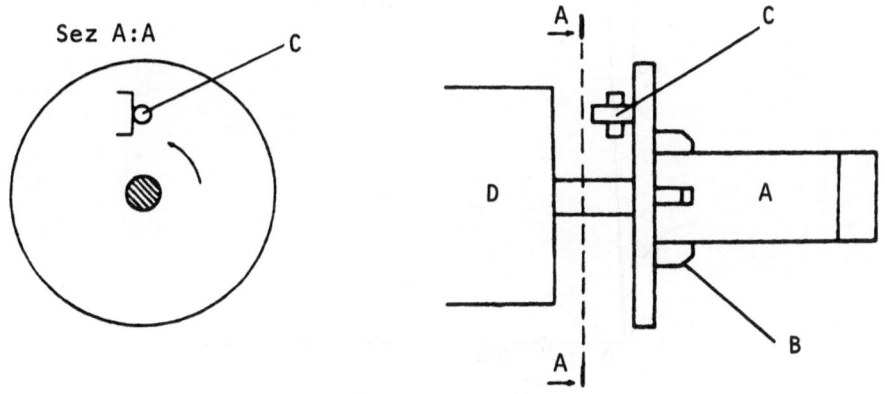

Fig. 2 Starting apparatus: A elastoviscometer, B block device,
        D starter.

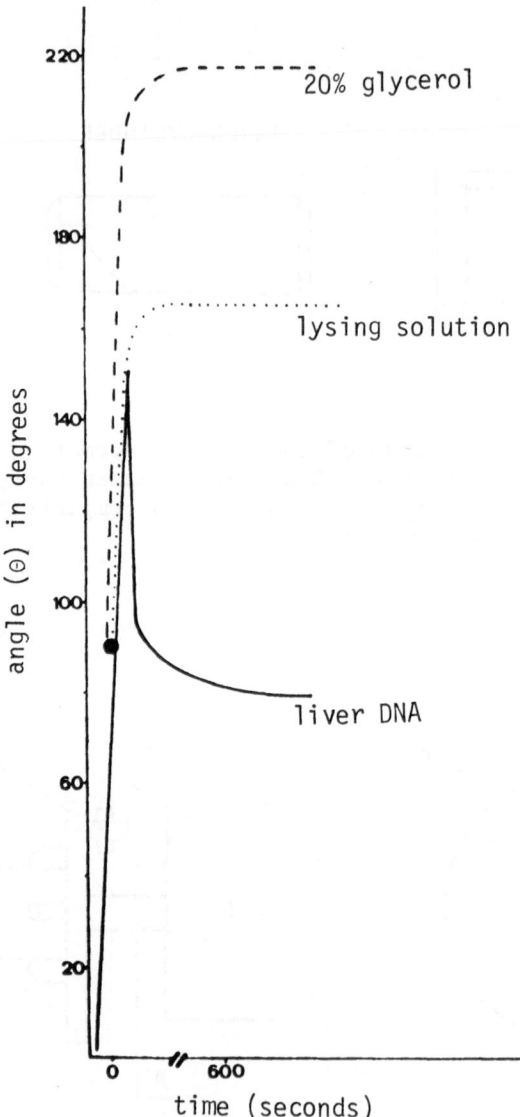

Fig. 3 Time-dependence of the rotation angle (with respect to
        the unperturbed position) of the buoyant inner cylinder,
        when the outer cylinder is rotated of 90° and the viscometer
        is filled with: a) glycerol 20%, b) lysing solution, c) DNA
        suspension from liver nuclei of an untreated rat.

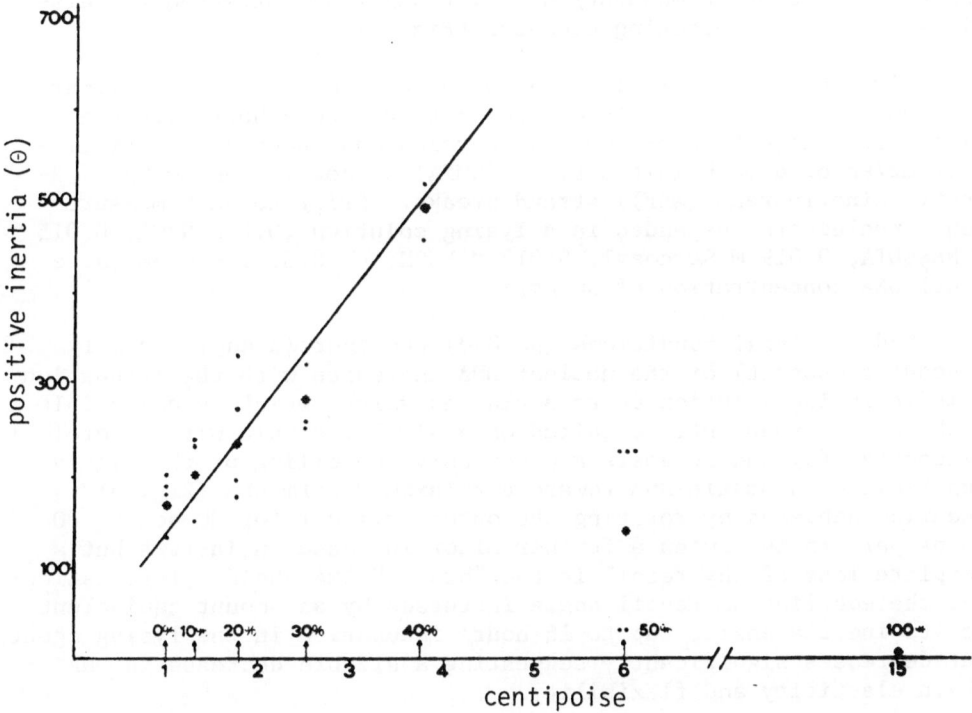

Fig. 4 Equilibrium inertia for various glycerol concentration
of known intrinsic viscosity.

the viscosity is so high that the inner and outer cylinders move like a single rigid body. The forward positive rotation (inertia angle) is then related (in the 1-5 cp range) to the intrinsic viscosity, and the recoil angle is present only with suspended DNA having an elastic component.

EFFECT OF CHEMICAL CARCINOGENS

The time dependence of equilibrium values of both the recoil angle (predominantly elastic component) and the inertia angle (predominantly viscous component) of liver DNA from untreated rat displays a rather interesting behavior (Fig. 5).

Liver nuclei are isolated as previously described (8) either from untreated control rats or from rats killed 4 hours after a single i.p. injection of chemical carcinogens inducing DNA single- (1.2 mg/kg of dimethylnitrosamine (DMNA) or double-(50 mg/kg of 2-acetylaminofluorene (AAF)) strand breaks. Prior to each measurement, nuclei are suspended in a lysing solution (0.8 M NaCl, 0.015 M Na_2EDTA, 0.019 M Sarcosyl, 0.015 M NaOH; pH 8.0; I = 0.88) at a final DNA concentration of 50 µg/ml.

Under neutral conditions (pH 8.0) the inertia angle (mostly viscous component) of the nuclear DNA increases with the incubation time in lysing solution up to a plateau value, which is compatible with data independently acquired on a similar sample with a toroidal viscometer (5) and suggests a progressive uncoiling of the highly supercoiled chromatin-DNA toward a relaxed B-form DNA (Fig. 5). Shearing achieved by rotating the outer cylinder for 30 sec at 80 turns per minute causes a further minor increase in inertia but a complete loss of any recoil in the "broken" DNA chain. Interestingly, the equilibrium recoil angle increases by an amount equivalent to its inertia angle, up to 16 hours incubation in the lysing agent, but decreases significantly suggesting a sizable decrease in DNA chain elasticity and flexibility.

The high reproducibility of these data, despite the empirical means used to apply a torque force, is apparent (Table I) by comparing the values obtained either with a manual rotation or with a mechanical device (see Fig. 2.) yielding a fixed torque. The same degree of reproducibility is apparent also in a DNA sample obtained from a rat exposed to a carcinogen (Table 2).

Figure 6 shows negative recoil angle and positive inertia angle for nuclear DNA either after single- (1.2 mg/kg of DMNA) or double-(50 mg/kg of AAF) strand breaks. It is comforting to note a substantial decrease in elasticity for both type of DNA damage, but the damage is more pronounced with the carcinogen inducing double-strand breaks, most likely because of a larger disruption of the chromatin fibers. Interestingly, an increased viscosity always accompanies a

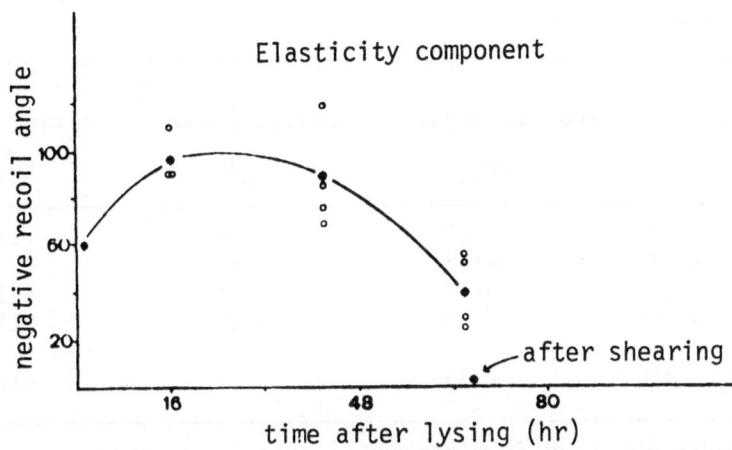

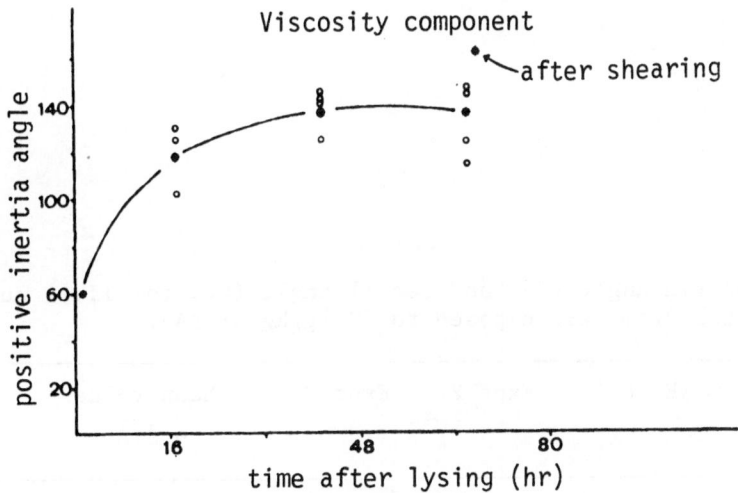

Fig. 5. Time Dependence of negative recoil angle (predominantly
elastic component) and positive inertia angle (predominantly
viscous component) of a DNA suspension from liver nuclei of
an untreated rat.

Table 1

Recoil and inertia measurements are taken using as source of constant 90º pulse to the outer cylinder either our hands (H) or a
spring (S) (see Fig. 2).

	H recoil angle (Θ_R)	H inertia angle (Θ_I)	S recoil angle (Θ_R)	S inertia angle (Θ_I)
Expt I	− 55	+115	− 75	+135
Expt II	− 25	+145	− 65	+130
Expt III	− 25	+145	− 40	+125
Expt IV	− 55	+125	− 25	+115
Mean value	− 40	+135	− 48	+127

These data were obtained from untreated rats liver nuclei 66 hours
after being suspended in a lysing solution.

Table 2

Excess inertia angle (Θ_I) and recoil angle (Θ_R) for liver nuclear
DNA isolated from rats exposed to 50 mg/kg of AAF.

	Expt 1	Expt 2	Expt 3	Mean value $\pm$ S.D.
Θ_I (degrees)	+ 63	+ 113	+ 162	+ 113.0 $\pm$ 23
Θ_R (degrees)	− 18	− 14	− 27	− 20.1 $\pm$ 3

All data are normalized to a constant pulse of 90° rotation
given to the outer cylinder.

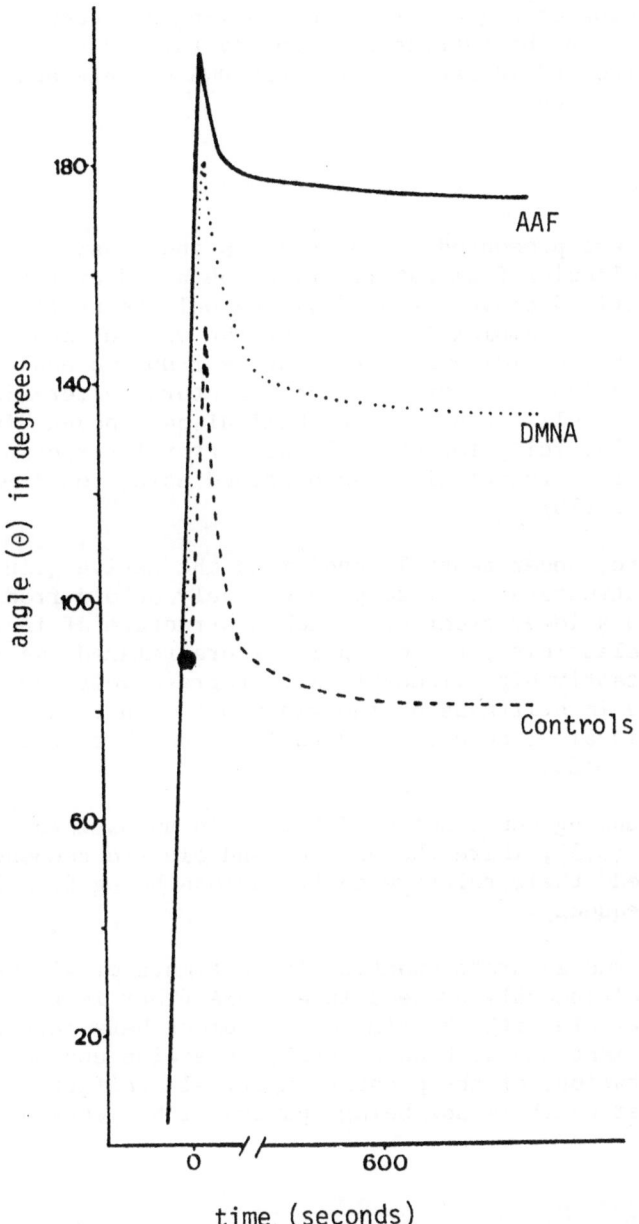

Fig. 6. Positive inertia angle and negative recoil angle of a DNA
suspension from liver nuclei obtained from (a) a control
rat, (b) a rat treated with 1.2 mg/kg of DMNA (single-strand
breaks, (c) a rat treated with 50 mg/kg of AAF (double-
strand breaks).

decrease in elasticity, as expected from the above explanation in terms of unfolding of higher-order DNA packing and compatible with previous results on the intrinsic viscosity (5) and structural alterations (2,9) induced in native chromatin-DNA by interactions with a chemical carcinogen.

CONCLUSION

The data here presented on the viscous and elastic properties of giant DNA molecules from rat liver, as obtained by the simple instrument described above, even if viewed only as preliminary, give new insights on the complex interplay of the viscous and elastic components in the unfolding of native nuclear DNA molecules exposed to a lysing solution "in vitro," or on structural alterations occurring in DNA from cells exposed to a chemical carcinogen "in vivo." The decreased elasticity for DNA molecule after interaction with a carcinogen confirms recent findings obtained using the Zimm-Crothers viscoelastometer (10).

Furthermore, under neutral conditions the native quintenary chromatin-DNA structures seem to progressively unfold from a highly packed fiber to a lower order of unpacked structure of increasing viscosity and elasticity, up to a point where relaxed DNA fibers appear of constantly high viscosity but progressively lower elasticity. A change in stiffness of the giant DNA with time of lysis was apparent also in alkaline elution data (11) best fitted to a rigorous physicochemical model.

This uncoupling could not be detected in an oscillating crucible viscometer (3,5), where the viscous and elastic components cannot be discriminated, their relative contributions being functions of the oscillation frequency.

The quick and separate quantitative estimate of viscosity and elasticity simultaneously present in any DNA fiber is readily (within minutes) feasible with the simple instrument here introduced by a single experiment and with an accuracy otherwise unattainable (despite the limitations of the present empirical configuration of our elastoviscometer which is now being updated with electronic devices.)

ACKNOWLEDGEMENTS

C.Nicolini was supported by Research and Study Leave Award from Temple University and by the Finalized Project "Control of Neoplastic Growth," National Research Council, Italy. The authors thank Drs. Carlo, Finollo, and Martelli for assistance in providing liver nuclei.

REFERENCES

1. Peterson A., Fox B. and Fox M. Biophys.Biochim.Acta 299: 385-396,1973.
2. Nicolini C., Ramanathan R., Kendall F., Murphy J., Parodi S. and Sarma D.S.R. Cancer Res. 36: 1725-1730,1976.
3. Parodi S., Carlo P., Martelli A., Taningher M., Finollo R., Pala M. and Giarretti W,J.Mol.Biol. 147:501-521,1981.
4. Kohn,K.W., Erickson L.C.,Ewig R.A.G. and Friedman C.A. Biochemistry 15: 4629-4637,1976
5. Nicolini C. et al., in this volume, page 381.
6. Chapman R.E., Klotz L.C.,Thompson D.S. and Zimm B.H. Macromolecules 2: 637-643,1969.
7. Carr M., Shen L. and Hermans J. Anal. Biochem. 72:202-211,1976.
8. Carlo P.,Martelli A.,Brambilla G., Nicolini C. Internal Report 1/81,Gruppo di Biostruttura,University of Genova,1981.
9. Nicolini C., Martelli A., Grattarola M. and Viviani R. Basic and Applied Histochemistry(1982) in press.
10. Shafer R.G. and Chase E.C. Cancer Res. 40: 3186-3193,1980.
11. Nicolini C., Belmont A., Zeitz S., Maura A., Pino A., Robbiano L. and Brambilla G., J.Theoret.Biology, in press and in this volume, page 93.

INITIATION OF EXPERIMENTAL LIVER CARCINOGENESIS BY CHEMICALS: ARE THE CARCINOGEN ALTERED HEPATOCYTES STIMULATED TO GROW INTO FOCI BY DIFFERENT SELECTION PROCEDURES IDENTICAL?

A. Columbano,* G.M. Ledda,* P.M. Rao, S. Rajalakshmi and D.S.R. Sarma

Department of Pathology, University of Toronto, Medical Sciences Building, Toronto, Ontario, Canada M5S 1A8

The multi-stage nature of the carcinogenic process has been demonstrated in many tissues including skin (1-3), liver (4, 5), mammary gland (6), urinary bladder (7) and vagina (8). However, the molecular mechanisms underlying this complex process are not yet understood clearly. The development of several experimental model systems for the sequential analysis of chemical carcinogenesis in rat liver has opened up new avenues for investigating this complex process. Our experimental approaches have two main objectives (i) to understand the mechanisms underlying the initiation phase of liver carcinogenesis and (ii) to characterize the initiated hepatocytes stimulated to grow into enzyme altered foci by some of the selection procedures. The experimental design was guided by the hypothesis shown in Figure 1.

The hypothesis predicts that carcinogens cause DNA damage either by direct interaction or otherwise. By and large the damage may be repaired. However, if the cell proliferates prior to the repair of such damage, then such proliferation might result in a carcinogen-induced "altered" cell representing probably an "initiated" cell; the implication of this would be that replica-

---

*Present Address: Cattedra di Patologia Generale I, Universita di Cagliari, Cagliari 09100, Italy.

This work was supported in part by U.S. PHS research grants CA-23958, CA21157 from the National Cancer Institute and from the National Cancer Institute of Canada.

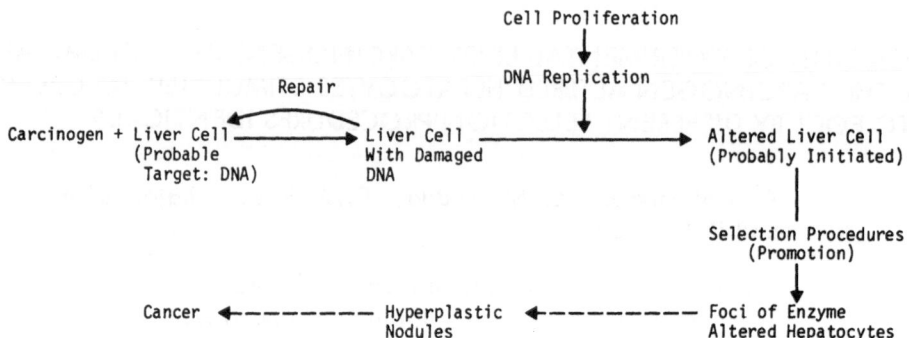

Fig. 1.   Schematic representation of the working hypothesis to study
           initiation in experimental liver carcinogenesis.

tion of carcinogen-damaged DNA during cell proliferation is an important
step in the initiation event. In the recently developed model systems for
liver carcinogenesis, such initiated hepatocytes can be selectively stimulated to grow into islands of enzyme altered hepatocytes using several dietary
regimens; the question therefore arises whether these various selecting
regimens promote the growth of identical or different population of initiated
hepatocytes. The results of our experiments aimed at answering some of the
questions raised by the hypothesis are presented here.

In the present discussion, initiated hepatocytes are defined as those
carcinogen-altered cells that can be selectively stimulated to grow into
islands of enzyme-altered hepatocytes. The validity of this definition lies
in the fact that the selection regimens, especially those described by Solt
and Farber (9) and Peraino et al. (10), not only promote the growth of
carcinogen-altered cells into foci but also cause an increase in cancer incidence (4, 5, 11). In addition, using the former procedure, a material
continuity has been established between the focal islands and liver cancer
by demonstrating the presence of cancer within the nodule (12). Since over
90% of the islands are γ-glutamyltransferase (γ-GT)-positive (13), quantitation of the γ-GT-positive foci can be used as an assay for initiation.

Using Solt and Farber's assay evidence was obtained to indicate that cell proliferation, prior to the repair of a carcinogen-induced critical lesion(s) is essential for the induction of initiated hepatocytes (14, 15). Exogenous cell proliferative stimulus, however, seems to be obviated when a necrogenic dose of the carcinogen is administered (15), probably because of the compensatory liver cell proliferation induced as a result of liver cell necrosis.

Our observation that hydrocortisone, an agent that inhibits liver DNA synthesis, inhibited the formation of γ-GT-positive foci only when given during the 'S' phase of the cell cycle (16) is consistent with the formulation that replication of carcinogen-damaged DNA during cell proliferation is an essential critical step for initiation. The similarity between the induction of foci of enzyme-altered hepatocytes by chemicals and cell transformation by chemicals, radiation and viruses is noteworthy in that they both require at least one round of cell proliferation (17-19).

If the above formulation is indeed correct, then the question arises what is the molecular mechanism(s) by which replication of carcinogen-damaged DNA induces "initiation." Three possibilities merit consideration : (i) Does the presence of a carcinogen-modified base in the template DNA strand cause misbase pairing (ii) Does replication on a carcinogen-damaged template result in gaps in the daughter strand which are subsequently filled in by some recombinational events that may be error prone and (iii) Does replication of carcinogen-altered DNA induce some "transposon"-like activity.

Our results on the replication in vivo of rat liver DNA containing methylated bases induced by the hepatocarcinogen dimethylnitrosamine (DMN) show that N-7-methylguanine and O^6-methylguanine and possibly some phosphotriesters do permit replication (Table 1). However, what is perhaps of greater significance is the presence of some of the methylated bases in the newly made daughter strand. Since the administered DMN was not detectable either in the blood or in the liver at the time of synthesis of the new strand, de novo methylation of the daughter strand was considered unlikely. Contamination by any methylated RNA was ruled out because of the methylated bases in the daughter strand even under alkaline conditions which would have hydrolyzed any RNA, if present. The possibility of reutilization of methylated DNA products for new DNA synthesis was excluded because administration of (^{14}C)-DMN methylated DNA in the form of bases, nucleosides, nucleotides or oligonucleotides during the 'S' phase, did not result in labelling of the replicated DNA. On the other hand, the data suggest that the methylated purines in the daughter strand might have arisen by way of transfer from the parental strand, mediated by some type of recombinational events. Such recombinational events may induce altera-

Table 1. Presence of (^{14}C)-DMN Induced Methylated Purines in the S$_1$-Nuclease Resistant, Hybrid Rat Liver DNA and in the Parental and Daugter Strands of the Hybrid.[a]

Methylated Purines	Methylated purines in the hybrid DNA[b] (pmoles/mg DNA)	% Distribution in	
		Parental Strand[c] (light)	Daughter Strand[c] (heavy)
N-7-Methyl-guanine	146.0 ± 7.6	88	12
O^6-Methylguanine	9.3 ± 1.4	66	34

[a]Male Fischer 344 rats weighing 120 to 140 g were given i.p. (^{14}C)-DMN (100 µCi/0.5 mg/100 g body weight). Four hours afterwards, at a time when the administered carcinogen could no longer be detected either in the blood or in the liver, the rats were subjected to partial hepatectomy (PH). Fifteen hours later a tablet of 5-bromo-2-deoxyuridine (300 mg) was implanted subcutaneously on the back of the rat. Twenty-four hours later the rats were sacrificed and liver DNA was isolated and centrifuged in neutral CsCl gradients (20).

[b]Hybrid DNA of density 1.727 g/cm^3 or greater was treated with S$_1$-nuclease to digest any single stranded regions probably representing un-replicated parental DNA. The S$_1$-nuclease resistant hybrid DNA was acid hydrolyzed and fractionated (20).

[c]The S$_1$-nuclease-resistant hybrid DNA was treated with formamide-formaldehyde and the separated strands isolated on neutral CsCl gradients. The separated strands are 100% digestible by S$_1$-nuclease. The methylated purines in the isolated strands were quantitated.

The results are the mean ± S.E. of 4 experiments. In each experiment 2 to 3 rats were used. The dpm in the methylated purines in individual experiments ranged from 1300-1900 for N-7-methylguanine; and 50-60 for O^6-methylguanine.

tions in DNA sequence and/or increase the chances of expression of a recessive lesion. In addition, our studies also show that, following replication, some O^6-methylguanine containing regions of replicated DNA become susceptible to attack by the single strand specific S_1-nuclease (21). These results were interpreted to indicate the presence of locally denatured regions in the replicated DNA and are of interest because O^6-methylguanine is considered to be a miscoding lesion.

Taken together the results show that, while several of the carcinogen-induced lesions permit in vivo replication, they might do so by any one or a combination of several different mechanisms. It is quite conceivable therefore that the resulting cell populations may be heterogenous and respond differently to different dietary regimens and grow into islands of enzyme-altered hepatocytes. We therefore asked whether the different dietary regimens select the same or different populations of initiated hepatocytes.

Several dietary regimens have been described which stimulate the growth of initiated hepatocytes into islands of enzyme-altered cells, staining positive for γ-GT. These include feeding diets containing: 0.02% 2-acetylaminofluorene (2-AAF) coupled with a liver cell proliferative stimulus, PH (9) or CCl_4 (22); 0.05% phenobarbital (4); polychlorinated biphenyls (23, 24); 1% orotic acid (unpublished observations) and a diet deficient in choline and methionine (CMD) (25). However, in our experiments we have used only two of these viz. 2-AAF + CCl_4 and CMD diet to see if they select the same population of initiated hepatocytes or not. The experimental approaches used for this purpose were based on three principles:

(i) Resistance to the mitoinhibitory effect of 2-AAF: Since the carcinogen-altered hepatocytes are selectively stimulated to grow into foci by the method of Cayama et al. (22) (2-AAF + CCl_4) by virtue of their resistance to the mitoinhibitory effect of 2-AAF, we asked the question are the foci selected by feeding the CMD diet similarly resistant to the mitoinhibition by 2-AAF. The experimental protocol consisted of the following: The rats were subjected to PH 12 hours after the administration of 1,2-dimethylhydrazine (1,2-DMH), and a week later they were fed a CMD diet for 6 weeks to selectively grow the initiated hepatocytes into γ-GT-positive foci. After a 2-week period on basal diet the rats were exposed to a diet containing 0.02% 2-AAF. One week afterwards CCl_4 was given to stimulate liver cell proliferation. Twenty-four hours later (^{3}H)-thymidine was injected repeatedly every 4 hours for 24 hours while the rats continued to be on 0.02% 2-AAF diet. Twenty-four hours after the last injection the rats were killed and the livers were processed for auto-radiographic analysis and histochemical staining for γ-GT.

The rationale for the design is:if the foci cells selected by CMD diet are resistant to the mitoinhibitory effect of 2-AAF, they should respond to the liver cell proliferative stimulus (CCl$_4$) in the presence of 2-AAF, incorporate (^{3}H)-thymidine and appear as labelled foci in the autoradiograms; the surrounding liver being inhibited. It was found that over 95% of the γ-GT-positive foci had incorporated (^{3}H)-thymidine into their DNA indicating that they were resistant to the mitoinhibitory effect of 2-AAF. The results may be interpreted to indicate that both selection procedures can stimulate the growth of identical population of initiated hepatocytes. Alternatively, γ-GT positive foci grown up to a size or stage become resistant to the mitoinhibitory effect of 2-AAF irrespective of how they were selected.

(ii) Ability of the selection regimen to stimulate the growth of altered hepatocytes is related to the presence of carcinogen-induced critical lesions at the time of DNA replication.

The experimental protocol used was the following:

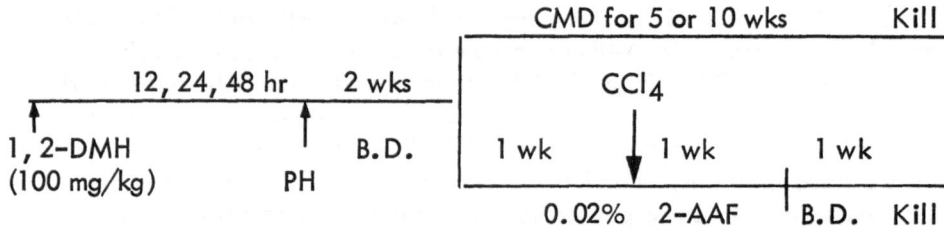

The rationale is based on the fact that delaying the PH would allow the carcinogen-induced lesions with shorter half-lives to be repaired before replication; therefore, hepatocytes replicated at different times after the carcinogen-treatment may differ in their ability to respond to the stimulatory effect of different selecting regimens. The data in Table 2 clearly show that carcinogen-damaged hepatocytes induced to proliferate 12 hours after 1,2-DMH-treatment yielded the highest number of γ-GT-positive foci when selected by either of the two regimens. However, when replication was delayed to 24 hours after 1,2-DMH, selection by CMD diet yielded far fewer foci while the 2-AAF + CCl$_4$ selection yielded essentially the same number of foci as at 12 hours. These results suggest that the two selecting regimens probably select different populations of initiated hepatocytes. However, the possibility that they might be selecting the same population but for different properties cannot be excluded.

(iii) Initiated hepatocytes once formed are stable and persist; therefore any time post-initiation, they should be stimulated to grow into γ-GT-

Table 2. Effect of Variation in the Time of Performance of PH on the Induction of γ-GT-Positive Foci Using Different Selecting Regimens.

Treatment	No. of γ-GT-Positive Foci/sq.cm		
	CMD for 5 wks	CMD for 10 wks	2-AAF + CCl_4[a]
1,2-DMH + PH (12 hr) (100 mg/kg)	14 ± 1.1 (10)	27 ± 3.2 (4)	19 ± 2.6 (16)
1,2-DMH + PH (24 hr)	7 ± 0.8 (8)	9 ± 1.8 (3)	15 ± 1.5 (26)
1,2-DMH + PH (48 hr)	5 ± 0.5 (12)	10 ± 1.3 (5)	6 ± 1.2 (10)
1,2-DMH + SH (12 hr)	2 ± 0.4 (6)	3 ± 1.2 (5)	4 ± 0.8 (14)
0.9% NaCl + PH (12 hr)	0.4 ± 0.2 (5)	0.3 ± 0.2 (5)	1 ± 0.2 (12)

Experimental protocol is given in the text and other details are given in Refs. 14 and 22.

[a]These values are taken from reference (16) for easy comparison. Numbers in parentheses represent number of rats used; values are mean ± S.E.

positive foci by any of the different selecting regimen.

We had earlier observed that subjecting the rats to 2-AAF + CCl_4 selection regimen 2 or 36 weeks after initiation by diethylnitrosamine, yielded essentially the same number of foci (26) and similar persistence of initiated hepatocyte was observed using N-methyl-N-nitrosourea as the initiating liver carcinogen. The question now asked was will CMD selection procedure also yield the same number of foci, irrespective of when it is applied after initiation. The experimental protocol was:

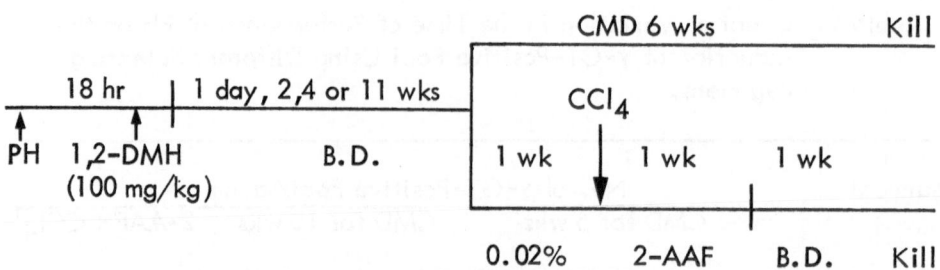

The results presented in Table 3 clearly show that the efficiency of the CMD diet to select the initiated hepatocytes falls down drastically if the selection regimen is started 4 or 11 weeks instead of 1 day or 2 weeks after the administration of 1, 2-DMH. In contrast, the 2-AAF + CCl$_4$ selection regimen can select the initiated hepatocytes at later time points with equal efficiency. These results again suggest that the two selection regimens are selecting different populations of initiated hepatocytes or they may be selecting the same population but using different properties by virtue of which the selecting regimen can select the initiated hepatocytes.

Table 3.   Effect of Delaying the Time of Starting the Selection Regimens on the Induction of γ-GT-positive Foci by 1, 2-Dimethyl-hydrazine

Treatment	Time of Starting the Selection Regimen		No. of γ-GT-positive foci/sq.cm.
	CMD (for 6 wks)	2-AAF + CCl$_4$	
PH + 1, 2-DMH (100 mg/kg)	1 day (5)		44 ± 3
PH + 1, 2-DMH	2 wks (5)		40 ± 5
PH + 1, 2-DMH	4 wks (6)		9 ± 2
PH + 1, 2-DMH	11 wks (5)		5 ± 1
PH + 1, 2-DMH		2 wks (5)	35 ± 4.2
PH + 1, 2-DMH		4 wks (4)	30 ± 3.2

Details of the experimental protocol are given in the text. Numbers in parentheses are the numbers of rats used; values are mean ± S.E.

The results of experiments (ii) and (iii) described above raise several interesting questions. For example, if initiation is irreversible as suggested from the data on skin (2, 27) and liver (26) carcinogenesis models why do the two selecting regimens, 2-AAF + CCl$_4$ and CMD diet, not elicit the same quantitative response from the initiated hepatocytes when applied at later time points after initiation? Secondly, why does the 2-AAF + CCl$_4$ selection give the same number of foci irrespective of whether liver cell proliferative stimulus was given 12 or 24 hours post 1, 2-DMH-treatment, while CMD diet selection is more effective when the liver cell proliferative stimulus was given at 12 hours rather than at 24 hours after the administration of 1, 2-DMH.

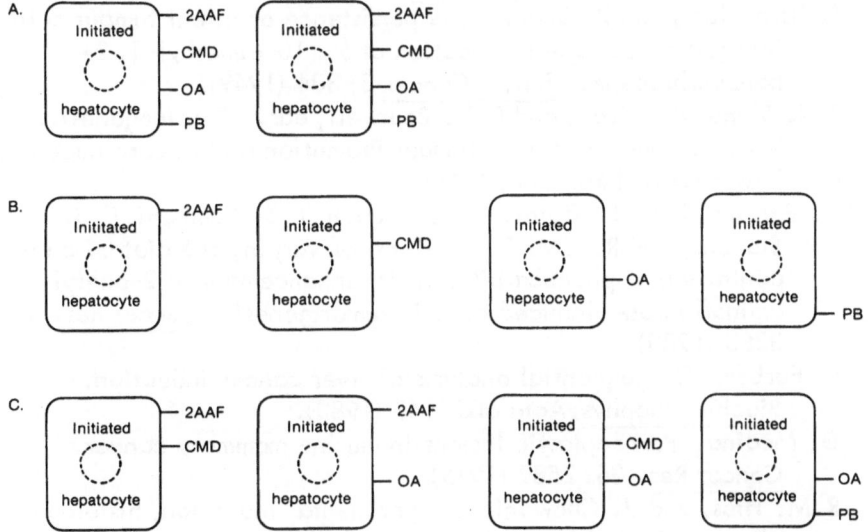

Fig.2.   Schematic representation of models of initiated hepatocytes with secondary lesions by virtue of which selection regimens can selectively stimulate them to grow into islands of enzyme altered hepatocytes. Model A: different selection regimens select the same population of initiated hepatocytes; Model B: each selecting regimen selects a different population of initiated hepatocytes; Model C: A selecting regimen selecting one or more populations of initiated hepatocytes.

It is tempting to speculate that there are at least two types of critical lesions: one a common primary lesion responsible for initiation and one or more secondary lesions that confer a property by virtue of which the selecting regimens can select the same or different initiated hepatocytes. Further, the primary lesion may also be responsible for the resistance of the initiated hepatocytes to the mitoinhibitory effect of 2-AAF. The secondary lesions, on the other hand, may have different half-lives and thus may account for the differences seen in the selection ability of the two selection regimens (see experiments Nos. ii and iii). Some of these possibilities are illustrated in Figure 2. Further work in this area should provide interesting insights into the nature of initiation.

References

1.   P. Rous and J.G. Kidd, Conditional neoplasms and subthreshold neoplastic states. J.Exp.Med. 73: 365 (1941).
2.   I. Berenblum, and P. Shubik, The persistence of latent tumour cells induced by a single application of 9, 10-dimethyl-1, 2-benzanthracene. Brit.J.Cancer 3: 384 (1949).
3.   T.J. Slaga, A. Sivak, and R.K. Boutwell, eds., Carcinogenesis. Vol. 2. Mechanisms of Tumour Promotion and Cocarcinogenesis. Raven Press, New York (1978).
4.   C. Peraino, E.F. Staffeldt, D.A. Haugen, L.S. Lombard, F.J. Stevens, and R.J.M. Fry, Effects of varying the dietary concentration of phenobarbital on its enhancement of 2-acetylaminofluorene-induced hepatic tumorigenesis. Cancer Res. 40: 3268 (1980).
5.   E. Farber, The sequential analysis of liver cancer induction. Biochim.Biophys.Acta 605: 149 (1980).
6.   D. Medina, Preneoplastic lesions in murine mammary cancer. Cancer Res. 36: 2589 (1976).
7.   R.M. Hics, and J. Chowaniec, Experimental induction, histology and ultrastructure of hyperplasia and neoplasia of the urinary bladder epithelium. Int.Rev.Exp.Pathol. 18: 199 (1968).
8.   A.L. Herbst, H. Ulfelder, and D.C. Poskanzer, Adenocarcinoma of the vagina. Association of maternal stilbestrol therapy with tumour appearance to young women. New Engl.J.Med. 284: 878 (1971).
9.   D.B. Solt, and E. Farber, New principle for analysis of chemical carcinogenesis. Nature 263: 701 (1976).
10.   C. Peraino, R.J.M. Fry and E.F. Staffeldt, Reduction and enhancement by phenobarbital of hepatocarcinogenesis induced in the rat by 2-acetylaminofluorene. Cancer Res. 31: 1506 (1971).

11. D. B. Solt, A. Medline, and E. Farber, Rapid emergence of carcinogen-induced hyperplastic lesions in a new model for the sequential analysis of liver carcinogenesis. Am. J. Pathol. 88: 595 (1977).

12. E. Farber and R. Cameron, The sequential analysis of cancer development. Adv. Cancer Res. 31: 125 (1980).

13. K. Ogawa, D. B. Solt and E. Farber, Phenotypic diversity as an early property of putative preneoplastic hepatocyte populations in liver carcinogenesis. Cancer Res. 40: 725 (1980).

14. A. Columbano, S. Rajalakshmi, and D.S.R. Sarma, Requirement of cell proliferation for the initiation of liver carcinogenesis as assayed by three different procedures. Cancer Res. 41: 2079 (1981).

15. T.S. Ying, D.S.R. Sarma, and E. Farber, Role of acute hepatic necrosis in the induction of early steps in liver carcinogenesis by diethylnitrosamine. Cancer Res. 41: 2096 (1981).

16. T.S. Ying, The role of DNA synthesis and of repair in the induction of putative preneoplastic lesions in rat liver by 1, 2-dimethylhydrazine (1, 2-DMH). Proc. Am. Assoc. Cancer Res. 21: 62 (1980).

17. C. Boreck, and L. Sachs, The number of cell generations required to fix the transformed state in X-ray involved transformation. Proc. Natl. Acad. Sci. (U.S.A.) 57: 1522 (1967).

18. T. Kakunaga, Requirement for cell proliferation in the fixation and expression of the transformed state in mouse cells treated with 4-nitroquinoline-1-oxide. Int. J. Cancer 14: 736 (1974).

19. G. J. Todaro and H. Green, Cell growth and the initiation of transformation by SV40. Proc. Natl. Acad. Sci. (U.S.A.) 55: 302 (1966).

20. S.E. Abanobi, A. Columbano, R.A. Mulivor, S. Rajalakshmi, and D.S.R. Sarma, In vivo replication of hepatic deoxyribonucleic acid of rats treated with dimethylnitrosamine: presence of dimethylnitrosamine-induced O^6-methylguanine, N-7-methylguanine, and N-3-methyladenine in the replicated hybrid deoxyribonucleic acid. Biochemistry 19: 1382 (1980).

21. G.M. Ledda, A. Columbano, P.M. Rao, S. Rajalakshmi, and D.S.R. Sarma, In vivo replication of carcinogen-modified rat liver DNA: Increased susceptibility of O^6-methylguanine compared to N-7-methylguanine in replicated DNA to S_1-nuclease. Biochem. Biophys. Res. Commun. 95: 816 (1980).

22. E. Cayama, H. Tsuda, D.S.R. Sarma, and E. Farber, Initiation of chemical carcinogenesis requires cell proliferation. Nature 275: 60 (1978).

23.   N. Ito, M. Tatematsu, M. Hirose, K. Nakanishi, and J. Muraski,
        Enhancing effect of chemicals on production of hyperplastic
        liver nodules induced by N-2-fluorenylacetamine in hepa-
        tectomized rat. Gann 69: 143 (1978).
24.   N.T. Kimura, T. Kanematsu, and T. Baba, Polychlorinated bi-
        phenyl(s) as a promoter in experimental hepatocarcinogenesis in
        rats. Z. Krebsförsch 87: 257 (1976).
25.   M.A. Sells, S.L. Katyal, S. Sell, H. Sinozuka and B. Lombardi,
        Induction of foci of altered γ-glutamyltranspeptidase-positive
        hepatocytes in carcinogen-treated rats fed a choline-deficient
        diet. Br. J. Cancer 40: 274 (1979).
26.   D.B. Solt, E. Cayama, D.S.R. Sarma, and E. Farber, Persistence
        of resistant putative preneoplastic hepatocytes induced by N-
        nitrosodiethylamine or N-methyl-N-nitrosourea. Cancer Res.
        40: 1112 (1980).
27.   J.C. Mottram, A developing factor in experimental blastogenesis.
        J. Pathol. Bacteriol. 56: 181 (1944).

INFLUENCE OF DNA CONFORMATION ON DNA METHYLATION AND THE DIRECT BINDING OF N-METHYL-N-NITROSO-N^1-NITRO-GUANIDINE *

S. Rajalakshmi, M. Jamaludin** and D.S.R. Sarma

Department of Pathology, University of Toronto
Medical Sciences Building
Toronto, Ontario, Canada M5S 1A8

INTRODUCTION

One of the attractive mechanisms by which chemicals can cause cancer is through somatic mutation. The theory of somatic mutation speculates that mutations relatable to carcinogenesis are induced by the presence of carcinogen modified base residue in an appropriate gene sequence during cell proliferation. This theory implies that the availability of base residues at specific genomic sites to the carcinogen for interaction is critical for the initiation of carcinogenic process. It is logical to presume that one of the major determinants for the exposition of gene sequence to the carcinogen may be the conformation of DNA. In order to gain an insight into whether DNA conformation and/or sequence can influence carcinogen-DNA interaction, we designed several studies on the effect of modulation of DNA conformation on DNA methylation by potent carcinogens. This study is concerned with the demonstration that (a) DNA structure and/or sequence affects DNA methylation by N-methyl-N-nitroso-N^1-nitroguanidine (MNNG) and (b) MNNG interacts directly with rat liver DNA forming DNA-MNNG complex prior to the transfer of its methyl group to DNA.

Principles Used in the Study

For the purpose of demonstrating that DNA conformation and/or

*This study was supported by grants from Medical Research Council, Canada.
**Present address: Sri Chitra Tirunal Medical Center; Trivandrum, India, 695012.

sequence affects DNA methylation we employed the technique of binding the ligand distamycin A to DNA to induce conformational changes. Distamycin-A induced unique conformational changes on binding to rat liver DNA; these changes were very similar to those reported for calf thymus DNA (1, 2). The technique of transient electric dichroism of rod-like DNA molecules developed by Hogan et al. (3) was used to follow the conformational changes.

To demonstrate the direct interaction of MNNG with DNA we utilised the technique of large zone gel exclusion chromatography. This method has been successfully employed to study the energetics of interaction of pApAp with poly U (4).

In general, gel exclusion chromatography carried out with systems in which one solute species in solution enters into complex formation with another results in a "reaction boundary" or zone which has transport characteristics different from those of the individual species. In addition to system parameters the elution profile of the interaction boundary is affected by the reaction rates and the rates of equilibration between the mobile and stationary phases (5), making it an extremely versatile method to detect interaction. Computer simulation studies have revealed that an interaction is often detected in large zone gel exclusion chromatography by alterations in the peak position and/or peak height of the concentration gradient at the leading edge of the boundary (5). Even though computer simulation studies have been limited only to equilibria in protein systems the chromatographic method is general and by the proper choice of experimental conditions can be used, in some cases, to study interactions of small molecules with macromolecules.

Materials and Methods

(^{14}C)-MNNG of specific activity 15 mCi/mmole was purchased from New England Nuclear, Boston, Massachusetts. Unlabelled MNNG was a product of Aldrich Chemicals and deoxy-guanosine-5'-phosphate was from P.L. Biochemicals. N-acetyl cysteine and glycine were purchased from Sigma Chemicals. Biogel P-2 was a product of Bio-Rad Laboratories and Sephadex gels were a product of Pharmacia, Uppsala, Sweden. Distamycin-A was obtained from Boehringer, Canada.

DNA Used in the Binding Studies

Rat liver DNA was isolated and purified by methods described in detail in our earlier publications (6, 7). The DNA was further purified by fractionation through Sephadex G-100 column after dissolving in 0.01 M sodium phosphate, pH 7.1 and the fraction excluding from the column was used for the binding studies.

DNA Used in the Methylation Studies

DNA of length 157 base pairs was used in the study on the effect of distamycin A on DNA methylation by MNNG. The purified DNA was sonicated and fractionated according to the procedure described by Hogan et al. (1). Methylation conditions are described under Table 1. The isolation of methylated DNA, hydrolysis of methylated DNA and the characterization of methylated bases have been described earlier (6, 7).

Sephadex G-50 Column Chromatography

A column (0.85 x 17.2 cm) of Sephadex G-50 (particle size 20-80 µ) equilibrated with 25 mM sodium phosphate buffer, pH 7.14 ± 0.01 was employed for the experiments. The column was pretreated by several passages of MNNG (10^{-4}M) in 25 mM sodium phosphate buffer, pH 7.1, to saturate any reactive groups in the gel. A molar absorbance of 6700 M^{-1} cm^{-1} at 260 nm was used to calculate the concentration of DNA in base-pair units. The molar absorbance of MNNG at 260 nm was 1.1×10^4 m^{-1} cm^{-1} under the conditions of the experiment. Freshly prepared aqueous solution of MNNG (1 mg/ml) was used in the experiment.

High Pressure Liquid Chromatography

The high pressure liquid chromatographic set up of Waters Associates (Milford, MA) was employed with a µBondapak C18 column. The eluting buffer was 0.05 M ammonium formate pH 5.0. A flow rate of 1.5 ml per min was used and the eluant was monitored at 254 nm and the absorbance was recorded automatically by means of the Data Module.

Results and Discussion

In Table 1 are presented the data on the effect of distamycin A on DNA methylation by MNNG. Distamycin A inhibits DNA methylation by MNNG in the concentration range of 0.125-0.5 µmole. The formation of both N-7-MeG and O^6-MeG were affected almost to the same extent. The formation of a complex between native DNA and distamycin A is necessary for the inhibition because dissociation of the complex by denaturing DNA with 50% DMSO abolished the inhibition of DNA methylation. The effect of distamycin A on DNA methylation induced by MNNG is very similar to that induced by N-methyl-N-nitrosourea (6-8). It is important to mention that no precipitation of DNA occurred on binding to distamycin A under the experimental conditions. We also could not detect any methylated deriva-

Table 1. Effect of Distamycin A on MNNG-Induced Formation
of N-7-Methylguanine and O^6-Methylguanine in rat
Liver DNA In Vitro

Concentration of Distamycin A (μmoles/ml)	nmoles methyl groups incorporated/mg DNA	
	N-7-MeG	O^6-MeG
0.00	20.8 ± 1.0	2.1 ± 0.12
0.125	14.2 ± 0.4 (32)	1.3 ± 0.03 (38)
0.250	9.0 ± 0.11 (57)	0.75 ± 0.03 (64)
0.500	2.0 ± 0.1 (90)	0.17 ± 0.02 (92)

The methylation of DNA was carried out by incubating sonicated
DNA (200 μg/ml) with 4 μmoles MNNG (specific radioactivity
1.4×10^6 DPM/μmole) in a total volume of 2 ml in the presence
of 10 mM Tris-HCl, pH 7.8 and glycine 10 mM for 4 hours at 37°.
The method for the isolation of methylated DNA, hydrolysis to
methylated bases and the identification of N-7-MeG, or O^6-MeG
was described in our earlier publications (6, 7). The specific
radioactivity was expressed as nmoles/mg DNA. Twenty absor-
bancy units at 260 nm were assumed to be equal to 1 mg DNA in
the calculation. Freshly made aqueous solution of distamycin A
at pH 7 was used at the concentration indicated in the Table.
The tubes were covered with foil to protect them from light during
incubation.
Values are the average of 4 experiments ± S.E.
Numbers in parentheses represent per cent inhibition.

tive of distamycin A under our experimental conditions.

Distamycin A inhibited specifically the methylation of DNA and not
that of deoxyguanosine-5-phosphate (dGMP). Whether distamycin A is
present or absent the amount of N-7-MeG formed was the same (6.1 ± 0.2

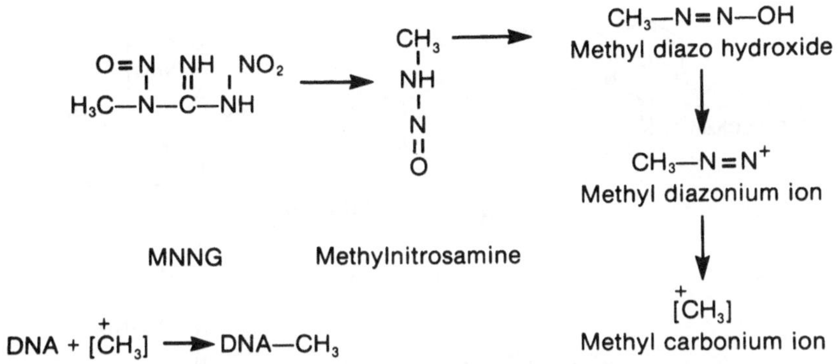

CH₃—N=N—OH
Methyl diazo hydroxide

O=N NH NO₂   CH₃
 | || | |
H₃C—N—C—NH   NH
                      |
                      N
                      ||
                      O

CH₃—N=N⁺
Methyl diazonium ion

MNNG   Methylnitrosamine

⁺
[CH₃]
Methyl carbonium ion

         +
DNA + [CH₃] ——► DNA—CH₃

Scheme 1.   Base catalyzed dissociation of MNNG and the
            interaction of methyl carbonium with DNA.

nmoles per mg dGMP). The lack of inhibition of dGMP methylation by distamycin A suggests that this antibiotic does not interfere with the release of active methylating species during the base catalyzed dissociation of MNNG. It is likely therefore that the inhibition of DNA methylation is due not to a lack of methylating intermediates but to the unavailability of methylatable sites. The fact that distamycin A does not bind to poly dG-dC and denatured DNA suggests that its effect on DNA methylation is unlikely to be due to non-specific binding to phosphates (9).

In a model proposed recently one molecule of distamycin A extends over 5 base pairs in the minor groove of DNA and is attached to an A-T cluster through four hydrogen bonds connecting the amide groups of the oligopeptide and the carbonyl groups of thymine and N-3 atom of adenine exposed in the minor groove. The structure of the complex is also stabilized by two hydrogen bonds linking the positively charged propionamidino group of the antibiotic and the negatively charged oxygens in the phosphate group (10).

These observations are in support of the interpretation that in the

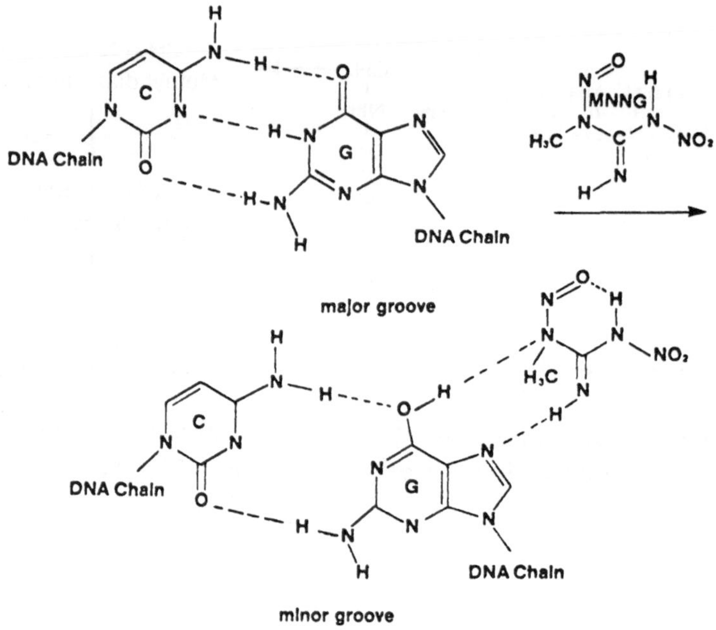

Scheme 2.   Schematic representation of interaction of MNNG
with DNA-guanines. A hydrogen-binding interaction of the N-7 of guanine with the amino group
of MNNG is visualized to favour the enolization
of the guanine. The feasibility of this is indicated
by the fact that the electronic spectrum of N-7-
methylguanine resembles more closely that of O^6-
methylguanine, the enolic analogue of guanine,
than that of guanine itself (unpublished observations).

conformation DNA assumes on binding to distamycin A, the methylatable
sites are rendered inaccessible to MNNG. However, this interprretation is
not consistent with what is believed to be the mechanism for DNA methylation by MNNG. According to current thinking MNNG methylates DNA
according to Scheme 1. The base catalyzed dissociation of MNNG

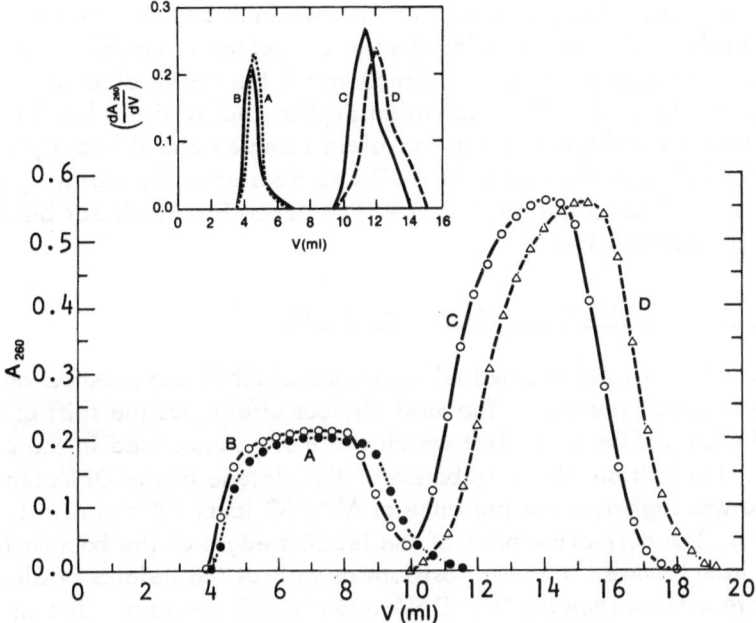

Fig. 1.   The mutual influence of DNA and MNNG on their respective elution profiles from a Sephadex G-50 column.   The
sample volume was 5 ml and contained 6.83 x 10^{-5}M base-
pair unit of rat-liver DNA and 1.1 x 10^{-4}M MNNG in 25
mM sodium phosphate buffer, pH 7.14 ± 0.01.   The temperature of the experiment was 21.5°C.   The column (0.85 x 17.2
cm) was eluted at a flow rate of 12 ml per hr and fractions
of 0.427 ml were collected automatically using an ISCO
fraction collector.   The fractions were kept in ice as they
emerged from the column, diluted with 0.5 ml of water and
their A_{260} measured. Curves A and B are the elution profiles
of DNA in the absence and in the presence of MNNG,
respectively.   Curves C and D are the elution profiles of
MNNG in the presence and in the absence of DNA, respectively.   The derivative plots of the curves are shown in the
inset.

liberates active short-lived intermediates which are electrophiles; these interact with DNA predominantly by SN_1 mechanism.

The question therefore arises as to what mechanism will be consistent with the observed inhibitory effect of distamycin A on DNA methylation even when the active methylating species are released normally from MNNG. The mechanism that will account for the above observations is depicted in Scheme 2. This mechanism implies: (a) a direct binding of MNNG with DNA-forming a non-covalent complex and (b) catalysis either by DNA or buffer of the bound MNNG and transfer of the methyl group to guanine at or close to the binding site. Evidence for the direct binding of MNNG is presented in Fig. 1.

DNA and MNNG Interact to Form a Complex

Fig. 1 illustrates the mutual influence of DNA and MNNG on their respective elution profiles. The most obvious effect was the shift of the entire elution profile to the left which was more pronounced in the case of MNNG. In addition, the absorbance at the plateau of the DNA region of the curve was higher in the presence of MNNG (curve B) than in its absence (curve A). The derivative plots of the leading edges of the boundaries (Fig. 1, inset) showed that the positions as well as the heights of elution peaks were altered showing that DNA and MNNG interact. The increased absorbance at the plateau region showed binding of MNNG to DNA to form a relatively stable complex.

The Products of Degradation of MNNG of the DNA–MNNG Complex are Different from Those Formed by Buffer Alone

In order to have an idea about the nature of MNNG in the DNA–MNNG complex, most of the DNA along with the MNNG still bound to it was separated from any of the products of degradation of MNNG by a modification of the rapid gel-filtration method of Neel and Folini (11).

A Beckman cellulose nitrate centrifuge tube (9/16" x 3 1/2") was perforated at the bottom by a fine needle. A plug of glass wool with a piece of filter paper above it were placed over the perforation inside the tube. This tube was in turn placed into a wider conical centrifuge tube with a hole at one side near the bottom. Ten ml of a suspension of 20 g of Biogel P-2 equilibrated in 100 ml of 0.05 M ammonium formate buffer, pH 5.0 at 4°C was poured into the inner centrifuge tube. After draining off the excess buffer collected in the outer centrifuge tube, the tubes were centrifuged at 700 x g for 5 min at 4°C. The liquid which collected in the conical centrifuge tube was discarded. 1.5 ml of the pooled DNA

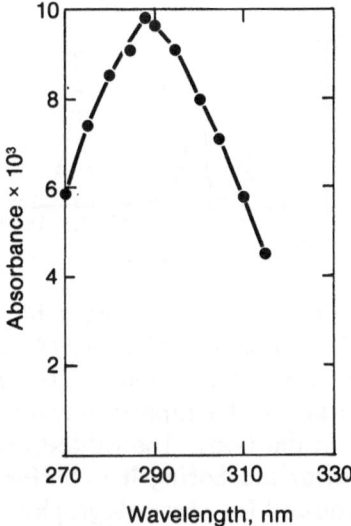

Fig. 2.   Ultraviolet absorption spectrum of the products of
decomposition of MNNG derived from DNA–
MNNG complex. Experimental details are given
in the text.

fraction (elution volumes 4.7 to 8.11; Fig. 1) was poured on the gel
column and centrifuged again as before. In this way 80–85% of the larger
molecular weight DNA was separated and obtained in the outer conical
centrifuge tube while the smaller molecular weight fragments derived from
MNNG along with 15–20% of the DNA initially present were retained in
the gel matrix of the inner tube. The gel matrix was then washed with 0.5
ml of cold water and centrifuged again as before. This liquid which now
collected in the outer centrifuge tube contained the fragments from MNNG
and some DNA. The ultraviolet absorption spectrum of this eluate shown in
Fig. 2 had a peak between 285 nm and 290 nm. MNNG under the same
conditions had an absorption maximum at 277.5 nm. None of the methylated DNA bases has a λ max beyond 280 nm.

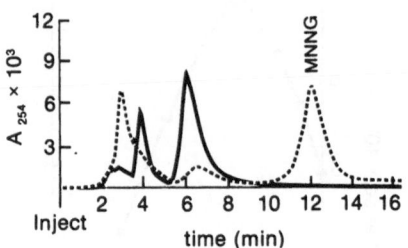

Fig. 3.   High pressure liquid chromatographic patterns of the
decomposition products of DNA-MNNG complex
(solid line) and MNNG (broken line). The material
(1.5 ml) used for the experiment was obtained as
described in the text. The MNNG sample was
obtained after incubating it in buffer for the length
of time required for chromatography of DNA-MNNG
mixture and then taken through the same treatment.

Examination of the material by high pressure liquid chromatography
showed two relatively major ultraviolet absorbing peaks which eluted
earlier than MNNG (Fig. 3, solid curve). Only negligible amounts of
these peaks were found when MNNG was degraded by buffer alone under
the same experimental conditions (Fig. 3, broken line). These results
showed that what had been a minor pathway of degradation of MNNG in
the absence of DNA became a major one in its presence.

The most nucleophilic centre in native double helical DNA is the
N-7 position of guanine. Since nucleophilicity can be regarded as a
measure of electron density, the N-7 position of guanine located in the

major groove of B form of DNA is the best candidate to participate in strong hydrogen-bonding interactions with appropriate donor groups. The amino group of MNNG constitutes such a hydrogen bond donor. A plausible specific hydrogen bonded structure of MNNG with a guanine residue in DNA is shown in Scheme 2. A hydrogen-bonding interaction of the N-7 of guanine with the amino group of MNNG is visualized to result in a redistribution of electrons which finally lead to the guanine's undergoing a tautomeric shift lowing in the process a hydrogen bond with cytosine. This loss of hydrogen bond is more than compensated for by the overall free energy change of the reaction depicted in Scheme 2 which results in a net gain of two hydrogen bonds and the energy of aromatization of the six-membered ring of guanine.

The methyl group of the bound MNNG projects out of the average plane of the atoms linked by hydrogen bonds and is exposed to attack by nucleophiles. In one of the two possible orientations, the methyl group can fall in between the N-7 and O^6 on an adjacent guanine at the 5'-side. The N-7 or O^6 could attack the methyl group in accordance with their respective nucleophilic strength resulting in the methylation of one or the other of these sites. The electron flow across the $-N-N = O$ group could facilitate nucleophilic attack. The elution of the degradation products earlier than MNNG from the high pressure liquid chromatographic column (Fig. 3) is consistent with the proposed mechanism because the demethylated product is expected to be less hydrophobic than MNNG. Finally, CPK model building studies show that both the cyclization of MNNG and its interaction with DNA as proposed in Scheme 2 are stereochemically feasible. The most important aspect of the proposed mechanism is that it predicts methylation of specific guanines in DNA sequence.

In the light of the observation (1, 2) that distamycin A induces unique conformational changes we propose that in the conformation DNA assumes on binding to the ligand, the guanine residues required for the binding of MNNG are inaccessible to MNNG. Since this step is essential for the transfer of methyl group, interference with this step arrests the guanine methylation. The new mechanism postulated in Scheme 2 may be useful in explaining certain puzzling aspects of mutagenesis such as the increased propensity of MNNG to mutate preferentially in the vicinity of replication fork with an intensity that frequently produces multiple closely-linked mutations (12). The susceptibility of proliferating cells for neoplastic transformation may also at least in part be due to the accessibility of certain gene sequences during cell replication that are not accessible in the resting cell. The study provides evidence which although circumstantial, yet directs our attention to new and novel ways of looking at carcinogen-DNA interaction. However, the validity of these concepts has to be critically examined in future studies.

References

1. M. Hogan, N. Datta Gupta and D.M. Crothers, Transmission of allosteric effects in DNA. Nature 278: 521 (1979).

2. S. Rajalakshmi, N. Datta Gupta and D.M. Crothers, (Unpublished data, 1980).

3. M. Hogan, N. Datta Gupta and D.M. Crothers, Transient electric dichroism of rod-like DNA molecules. Proc. Natl. Acad. Sci. (U.S.A.) 75: 195 (1978).

4. S.E. Bresler, V.M. Chernajenko and E.M. Saminski, Study of the interaction of polynucleotide chains with olgiomers by means of chromatography. Bio-polymers, 11: 1541 (1972).

5. P.W. Chin and M.C.K. Yang, Scanning molecular sieve chromatography of interacting protein systems. Simulation of large zone behaviour for self-associating solutes undergoing rapid chemical equilibration under kinetic control. Biophysical Chemistry 7: 347 (1978).

6. S. Rajalakshmi, P.M. Rao and D.S.R. Sarma, Studies on carcinogen chromatin-DNA interaction. Inhibition of N-methyl-N-nitroso-urea-induced methylation of chromatin-DNA by spermine and distamycin A. Biochemistry 17: 4515 (1978).

7. S. Rajalakshmi, P.M. Rao and D.S.R. Sarma, Differential effects of distamycin A and spermine on the formation of 7-methyl-guanine in DNA by N-methyl-N-nitrosourea, methylmethane-sulfonate and dimethyl sulphate. Tertogenesis, Carcinogenesis and Mutagenesis, 1: 97 (1980).

8. S. Rajalakshmi, P.M. Rao and D.S.R. Sarma, Carcinogen-DNA interaction: Complexing of distamycin A with DNA is necessary for its inhibitory effect on the N-methyl-N-nitroso-urea induced methylation of DNA. Chem.-Biol. Interact. 35: 125 (1981).

9. C.I. Zimmer, Effects of antibiotics netropsin and distamycin A on the structure and function of nucleic acids. Prog. Nucleic Acid Res. Mol. Biol. 15: 285 (1975).

10.   G.V. Gursky, V.C. Tumanyan, A.S. Zasedatelev, A.L. Zhuze,
       S.L. Gorklovsky and B.P. Gottikh, A code controlling
       specific binding of proteins to double-helical DNA and RNA,
       in: "Nucleic Acid-Protein Recognition," H.J. Vogel, ed.,
       Academic Press, London/New York, p. 189 (1977).

11.   M.W. Neel and J.R. Folini, A rapid method for desalting small
       volume of solution. Anal. Biochem. 55: 328 (1973).

12.   J.W. Drake and R.H. Baltz, The biochemistry of mutagenesis.
       Ann.Rev. Biochem. 15: 20 (1976).

GENOTOXIC EFFECTS OF DRUGS: EXPERIMENTAL FINDINGS CONCERNING SOME CHEMICAL FAMILIES OF THERAPEUTIC RELEVANCE

G. Brambilla*, M. Cavanna* and S. De Flora**

Institutes of Pharmacology and *Hygiene***
School of Medicine, University of Genoa
I-16132 Genoa, Italy

1 INTRODUCTION

Among the multiple possible interactions of drugs with cellular macromolecules, the one with DNA is of paramount importance, since it may be followed either by cell death or by heritable alterations of the genetic code. Cell death can be the aim of a therapeutic approach, as indeed is the case for antiproliferative agents (antineoplastic and immunosuppressive drugs). Conversely, a drug-induced heritable alteration of DNA must be considered a toxic effect. If this alteration concerns somatic cells (somatic mutation), a possible consequence is cancer induction; aging and atherosclerosis have been also related to DNA damage. When this alteration concerns germinal cells (germinal mutation), birth defects and the gradual accumulation in the human gene pool of subtle but essentially irreversible deleterious mutations are likely to take place.

Considering that drugs, unlike other agents, are often administered in high doses and/or for prolonged periods of time (in some cases every day for many years!), it is perhaps surprising that our experimental knowledge on their possible genotoxic activity is rather scanty. This statement is confirmed by the conclusions reached by IARC: of 16 pharmaceutical drugs considered in vol. 24 of the Monographs on the Evaluation of the Carcinogenic Risk of Chemicals to

193

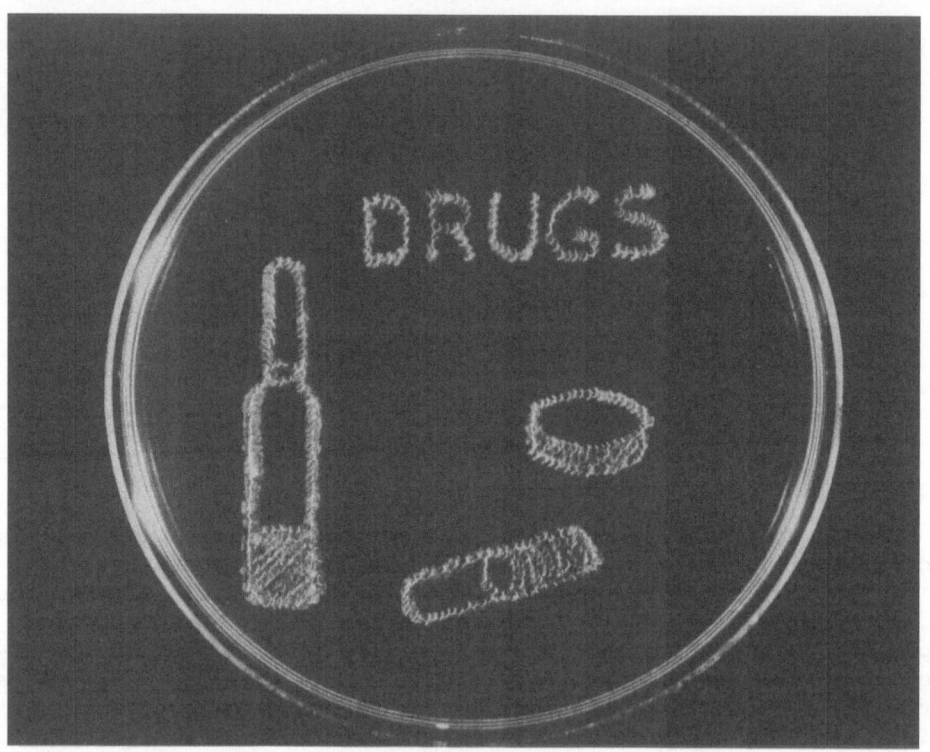

Fig. 1.   This *mutagenic drawing* was obtained by suitably streaking
          S. typhimurium, strain TA100, on the surface of top agar
          embedding nitrofurantoin. The 10^{-5} content of a commercial
          tablet containing this drug was found to be positive in the
          Ames test (De Flora, 1981a).

Humans (IARC, vol.24, 1980), for only 3 *sufficient* evidence of carcinogenicity in animals was achieved, which makes it reasonable for
practical purposes to regard actually such drugs as if they presented a carcinogenic risk for humans. For the other 13 drugs, the
evidence for carcinogenicity in animals was *limited* or *inadequate*,
which means that more experimental investigation is required. In
this framework it is evident that no evaluation can be made of the
benefit/risk ratio, being the second term of this ratio practically
unknown. The large majority of drugs now in use are in an even worse
condition in terms of the experimental evaluation of their genotoxic
effects, since evidence is neither limited nor inadequate, but minimal or totally absent. Consequently, the current estimate that
drugs would account for substantially less than 1% of all cancers
might perhaps be an underestimate (Smith and Jick, 1977; Maugh II,
1979).

     In this situation, because of the economical and temporal ob-
stacles which practically preclude a *sufficient* evaluation of carcinogenic activity of drugs with long-term assays, an extensive evaluation of genotoxic effects with a wide spectrum of short-term tests
should be useful to detect potentially hazardous drugs, which might
deserve further evaluation by life-time administration in laboratory
animals. In several Countries this point of view has recently had
a legal impact, since the evaluation of the genotoxic effects has
been added to the usual pharmacotoxicological assays required for
new drugs. In our opinion, independently of further long-term evaluation in animals, a clear evidence of genotoxic activity in a sufficiently wide and well balanced battery of short term tests should
be considered *per se* sufficiently predictive of a genotoxic risk for
humans. Quantification of this risk is at present impossible, as it
is for extrapolation of carcinogenicity data from animals to humans.

     After a rapid survey of the families of drugs for which expe-
rimental and/or epidemiological evidences suggest a potential genotoxic activity in humans, this article deals with experimental results obtained with some groups of chemicals of therapeutic interest.

2 PAST EVIDENCE AND FUTURE TRENDS

     From the many review articles (e.g.: Fraumeni and Miller, 1972;
Hoover and Fraumeni, 1975) on the subject *drug-induced cancer* it
appears evident that our knowledge in this field is mainly derived
from epidemiological studies. The drugs for which there is definite
evidence of carcinogenicity for humans are: some alkylating agents
(chlornaphazine, urinary bladder tumors; cyclophosphamide and melphalan, acute leukemia), immunosuppressive drugs (lymphoma), and
diethylstilbestrol (vaginal adenocarcinoma in young women whose
mothers had taken diethylstilbestrol during pregnancy). Far less
conclusive is the evidence of a carcinogenic activity in man for

other drugs: phenacetin (transitional cell tumors of renal pelvis), diphenylhydantoin (lymphoma), and chloramphenicol (leukemia).

The likelyhood to identify a cause-effect relationship from epidemiological studies can be reduced to a very small degree owing to several reason such as a low carcinogenic potency, a long latency period as opposed to a short duration of follow up, the simultaneous exposure to different carcinogenic agents (and to different drugs!). Moreover, if a drug increases the incidence of a type of tumor that is already relatively frequent, such an effect could be easily gone undetected. That is what would have been likely to occur for diethylstilbestrol, unless vaginal adenocarcinoma had been virtually unknown in young women. On the other hand, the epidemiological evidence linking certain drugs to cancer in humans leads to concern that other drugs may also be carcinogenic and in a broader sense genotoxic. This possibility is stressed by the results of a recent screening for carcinogenicity in humans of 95 commonly used drugs (Friedman and Ury, 1980), which showed that, in relation to 56 primary cancer sites, significant positive or negative associations with at least one site were found for 53 drugs.

With these considerations in mind about the limits inherent to epidemiological investigations (from which the results even if conclusive are unfortunately found after the right time), it is evident that future studies about drugs as inducers of cancer should be pursued also with a different type of approach, suitable to define the potential genotoxic effects for humans. It must be stressed that there are also carcinogens, such as compounds with hormonal mechanism, tentativelly classified as "epigenetic carcinogens", for which no evidence of genotoxicity (interaction with and alteration of DNA) has been found until now and consequently would require a different type of approach. However, this problem is beyond the aim of this article.

Studies on chemical carcinogenesis have shown that oncogenic potential is often linked to a peculiar chemical structure (direct alkylating agents, polycyclic hydrocarbons, N-nitroso compounds, aromatic amines or amides, etc.). Since most drugs belong to a certain number of chemical families, a reasonable approach to the study of their genotoxicity would be to make use of a series of tests to assess mutagenic-carcinogenic activity in a limited number of compounds from each class. The results could suggest which classes present a greater human risk. The drugs in the suspected classes should be subsequently investigated for confirmation of carcinogenicity with wider and more direct experiments as well as with *aimed* epidemiological studies. Although until now genotoxicity of drugs, and in particular of established drugs, has been sought rather randomly, the data from isolated case reports and epidemiological studies and those collected from chemical carcinogenesis studies just now suggest that some chemical families of drugs are highly suspected of genotoxic effects.

A first example of a family of drugs for which there is a consistent experimental evidence as to their capability to elicit genotoxic effects is that of nitroheterocycle derivatives (nitrofurans, nitroimidazoles and nitrothiazoles). Various chemotherapeutic agents belong to this group. Among them, we list antibacterial drugs (nitrofurantoin (Fig. 1), furaltadone, nitrofurazone, nifuradene, furothiazole and dihydroxymethylfuratrizine), antiprotozoal (metronidazole) and schistosomicidal agents (niridazole). For several compounds of this chemical group, their capability to elicit DNA damage in mammalian cells (Olive and McCalla, 1975), bacterial mutations (Wang et al., 1975) and induction of tumors in rodents (IARC, vol. 7, 1974) has been evidenced. Another highly suspected family is that of hydrazine derivatives, whereas an outstanding case is represented by drugs carrying amine groups and susceptible to form N-nitrosoderivatives in gastric environment. About both hydrazine and N-nitrosatable drugs we shall go into some details below. As a family of drugs, thiouracil derivatives (methylthiouracil, propylthiouracil and thiouracil),used as antithyroid drugs, produce tyroid tumors in a variety of experimental animals (IARC, Vol. 7, 1974), especially with a frequency inversely related to the amount of dietary iodine. The ultimate cause appears to be a hormonal imbalance of the hypothalamo-pituitary-thyroid system. Like carcinogenic hormones, the thiouracils affect endocrine system balance and could be categorized as epigenetic rather than genotoxic carcinogens.

Rather limited is the experimental evidence about other chemical families of therapeutic relevance, since often genotoxicity evaluation concerns a single compound. Space limitation, however, precludes a systematic review on this subject. Therefore, we shall limit the consideration only to give some relevant evidence. DNA damaging, mutagenic and carcinogenic activity have been found for two antischistosomal thioxanthenone derivatives (lucanthone and hycanthone) (Bueding and Batzinger, 1977); mutagenic activity was reported for some anthraquinones (Brown and Dietrich, 1979) and at least one antipsychotic phenothiazine (fluphenazine) (Rao and Rao, 1981). Proflavine and acriflavine (acridine derivatives once often represented as drugs, but now generally being phased out) were irregularly reported to be carcinogenic whereas they appear to be mutagenic; nafenopin, clofibrate, dapsone, phenazopyridine, reserpine, rifampicin, ethionamide, phenobarbital, phenytoin and pronetalol showed experimental carcinogenicity (IARC: Vol. 13, 1977; Vol. 24, 1980).

3 HYDRAZINE DERIVATIVES

3.1 Foreword

Hydrazine derivatives (hydrazines, hydrazides, and hydrazones) of synthetic and natural origin have been shown to induce cancer in laboratory animals. At present, 40 out of 40 hydrazine derivatives tested were found to be in various degree tumorigenic in rodents (Toth, 1975 and 1980). Even so, several hydrazine derivatives have been used in the past, are currently used, or are considered for future use as antidepressive, antihypertensive and antitubercolar drugs, in many cases in the absence of experimental data on their carcinogenic activity. When these data are available from literature, they appear to have been published after such drugs have come into medical use. This harmful situation is probably to be ascribed to the long time and to the large expense required for reliable long-term tests of oncogenic activity in rodents. Consequently we deemed important: a) preliminarly to evaluate whether or not a satisfactory correlation exists for this class of chemicals between the carcinogenic activity in laboratory animals and the biological activity in some short-term tests; b) subsequently, if this relationship were positive, to examine by the use of these tests the genotoxic potential of a series of pharmaceutical hydrazine derivatives.

In the following pages we summarize the results already obtained for hydrazine drugs by the use of the following battery of *in vivo* and *in vitro* tests: 1) evaluation of DNA damage in some tissues of treated mice; 2) analysis of sister chromatid exchanges in bone marrow cells of treated mice; 3) assessment of the mutagenic response in five his^- *S. typhimurium* strains both in the absence and in the presence of three metabolic systems; 4) evaluation of the toxic activity toward a series of five trp^- *E. coli* strains lacking a variety of repair mechanisms. Although this work is still in progress, the data available up to now confirm the general genotoxic potential of the hydrazine structure and strongly suggest that some drugs still untested for carcinogenicity are likely to own such an activity.

3.2 DNA Damage *In Vivo*

Another chapter of this book describes the scientific basis of alkaline elution technique, which provides a sensitive measure of DNA single-strand length distribution in mammalian cells and is applicable also to measure DNA damage in various tissues of a treated animal. In the same chapter is shown that a satisfactory correlation exists for a number of carcinogens between DNA damaging and carcinogenic potencies. Concerning eleven carcinogenic hydrazines a regression analysis between their potency in inducing lung tumors in mice and their potency in damaging liver and lung DNA was carried out (Parodi et al., 1981b). With both tissues, the correlation was statistically very significant ($p < 0.005$).

Table 1. DNA-damaging potency of hydrazine derivatives of
therapeutic interest in various tissues of mice

Compound	DNA-damaging potency[a]			
	Liver	Lung	Kidney	Spleen
Procarbazine	40.6*	35.5*	19.3*	8.4*
Isocarboxazid	29.9*	49.5*		
Nialamide	5.5*	4.1*		
Mebanazine	2.5	3.6*		
Phenelzine	7.5*	5.9*		
Iproniazid	0.4	0.6		
Hydralazine	26.2*	26.2*	18.1*	11.9*
Dihydralazine	4.5	15.6*	23.6*	20.0*
Endralazine	8.5*	1.0	4.5*	12.7*
Isoniazid	5.0*	10.0*		
1,2-Dimethylhydrazine	75.5*	8.3*		

[a] The DNA-damaging potency was calculated by the formula:

$$\frac{(K_t - K_c)}{mmol/Kg} \times 1000$$

where $(K_t - K_c)$ is the average elution rate over controls. K is given by the
formula:

$$K = ln \frac{1}{\text{(fraction of DNA retained on potter)}} \times \frac{1}{V}$$

where V is the eluted volume in ml.

* The increase in DNA elution rate over the corresponding controls was
statistically significant ($P < 0.05$).

Table 1 shows DNA damaging potency in mice for each of the 10
pharmaceutical hydrazines studied and for each tissue so far considered. Since for each drug the assay was performed with different
dosage schedules and killing animals at various times from administration, in each case computation of DNA damaging potency was based
only on the most effective treatment. Five of these 10 hydrazines
have already been tested for oncogenic activity. Their potency in
inducing pulmonary tumors in mice (Parodi et al., 1981b), which varies over an ∼ 3,400-fold range, decreases in the following order:
procarbazine, 379; iproniazid, 1.5; phenelzine, 1.0; isoniazid, 0.52;
hydralazine, 0.11. Out of the same 10 hydrazines, 6 elicited a significant increase in both liver and lung DNA elution rate, procarbazine, isocarboxazid and hydralazine resulting clearly more potent
than phenelzine, isoniazid and nialamide. Dihydralazine and

mebanazine apparently damaged only lung DNA, and endralazine only
liver DNA. Iproniazid, was the only one apparently inactive in both
organs. The evaluation of DNA damage in kidney and spleen until now
has been carried out only for 4 of the 10 drugs but the positive results obtained suggest that DNA fragmentation induced by hydrazine
derivatives is not limited to a specific target organ, but can take
place, although in variable degree, in several tissues. This hypothesis is strengthened by the demonstrated capacity of procarbazine
of damaging also bone marrow and thymus DNA (Brambilla et al., 1981b),
and of 1,2-dimethylhydrazine of causing DNA fragmentation in liver,
lung, kidney, colon and stomach mucosa (Brambilla et al., 1978).

     DNA alkaline elution, the technique employed to monitor DNA frag-
mentation, has been shown to be capable in our experimental conditions of detecting 0.5-1 breaks x 10^{-9} daltons. Therefore, it can
be inadequate to reveal a minimal degree of DNA damage, as for instance that possibly induced by iproniazid, which resulted negative
in our test despite its ability of increasing the incidence of pulmonary tumors in mice. With the double aim of testing this possibility, and of verifying with an independent method the results obtained
by the use of alkaline elution, we carried out some experiments with
a new viscoelastometric technique, recently developed by our group
(Parodi et al., 1981a), which allows the detection of approximately.

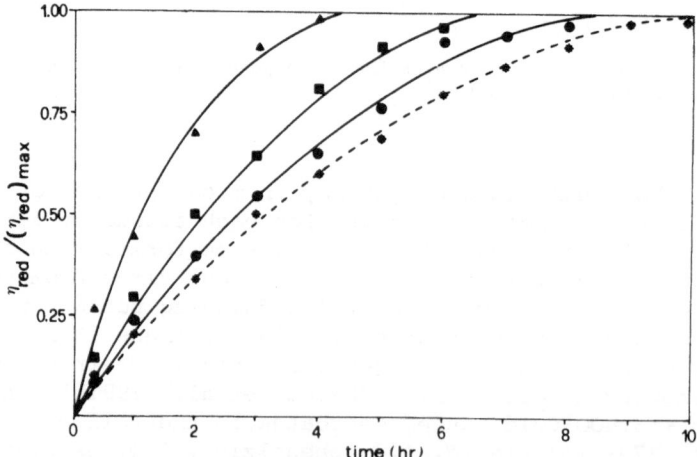

Fig. 2.   Ratio |reduced viscosity (η_{red})/reduced viscosity at plateau
          level (η_{red})max| plotted against time. Liver DNA from con-
          trol rats ✳--✳, and from rats treated with iproniazid ●──●,
          isoniazid ■──■, and phenelzine ▲──▲ .

0.3 single-strand breaks x 10^{-10} daltons. With this technique the time required by DNA to reach maximum plateau viscosity in alkaline conditions decreases with the decrease of DNA molecular weight. Because of problems in obtaining cellular suspensions without causing a *technical* DNA damage, this technique can be at present applied only to rat liver cells.

Fig. 2 shows, as ratio [reduced viscosity (η_{red}) /reduced viscosity at plateau level $(\eta_{red})max$] plotted against time, the results obtained with LD50 of iproniazid, isoniazid, and phenelzine. From these preliminary viscometric results, which need to be confirmed by alkaline elution assay in rats, it seems that fragmentation of liver DNA was, respectively, practically absent in rats treated with iproniazid, minimal with isoniazid, and clearly evident but of limited extent with phenelzine. A comparison in terms of single-strand breaks with liver DNA fragmentation induced by equitoxic doses of isoniazid and phenelzine in mice suggests that the rat is less sensitive to the DNA-damaging activity of these two drugs. For isoniazid, this finding seems in good agreement with the negative effects obtained in several long-term carcinogenicity tests in rats (IARC, vol. 4, 1974) and by metabolic studies in the Ames test (see 3.5).

3.3 Sister Chromatid Exchanges *In Vivo*

Sister chromatid exchange (SCE) analysis, although the molecular basis of SCE formation and their biological significance are not completely understood, is being extensively used to evaluate the impact of mutagens and carcinogens on chromosomes. Even if the validity of this test for the screening of genotoxic compounds is still under investigation, it has been observed that several agents known to cause DNA damage elicit a significant increase in SCE frequency at doses lower than those necessary to induce an appreciable increase in chromosome aberrations. A recent review on the methodologies for SCE detection, and on the relationships among SCE induction , DNA damage and repair, mutagenicity and carcinogenicity has been published by Latt et al. (1978).

SCE analysis has been carried out according to Allen et al. (1977) in bone marrow cells of Swiss male mice treated i.p. with 8 of the 10 pharmaceutical hydrazines considered (isoniazid is still to be tested, and mebanazine is no longer available). The results obtained are shown in Table 2. Since for some drugs the assay was performed with different dosage schedules, in these cases computation of the potency in inducing SCE was based only on the most effective treatment. All the 8 hydrazine drugs tested significantly increased the SCE frequency in bone marrow cells, their relative potency in inducing this genotoxic effect varying over a 7-fold range and decreasing in the following order: isocarboxazid, 7.0; dihydralazine, 6.5; endralazine, 4.3; procarbazine, 3.4; hydralazine, 2.5; phenelzine, 1.5; nialamide, 1.1; iproniazid, 1.0.

Table 2. Potency of hydrazine derivatives of therapeutic
          interest in increasing SCE frequency in bone
          marrow cells of mice

Compound	Potency in inducing SCE[a]
Procarbazine	105
Isocarboxazid	217
Nialamide	34
Phenelzine	47
Iproniazid	31
Hydralazine	79
Dihydralazine	202
Endralazine	132

[a]The potency in inducing SCE was calculated according to the formula:

$$\frac{\% \text{ increase of SCE over controls}}{\text{mmol/Kg}}$$

3.4 DNA Damage and Repair in Bacteria

Five antidepressant monoamine oxidase inhibitors (nialamide,
phenelzine, mebanazine, isocarboxazid and iproniazid) and three
antihypertensive hydrazine derivatives (hydralazine, dihydralazine
and endralazine) were assayed for their genotoxic activity in a selective lethality test in repair-deficient or -proficient $E.coli$.
Bacterial tester strains have the following genetic markers:

WP2:	trp^-
WP2uvrA:	trp^- $uvrA^-$
WP67:	trp^- $polA^-$
CM871:	trp^- $uvrA^-$ $recA^-$ $lexA^-$
TM1080:	trp^- $polA^-$ $lexA^-$ plasmid R391

The toxic activity of compounds was determined by filling wells at
the centre of agar plates, incorporating each of the 5 $E.coli$
strains, with 50 µl of their appropriate solutions.

The results obtained are summarized in Table 3. All the hydrazine derivatives tested, with the exception of isocarboxazid and
iproniazid, were found to be more toxic in repair-deficient strains
than in WP2, this showing their ability in directly interacting with
bacterial DNA. Although not very pronounced, the differences observed were statistically significant, dose-dependent and reproducible in separate experiments.

Table 3. Diameter of the zone of inhibition of bacterial growth (mean of triplicates) produced by various compounds in repair-deficient or -proficient *E.coli*, in the absence of S-9 mix. Confidence limits were comprised within the 10% of mean values. Significant increases in repair-deficient strains are underlined. Similar patterns were observed at least at two other dose levels for each compound

Compound	Amount per plate (mg)	E. coli strain				
		WP2	WP2uvrA	WP67	CM871	TM1080
HYDRAZINE DERIVATIVES						
Nialamide	8	14.9	13.2	_17.7_	_21.1_	14.2
Phenelzine·H₂SO₄	1	10.1	12.3	_22.8_	_17.9_	_14.8_
Mebanazine oxalate	0.5	23.9	25.2	_29.5_	_29.0_	_26.3_
Isocarboxazid	20	15.1	14.2	15.7	13.8	15.9
Iproniazid	20	8.8	8.6	8.3	9.5	8.4
Hydralazine·HCl	5	25.9	26.2	_32.3_	_40.8_	_38.1_
Dihydralazine.H₂SO₄	5	24.5	23.2	23.7	_28.6_	_28.0_
Endralazine mesilate	5	15.3	15.9	14.9	_21.1_	_20.2_
ICR COMPOUNDS						
ICR 191	0.2	10.8	11.2	9.5	_16.3_	_21.3_
ICR 170	0.2	8.3	8.8	8.9	_15.4_	_18.1_
N-NITROSODERIVATIVES						
Cimetidine	2.5	–	–	–	–	–
Ranitidine	2.5	–	–	–	–	–
Na nitrite*	2.5	–	–	–	–	–
(Na nitrite + Cimetidine)*	2.5 + 2.5	13.1	_17.8_	_17.2_	_28.3_	_23.4_
(Na nitrite + Ranitidine)*	2.5 + 2.5	20.3	21.2	_23.0_	_28.7_	20.9
MNNG	0.01	17.7	16.8	_35.1_	_35.8_	_34.2_

– = no halo of bacterial killing

* Acidified to pH 3.0 and kept for 60 min at 37°C.

As shown in Table 3, the excision repair system (*uvrA*) was not involved in repairing the DNA damage determined by any of the hydrazine derivatives tested, while polymerase I activity (*polA*) was important in repairing the damage induced by nialamide and hydralazine and, to a greater extent, by the two isomers of phenylethylhydrazine, i.e. phenelzine and mebanazine. With these two exceptions, strain CM871, lacking recombination (*recA*) and post-replication (*lexA*) repair mechanisms, in addition to the excision repair system, was the most sensitive in revealing the genotoxic activity of compounds in this chemical class. TM1080, which was found to be the most sensitive repair-deficient strain with other compounds tested in the same laboratory, e.g. ICR 191 and ICR 170 (Table 3), methylmethane sulfonate, Na dichromate and Pb chromate (De Flora, unpublished data), surprisingly showed a greater survival than WP67 in the case of the 3 antidepressant hydrazine derivatives. This indicates that for some chemical compounds the polymerase I activity is decreased, rather than being reinforced, by combination with the *lexA* mutation and/or with plasmid R391.

3.5 Bacterial Mutagenicity

The results of the study of 17 hydrazine derivatives in the Ames reversion test are summarized in Table 4. Fourteen of them (82.3%) could be classified as clearcut or borderline mutagens in this prokaryotic test system. The results were in total agreement with those of the selective lethality test in *E.coli* for the 8 hydrazine derivatives reported in Table 3.

From a qualitative standpoint, the correlation with homogeneous carcinogenicity data (induction of pulmonary tumors in mice chronically treated p.o.), which were available for 11 compounds, was quite satisfactory (81.8%). Conversely, the quantitative correlation between these two biological systems was poor (Parodi et al., 1981b).

The mutagenic potency varied over a 3.2×10^3-fold range in assays performed without S-9 mix and over a 7.2×10^3-fold range in the presence of S-9 mix containing rat liver (Aroclor) S-9 fractions. For comparison, the mutagenic potency calculated in a study with 121 compounds of various chemical classes, tested in the same laboratory, varied between 0.0003 and 2,880 revertants per nmole, i.e. over a 10^7-fold range (De Flora, 1981b). Indeed, none of the positive hydrazine derivatives can be considered as a potent mutagen, while some of them were very weak or borderline, either because of the low figures of induced revertants over background and/or because of the high doses of compounds needed to elicit a mutagenic response.

The same 17 hydrazine derivatives were tested in the presence of S-9 mix containing not only liver S-9 fractions from Aroclor-treated Sprague-Dawley rats, but also liver and lung S-9 fractions from Aroclor-treated Swiss albino mice. The liver preparations from these two animal species showed similar metabolic effects. However, rat liver was generally somewhat more efficient than mouse liver S-9 in decreasing the mutagenicity of some hydrazine derivatives, e.g. isoniazid, which might account for the conflicting results of carcinogenicity assays in rats and mice with this compound (Wade et al., 1981). An interesting exception was nialamide, whose activity was lowered by rat liver and mouse lung S-9 and conversely increased by mouse liver S-9, through NADPH-requiring mechanisms.

Table 4. Activity of 17 hydrazine derivatives in the *Salmonella*/ microsome test

Compound	Reverted strains					Potency (revs./ nmol)	Metabolic effect (Aroclor rat liver S-9)
	TA1535	TA1537	TA1538	TA98	TA100		
Hydrazine hydrate	+	-	-	-	-	0.007	decrease
1,1-Dimethylhydrazine	-	-	-	±	-	0.0008	slight increase
1,2-Dimethylhydrazine	-	-	-	-	+	0.009	no change
Carbamylhydrazine	+	-	-	-	-	0.0009	decrease
Phenylhydrazine	-	+	-	-	-	0.033	slight decrease
1-Carbamyl-2-phenylhydrazine	-	-	-	-	-		
2,4-Dinitrophenylhydrazine	-	+	+	+	+	0.96	decrease
Mebanazine oxalate	-	-	w	w	-	0.07	no change
Phenelzine·H$_2$SO$_4$	+	-	-	-	+	0.19	decrease
Procarbazine·HCl	-	-	±	w	-	0.0005	slight increase
Isoniazid	w	-	-	-	±	0.0004	decrease
Iproniazid	-	-	-	-	-		
Nialamide	+	-	-	-	+	0.62	decrease
Isocarboxazid	-	-	-	-	-		
Hydralazine·HCl	+	-	-	+	+	0.05	no change
Dihydralazine·H$_2$SO$_4$	-	+	+	+	+	0.03	no change
Endralazine mesilate	-	-	+	+	-	0.003	no change

+ more than 3-fold, dose-related and reproducible increase of revertants

w 2 to 3-fold increase

± reproducible but less than 2-fold increase of revertants

At the same time, nialamide was more efficient in inducing DNA fragmentation in mouse liver than in the lung (Parodi et al., 1981b; Brambilla et al., 1981a). Apart from an aspecific deactivating effect on phenelzine, mouse lung preparations showed poor metabolic effects, compared with the liver preparations of the same animal species.

3.6 Structure-Activity Relationships

Out of a number of families of chemical compounds investigated in this laboratory (De Flora, 1981a and 1981b), the class of hydrazine derivatives appears to be the only one showing a poor homoge-

nicity of all the three parameters evaluated in the Ames test, i.e.
a) the mechanism of reversion, b) the mutagenic potency and c) the
in vitro metabolic behaviour.

However, as discussed more in detail in another paper (De Flora
and Mugnoli, 1981), these apparent discrepancies can be settled by
considering some chemical features of test compounds, such as their
structures or the addition of a variety of radicals to the H_2N-NH_2
group.

The assessment of structure-activity relationships under controlled *in vitro* conditions was facilitated by the circumstance that
almost all the positive hydrazine derivatives were directly active
in *S. typhimurium his⁻* strains.

In fact, the only two derivatives undergoing a slight increase
of activity in the presence of S-9 mix were the borderline frameshift mutagens 1,1-dimethylhydrazine (carrying geminal methyl groups)
and procarbazine (carrying an isopropyl group bonded to a nitrogen
atom). As also inferred from the study of compounds of other chemical classes (De Flora, 1981b), geminal methyl groups seem to determine a decrease of mutagenicity, irrespective of the atoms bearing
them. They are present either in negative compounds (e.g. iproniazid
among hydrazine derivatives) or in borderline mutagens whose activity
is slightly enhanced by S-9 mix, or in weak mutagens requiring liquid preincubation with S-9 mix and bacteria. In the case of 1,1-
dimethylhydrazine and procarbazine, no further increase of revertants
could be observed following liquid preincubation.

An opposite example is provided by NO_2 groups, which, as shown
on a large series of compounds (De Flora, 1981b), clearly favour the
mutagenic response a) by broadening the spectrum of sensitive strains,
b) by enhancing the mutagenic potency and c) by affording a direct
mutagenicity to polycyclic compounds. The comparison of 2,4-dinitro-
phenylhydrazine with phenylhydrazine (see Table 4) is consistent
with the general assumptions made in points a) and b).

It is noteworthy that all the hydrazides tested were either negative (1-carbamyl-2-phenylhydrazine, iproniazid and isocarboxazid)
or induced only base-pair substitutions which were clearly decreased
by S-9 mix (carbamylhydrazine, isoniazid and nialamide).

Some systematic trends of structural parameters could be also
pointed out. In fact, by examining the structures of test compounds
available in the literature, the molecules of frameshift hydrazines
appear to be remarkably planar. Conversely, the molecules of hydrazides appear to significantly deviate from planarity, and the values
of their torsion angles seem to be related to the mutagenic potency
of these compounds (De Flora and Mugnoli, 1981).

4   ICR ANTITUMOR COMPOUNDS

4.1 Foreword

ICR compunds (Table 5), consisting of an acridine and of a
nitrogen mustard moiety were synthesized 20 years ago as antitumor

agents (Creech et al., 1972). Since their development, some of them
were recognized to possess genotoxic properties and became an important tool of research in mutagenesis laboratories, using a variety
of eukaryotic and prokaryotic test systems. For instance, as many
as 154 specific references where available for ICR 170(1965-1980)
and 157 for ICR 191(1966-1980) in the bibliography of the Environmental Mutagen Information Center (EMIC, Oak Ridge, Tennessee; Mary
W. Francis, personal communication).

Therefore, ICR compounds provide an interesting example of antineoplastic drugs undergoing a very extensive evaluation of genotoxicity prior to their clinical use. Another element of interest is
that these structurally related chemicals show distinctive mutagenic,
metabolic, carcinogenic and antineoplastic properties, which can be
tentatively explained on the basis of their mutual interplay.

4.2 DNA Damage and Mutagenicity in Bacteria

ICR 170 and ICR 191 interacted with $E.coli$ DNA by inducing a
greater lethality only in the two strains carrying multiple genetic
defects (CM871 and 1080) (Table 3). The same compounds potently
induced frameshift errors in his^- $Salmonella$ strains TA1538, TA98,
TA100 and especially TA1537 ($his3076$ mutation), which is consistent
with the conclusion of genetic studies, indicating that ICR compounds
induce +1 or -1 mutations in runs of G·C base pairs (Isono and
Yourno, 1974). In the absence of S-9 mix, ICR 191 displayed a wider
range of activity and was more potent than ICR 170 (Table 5) (De
Flora, 1981a and 1981b; De Flora et al., 1981a).

Though showing a very narrow range of activity, only in strain
TA1537, and a far lower potency, the two compounds carrying the
hydroxyethyl group (ICR 191-OH and ICR 170-OH) were also directly
mutagenic. This finding was rather unexpected since both these compounds had been found to be inactive in the CHO/HGPRT forward mutation system, where the corresponding chloroethyl ICR compounds are
clearly positive (O'Neill et al., 1978; Fuscoe et al., 1979), and

Table 5. Flow diagram showing mutagenic activity in *S. typhimurium* and *in vitro* metabolic behaviour of ICR compounds (De Flora et al., 1981a) as related to their ability in inducing lung adenomas in strain A mice when administered i.p. (Shimkin et al., 1966) or i.v. (Peck et al., 1976) and to their activity against ascites tumors in ICR Swiss albino mice (Creech et al., 1972)

Compound	R	Mutagenicity (TA1537)		Meta-bolic deactiv.	Carcino-genicity		Anti-neoplastic activity
		activ. range (nmoles/plate)	potency (revs./nmol)		i.p.	i.v.	
ICR 170	N< CH_2CH_3 / CH_2CH_2Cl	10–200	270	+	−	++	++
ICR 170-OH	N< CH_2CH_3 / CH_2CH_2OH	100–200	3	+			
ICR 191	N< H / CH_2CH_2Cl	1–200	480	++	−		+
ICR 191-OH	N< H / CH_2CH_2OH	50–250	14	++	−		−

− inactive

+ moderately active

++ highly active

ICR 191-OH did not revert *Salmonella* strains TA1535, TA100, TA1538 and TA98 (McCann et al., 1975) nor induced lung adenomas in strain A mice (Peck et al., 1976b). HPLC analysis provided evidence that no cross-contamination existed between any of the four ICR compounds tested, while all the four commercial products were found to contain, in variable amounts (0.4 to 16.6%), a common impurity itself reverting TA1537 and undergoing an efficient deactivation in the presence of S-9 mix. Although such a circumstance might have influenced the quantitative mutagenicity data of all the four ICR compounds, the actual genotoxicity of both ICR 191-OH and ICR 170-OH could be convincingly demonstrated by examining the eluates of the corresponding HPLC peaks (De Flora et al., 1981a).

4.3 Metabolic Deactivation *In Vitro*

The direct mutagenicity of ICR 191 was decreased in the presence of a variety of rat, mouse and human S-9 fractions (Fig. 3). Liver S-9 fractions were the most efficient in producing such a metabolic effect, which was strongly enhanced by pre-treatment of

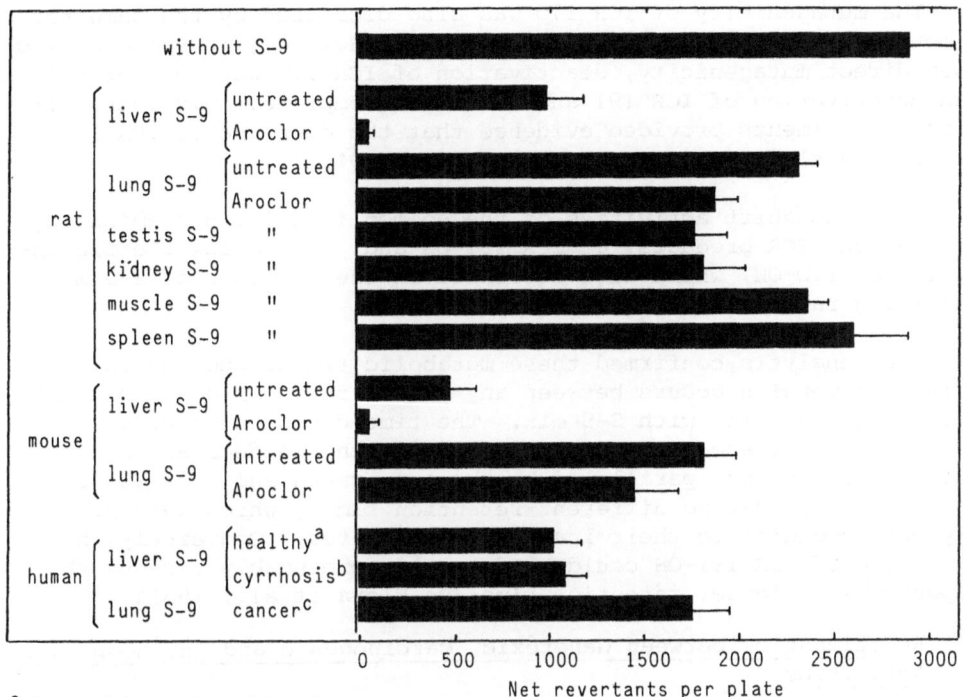

a Pool of 4 surgical biopsies

b Pool of 3 surgical biopsies

c Pool of 3 biopsies of peripheral tissue surrounding the neoplasia

Fig. 3. Mutagenicity of ICR 191 (20 nmoles/plate) for *S. typhimurium*,
strain TA1537, either without S-9 mix or following preincubation (1 hr at 37 C) with S-9 mix containing S-9 fractions
(100 μl/plate) from rat, mouse or human tissues

animals with Aroclor 1254, practically resulting in a complete re-
versal of mutagenicity. Mouse preparations were even more active
than the corresponding rat preparations.

S-9 mix cofactors, without S-9 fractions, did not affect the
mutagenicity of ICR 191. Heated metabolic systems were ineffective
as well. S-9 mix lacking NADP$^+$ had some activity, especially in the
case of liver preparations, but addition of this coenzyme strongly
increased their deactivating ability. The poor metabolic effect
observed in the absence of added NADP$^+$ may be ascribed either to
traces of endogenous NADPH in tissue homogenates or to some aspecific
reaction. However, it is noteworthy that no statistically significant correlation existed between the protein concentration of S-9
fractions and their deactivating ability.

The mutagenicity of ICR 170 was also decreased by the same rat or mouse S-9 fractions reported in Fig. 3. However, in spite of its lower direct mutagenicity, deactivation of ICR 170 was less efficient than deactivation of ICR 191 and was never complete. Moreover, time-course experiments provided evidence that the decrease of ICR 170 activity is slower than in the case of ICR 191.

The frameshift activities of the common impurity contaminating all the four ICR products, of ICR 191-OH and, with a lower efficiency, of ICR 170-OH, where also decreased in the presence of S-9 mix containing rat liver (Aroclor) S-9 fractions.

HPLC analysis confirmed these metabolic trends and showed that no interconversion occurs between any of the four ICR compounds following preincubation with S-9 mix. The time-dependent decrease of ICR 191, ICR 170 and ICR 170-OH, together with the decrease of their common impurity, was paralleled by the appearance and increase of new HPLC peaks, having different retention times, which were presumably corresponding to their inactive metabolites. Conversely, no metabolite of ICR 191-OH could be detected, presumably because this compound had a longer retention time (De Flora et al., 1981a).

4.4 Relationships between Genotoxic, Carcinogenic and Antineoplastic Activities

Although the inactive metabolites of ICR compounds have not been chemically identified, the metabolic findings of this study seem to provide a possible clue to their different activity in various mutagenicity test systems and especially to their differential behaviour *in vivo*.

In fact, the more efficient detoxification of ICR 191 by cytoplasmic enzymes, compared with ICR 170, might justify the more potent activity of the latter compound in systems such as *Neurospora* and *Drosophila* (Creech et al., 1972) and the CHO/HGPRT forward mutation assay (O'Neill et al., 1978), which contrasts with the higher activity of ICR 191 in simple bacterial targets, such as *E.coli* and *S.typhimurium*.

The efficient metabolic deactivation of both ICR 191 and ICR 191-OH is consistent with their lack of carcinogenicity (Table 5). On the other hand, the incomplete and slower deactivation of ICR 170 might explain why this compound was able to induce lung adenomas when injected i.v., while it did not induce any tumor when administered i.p., a route involving a slower absorption and distribution of chemicals prior to reaching the lungs. Since also lung preparations showed a moderate deactivating ability, it can be expected that local tumors may be initiated only by doses overcoming the biotransformation capacity of lung cells.

Finally, since the ability of ICR compounds of intercalating
into nucleic acids and becoming covalently bound appears to be necessary for both antitumor and microbial mutagenic activities (Creech
et al., 1972), the conclusions drawn in the present study may also
be useful to interpret their pharmacologic activity or even to predict their efficacy in different tissues. In fact, ICR 170 showed
a pronounced degree of activity against ascite tumors, while ICR 191
was only moderately active and ICR 191-OH totally inactive (Table 5).

5   NITROSATABLE DRUGS

5.1   Foreword

Many N-nitroso compounds have been shown to be carcinogenic
in experimental animals (IARC, vol. 17, 1978). By grouping them together, nitrosamines and nitrosamides appear to be, as a class, among
the most carcinogenic agents. Since N-nitroso compounds are possibly
formed from all compounds that contain amino groups, it is a sound
policy to exert a control on every industrial process concerning
nitrosatable chemicals in the human environment. If such chemicals
are medicinal drugs, the control should be still closer because they
can be used on a long-term basis. In the last decade, many N-nitroso
compounds have been shown to be formed from a variety of drugs by
reacting with nitrite (Mirvish, 1975), according to the chemistry
of N-nitrosation. Moreover, the concern has been increasing since
it was first discussed (Druckrey and Preussmann, 1962) and later
demonstrated that N-nitrosation reactions can occur *in vivo* mainly
in the acid gastric milieu in the presence of nitrite taken in as
such or as a precursor in food or in drinking water (Mirvish, 1975).

The induction of tumors in experimental animals by feeding a
drug with nitrite has been repeatedly observed, mostly in rats and
mice (IARC, vol. 24, 1980), the nitrosatable drugs being secondary
or tertiary amines. Being administered as a drug combination, the
difficulties already present in a long term carcinogenicity test
were further increased owing to the necessity to plan experiments
meeting with a good experimental design.

In our laboratories we faced the problem of evaluating the hazard resulting from nitrosation of drugs *in vivo* by using two different experimental models.

The first one, operating *in vivo*, allows the administration of
nitrosatable drugs together with nitrite, in various molar ratios,
to ascertain the genotoxic effects of the N-nitroso compounds possibly formed in the gastric environment. This model is based on the
DNA damage in vivo/alkaline elution assay.

The second approach involves use of bacteria as targets of the genotoxic activity. Although studies on the formation of N-nitroso derivatives in bacterial test systems were performed *in vitro*, they were envisaged in such a way to simulate as much as possible a physiological situation in human stomach. With this aim, precursor compounds were allowed to react in an excess human gastric juice from healthy individuals. For some compounds, e.g. antiulcer drugs, gastric juice samples from treated patients, either with or without enrichment with nitrite, were also examined. Generally, various factors affecting the reaction rate (e.g. doses of precursor compounds, pH, time and temperature of preincubation, efficiency of inhibitors) were also investigated. For the evaluation of results, the number of revertants induced by nitrite (in strains sensitive to base-substituting agents) were subtracted from those induced by nitrite-precursor mixtures. Alternatively, nitrite was efficiently removed by adding equimolar sulfamic acid after the preincubation step. The results of studies on nitrosatable drugs in repair-deficient *E.coli* and in the *Salmonella*/microsome test are summarized in Tables 3 and 6, respectively.

5.2 Analgesic Pyrazolon Derivatives

5.2.1 DNA damage *in vivo*. The first nitrosatable drug under our investigation was aminopyrine (Parodi et al., 1980). Rats were fed with single or repeated high doses of aminopyrine and/or nitrite. The combination given for 20 days, caused liver DNA fragmentation, possibly due to the formation of N-nitrosodimethylamine (DMNA) from aminopyrine (Lijinski, 1974). Such a damage was of the order of that observed in positive control rats given orally 10-20 mg/kg of DMNA. Also the single dose of the combination was effective in eliciting DNA damage, though to a limited extent. The above study showed that liver fragmentation can follow the formation of N-nitroso compounds in the gastric environment (Table 7). Furthermore, liver DNA damage appears to be a sensitive index of the potential carcinogenic activity of N-nitroso compounds (Brambilla et al., 1981c).

5.2.2 Bacterial mutagenicity. The primary amine aminoantipyrine (AAP) readily reacted with an excess sodium nitrite in human gastric juice, to yield directly acting mutagenic derivatives (Table 6). Mutagenicity could be ascribed to the formation of the corresponding diazonium salt which, at variance with that formed upon nitrosation of another primary amine aniline, was quite stable (Boido et al., 1980). The case of AAP is of peculiar interest, because this compound, which is *per se* nonmutagenic, is considered to be carcinogenic on the basis of the positive results of an implantation technique in mouse bladder (Boyland et al., 1964). Studies are now in progress to check whether AAP nitrosation can also occur in human or mouse urine.

Table 6. Mutagenicity of some drugs following combination with nitrite in human gastric juice

Compounds	Rev. strains TA1535	TA1537	TA1538	TA98	TA100	Effect of S-9 mix (Ar. rat liver)	References
Sodium nitrite	+	-	-	-	+	slight decr.	De Flora, 1978 and 1981a
Aminoantipyrine (AAP)	-	-	-	-	-	-	Boido et al., 1980
Nitrite + AAP				+	+	slight decr.	
Aminopyrine (AP)	-	-	-	-	-	-	De Flora et al., 1980
Nitrite + AP				-	+	activation	
ICR 191	-	+	+	+	+	deactivation	De Flora and De Flora, 1981
Nitrite + ICR 191	-	w	+	+	+	activation	
ICR 170	-	+	+	+	+	deactivation	De Flora et al., 1981b
Nitrite + ICR 170	-	w	+	+	+	activation	
Cimetidine	-	-	-	-	-	-	De Flora and Picciotto, 1980
Nitrite + Cimetidine	+	w	w	w	+	no change	
Ranitidine	-	-	-	-	-	-	In preparation
Nitrite + Ranitidine	+	-	-	-	+	slight incr.	
MNNG	+	+	+	+	+	no change	De Flora, 1981a

+ more than 3-fold, dose related and reproducible increase of revertants

w 2 to 3-fold increase

     As previously discussed, aminopyrine (AP) or piramidone - a tertiary aromatic amine differing from AAP only for the presence of geminal methyl groups on the nitrogen atom - reacts with nitrite in acidic environment to form DMNA. As well known, the mutagenicity of DMNA is difficult to evidence in the Ames test, compared with *in vivo* systems, especially due to the high reactivity and short half-life of its N-dealkylated metabolites (Bartsch et al., 1975). Although the details of the nitrite-AP reaction were not explored, the formation of mutagenic derivatives in strain TA100 could be demonstrated by performing two preincubation steps: the first one involving combination of AP with nitrite in human gastric juice and the second one, after neutralization of the above mixture, involving addition of S-9 mix and bacteria prior to plating (De Flora et al, 1980).

Table 7. Liver DNA fragmentation by alkaline elution and by hydroxyl-
         apatite chromatography after various oral treatment sched-
         ules with aminopyrine, cimetidine, and ranitidine given
         alone or in equimolar combination with nitrite in rats

Compounds	DNA fragmentation according to treatment schedules				
	Single dose	P	5 daily doses	20 daily doses	P
Aminopyrine (AP)	–		NT	–	
AP and nitrite	+	<0.01	NT	+	≪0.01
Cimetidine (C)	–		–	–	
C and nitrite	–/(–)[a]		–	NT	
Ranitidine (R)	–		–	NT	
R and nitrite	–/(+)[b]		–	NT	

+ = positive   – = negative   NT = not tested

[a]Neither long term (60 hr) fasting nor fasting for 60 hr along with histamine
   injection 30 min before oral administration of the drug and nitrite elicited
   a significant DNA fragmentation

[b]Both fasting and histamine injection as in (a) elicited a significant DNA
   fragmentation (P <0.05 and P < 0.02, respectively)

5.3 Inhibitors of H-2 Histamine Receptors (Cimetidine and Ranitidine)

5.3.1. DNA damage in mammalian cells. Cimetidine (a drug used in
the therapy of peptic ulcer) and the occurrence of gastric cancer
have been suggested to be correlated. Cimetidine is readily nitrosatable *in vitro* and nitrosocimetidine appears to be mutagenic in
be Ames bacterial test (see 5.3.2) and to methylate DNA *in vitro*
(Jensen and Magee, 1981). In order to verify whether or not nitrosocimetidine could be possibly formed *in vivo*, hepatocytes were investigated for DNA damage after single or repeated high doses of
cimetidine and nitrite fed to rats (Table 7). Evidence of DNA damage was not found in any of the treated groups. The lowering of
gastric pH with fasting or histamine administration prior to administration of the combination did not enhance the induction of liver
DNA fragmentation (unpublished data). Studies on the possible DNA
damage in gastric mucosa cells are in progress.

The same concern which has arisen for cimetidine could be applied to ranitidine (a more recent inhibitor of gastric secretion)

since it presents like cimetidine nitrosatable groups, apart from structure-activity relationships. Therefore, we have in analogy investigated for the effects of ranitidine (unpublished results). The nitrosation derivative of ranitidine obtained *in vitro* induced a concentration-dependent increase in the amount of DNA fragmentation in cultured CHO mammalian cells (Table 8). DNA fragmentation was also measured *in vivo* in liver of rats fed simultaneously approximately equimolar amounts of ranitidine and nitrite (Table 7). In rats fed daily for five days, liver DNA fragmentation was not observed. After a single dose of the combination, no damage was observed in rats not fasted and in rats fasting for 12 hr. If the fasting (except for water and sucrose) was prolonged up to 60 hr significant liver DNA fragmentation was observed, as well as a lowering of gastric pH to about 2.5. If rats fasting for 60 hr were injected with histamine, an increase in DNA damage was elicited. Thus, the feeding of ranitidine and nitrite can elicit liver DNA damage in rats when gastric pH is sufficiently low.

5.3.2. <u>DNA damage and mutagenicity in bacteria</u>. Both cimetidine and ranitidine, either in neutral or acidic environment, are nontoxic and nonmutagenic for bacteria. However, they combine with nitrite in human gastric juice or in acidified 0.15M NaCl to form genotoxic N-nitrosoderivatives (Tables 3 and 6). Some examples of positive spot tests in *his⁻ S.typhimurium* and *trp⁻ E.coli* are represented in Fig. 4.

Although the study with ranitidine is still in progress, the results so far obtained allow some conclusions to be drawn and to point out some differences with the problem of cimetidine, which was investigated more in detail (De Flora and Picciotto, 1980).

Table 8. DNA fragmentation by alkaline elution and hydroxylapatite chromatography in CHO-K1 cells exposed to ranitidine and nitrosoranitidine

Incubation	% of eluted DNA over controls	% of single strand DNA over controls
Ranitidine (3 mM)	3	1
Nitrite (3 mM)	1	1
Nitrosoranitidine		
(~0.3 mM)	12	18
(~1 mM)	37	32
(~3 mM)	73	66

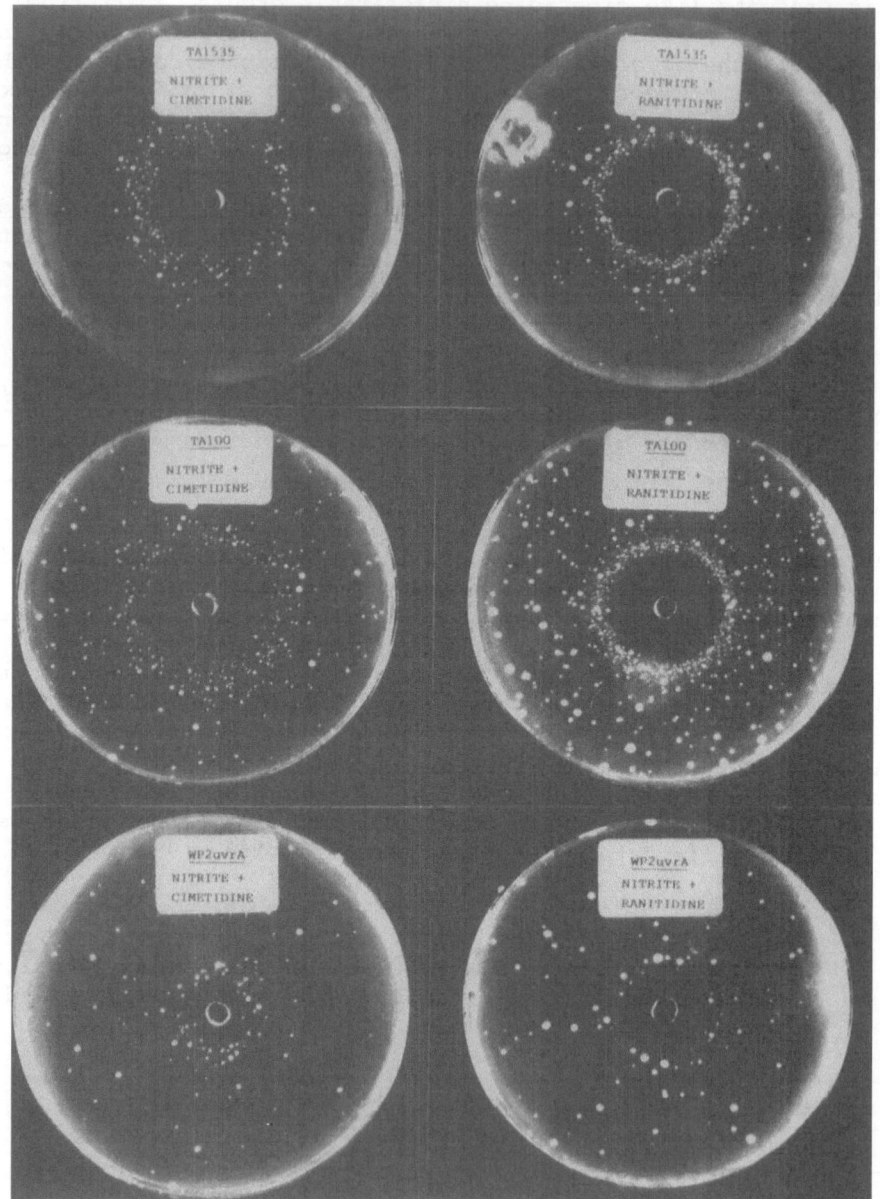

Fig. 4. Mutagenicity in the spot test of mixtures of nitrite (2.5
         mg) with cimetidine (2.5 mg) or ranitidine (2.5 mg), com-
         bined in human gastric juice, towards *his⁻ S.typhimurium*
         (TA1535 and TA100) and *trp⁻ E.coli* (WP2uvrA). Excess ni-
         trite was removed by adding equimolar sulfamic acid after
         preincubation of precursor compounds

For instance, the optimal reaction of nitrite with cimetidine occurs
at slightly lower pH values than with ranitidine. The product of
the nitrite-ranitidine reaction elicits only base-pair substitutions
in bacterial DNA, while combination of nitrite with cimetidine induces, though weakly, also frameshift errors (Table 6). This might
be ascribed either to the formation of more than one mutagenic N-
nitrosocimetidine under our experimental conditions or to the formation of a single N-nitrosoderivative eliciting a broad spectrum
of mutations, as it is the case for N-methyl-N-nitroso-N'-nitro-
guanidine (MNNG) (Table 6). This known gastric carcinogen is also
positive in the selective lethality test in *E.coli* (Table 3) and
has a methylating ability similar to that of N-nitrosocimetidine
(Foster et al., 1980; Jensen and Magee, 1981).

Another difference between the nitrosoderivatives of the two
antiulcer drugs is that the mutagenicity of N-nitrosocimetidine is
proportional to the amounts of precursor compounds (up to 20 mg cimetidine) and is neither disturbed by toxic effects nor varied in
the presence of rat liver (Aroclor) S-9 fractions. Conversely, the
optimal reaction of ranitidine with nitrite occurs at about 100 μg
per plate and thereafter the mutagenic effects are gradually converted into toxic effects. Killing of bacteria is reduced by S-9 mix,
which results in a better expression of the mutagenic response.
Such a metabolic effect is not further enhanced by liquid preincubation with S-9 mix and bacteria.

The study with cimetidine led to the suggestive evidence that
the simple addition of nitrite to gastric juice samples from patients treated with this drug, under physiological conditions, determines a mutagenic response in the Ames test. Therefore, the
only crucial question about its possible occurrence *in vivo* is
whether sufficient amounts of nitrite may reach the gastric environment containing cimetidine. Though taking into account the great
benefits resulting from the clinical use of these antiulcer drugs,
the recognized predictive value of the short-term tests used should
advise, at least for prudential reasons, to minimize as much as possible their reaction with nitrite. Such a task might be pursued
a) by suggesting diet and beverages poor in nitrites and nitrates,
b) by introducing the drugs at distance from meals and c) by simultaneously administering inhibitors of nitrosation. It is noteworthy,
with this respect, that ascorbic acid was quite efficient in preventing *in vitro* the nitrosation of cimetidine (De Flora and Picciotto, 1980).

5.4   ICR Antitumor Compounds (ICR 170, ICR 191)

5.4.1 Variations of frameshift mutagenicity and of metabolic behaviour. Although the formation of mutagenic N-nitrosoderivatives from
ICR compounds has probably no practical interest, their assessment
provides an elegant example of the sensitivity and flexibility of

the *Salmonella*/microsome test. In fact, at variance with the previously discussed nitrosatable compounds, both ICR 170 and ICR 191
are *per se* mutagenic, as extensively discussed in Section 4. Nevertheless, even without any chemical analysis, the formation of
other mutagenic products could be evidenced thanks to the suitabil-
ity of the Ames test in revealing the genetic mechanism of reversion and the metabolic trends of test compounds (Table 6).

Specifically, nitrosation of ICR 170 (tertiary amine on the
side chain) and, slightly more efficiently, of ICR 191 (secondary
amine - see Table 5), produced derivatives requiring metabolic activation instead of being deactivated by S-9 mix. Moreover, they
mainly reverted the *hisD3052* mutation of *S.typhimurium* (which is
close to a repetitive -C-G-C-G-C-G-C-G- sequence), while precursor
compounds mainly reverted the *hisC3076* mutation, corresponding to
a run of C's (Ames et al., 1975)

ACKNOWLEDGEMENTS

This study was supported by CNR grants (Finalized Project *Controllo della Crescita Neoplastica* and *Gruppo Cardiorespiratorio*),
and was performed under the auspices of the *Centro di Informazione
Farmacotossicologica* supported by region of Liguria.

REFERENCES

Allen, J.W., Shuler, C.F., Mendes, R.W., and Latt, S.A., 1977, A
    simplified technique for *in vivo* analysis of sister chromatid
    exchanges using 5-bromodeoxyuridine tablets, *Cytogenet.Cell
    Genet. (Basel)*, 18: 231-237.
Ames, B.N., McCann, J., and Yamasaki, E., 1975, Methods for detect-
    ing carcinogens and mutagens with the *Salmonella* /mammalian-
    microsome mutagenicity test, *Mutat.Res.*, 31: 347-364.
Bartsch, H., Malaveille, C., and Montesano, R., 1975, *In vitro* me-
    tabolism and microsome-mediated mutagenicity of dialkylnitro-
    samines in rat, hamster, and mouse tissues, *Cancer Res.*, 35:
    644-651.
Boido, V., Bennicelli, C., Zanacchi, P., and De Flora, S., 1980,
    Formation of mutagenic derivatives from nitrite and two prima-
    ry amines, *Toxicol. Lett.*, 6: 379-383.
Boyland, E., Busby, E.R., Dukes, C.E., Grover, P.L., and Manson, D.,
    1964, Further experiments on implantation of materials into
    the urinary bladder of mice, *Br.J.Cancer*, 18: 575-581.
Brambilla, G., Cavanna, M., Faggin, P., Pino, A., Robbiano, L., Ben-
    nicelli, C., Zanacchi, P., Camoirano, A., and De Flora, S.,
    1981a, Genotoxic activity of five antidepressant hydrazines
    in a battery of *in vivo* and *in vitro* short-term tests, *J.
    Toxicol. Environ. Health*, in press.

Brambilla, G., Cavanna, M., Parodi, S., Sciabà, L., Pino, A., and
    Robbiano, L., 1978, DNA damage in liver, colon, stomach, lung
    and kidney of BALB/c mice treated with 1,2-dimethylhydrazine,
    Int. J. Cancer, 22: 174-180.
Brambilla, G., Cavanna, M., Pino, A., and Robbiano, L., 1981b, DNA
    damage and repair in mouse tissues following procarbazine ad-
    ministration, *Pharmacol. Res. Commun.,* 13: 213-222.
Brambilla, G., Cavanna, M., Pino, A., and Robbiano, L., 1981c, Quan-
    titative correlation among DNA damaging potency of six N-nitro-
    so compounds and their potency in inducing tumor growth and
    bacterial mutations, *Carcinogenesis,* 2: 425-429.
Brown, J.P., and Dietrich,.P.S., 1979, Mutagenicity of anthraquinone
    and benzanthrone derivatives in the *Salmonella* /microsome test:
    activation of anthraquinone glycosides by enzymic extracts of
    rat cecal bacteria, *Mutat. Res.,* 66: 9-24.
Bueding, E., and Batzinger, R.P., 1977, Hycanthone and other anti-
    schistosomal drugs: lack of obligatory association between
    chemotherapeutic effects of mutagenic activity, in: *Origins
    of Human Cancer,* Hiatt, H.H., Watson, J.D., and Winsten, J.A.,
    (Eds.), Book A p. 445-464, Cold Spring Harbor Laboratory.
Creech, H.J., Preston, R.K., Peck, R.M., O'Connell, A.P., and Ames,
    B.N., 1972, Antitumor and mutagenic properties of a variety
    of heterocyclic nitrogen and sulfur mustards, *J. Med. Chem.,*
    15: 739-746.
De Flora, S., 1978, Metabolic deactivation of mutagens in the *Salmo-
    nella*/microsome test, *Nature (London),* 271: 455-456.
De Flora, S., 1981a, Study of 106 organic and inorganic compounds
    in the *Salmonella*/microsome test, *Carcinogenesis,* 2: 283-298.
De Flora, S., 1981b, Biotransformation and interaction of chemicals
    as modulators of mutagenicity and carcinogenicity, *Third Inter-
    national Conference on Environmental Mutagens,* Tokyo, Sept.
    21-24.
De Flora, S., Boido, V., and Picciotto, A., 1980, Metabolism of mu-
    tagens in the gastric environment, *Mutat. Res.,* 74: 187-188.
De Flora, S., and De Flora, A., 1981, Variation of the frameshift
    activity of a mutagen (ICR 191) following nitrosation in hu-
    man gastric juice, *Cancer Lett.,* 11: 185-189.
De Flora, S., Morelli, A., Zanacchi, P., Bennicelli, C., and De Flo-
    ra, A., 1981a, Selective deactivation of ICR mutagens as relat-
    ed to their distinctive pulmonary carcinogenicity, *Carcinogesis,*
    submitted for publication.
De Flora, S., and Mugnoli, A., 1981, Relationships between mutagenic
    potency, reversion mechanism and metabolic behaviour within a
    class of chemicals (hydrazines), *Cancer Lett.,* 12: 279-285.
De Flora, S., and Picciotto, A., 1980, Mutagenicity of cimetidine
    in nitrite-enriched human gastric juice, *Carcinogenesis,* 1:
    925-930.
De Flora, S., Zanacchi, P., Camoirano, A., and Bennicelli, C., 1981b,
    Mutagenicity patterns resulting from the reaction of nitrite

with ICR 170, *Mutat. Res. Lett.*, in press.

Druckrey, H., and Preussmann, R., 1962, Formation of carcinogenic nitrosamines in tobacco smoke (Ger.), *Naturwissenschafften*, 49: 498-499.

Foster, A.B., Jarman, M., and Manson, D., 1980, Structure and reactivity of nitrosocimetidine, *Cancer Lett.*, 9: 47-52.

Fraumeni jr, J.F., and Miller, R.W., 1972, Drug-induced cancer, *J. Nat. Cancer Inst.*, 48: 1267-1270.

Friedman, G.D., and Ury, H.K., 1980, Initial screening for carcinogenicity of commonly used drugs, *J. Nat. Cancer Inst.*, 65: 723-733.

Fuscoe, J.C., O'Neill, J.P., Peck, R.M., and Hsie, A.W., 1979, Mutagenicity and cytotoxicity of nineteen heterocyclic mustards (ICR compounds) in cultured mammalian cells, *Cancer Res.*, 39: 4875-4881.

Hoover, R., and Fraumeni jr, J.F., 1975, Drugs in clinical use which cause cancer, *J. Clin. Pharmacol.*, 15: 16-23.

Jensen, D.E., and Magee, P.N., 1981, Methylation of DNA by nitrosocimetidine *in vitro*, *Cancer Res.*, 41: 230-236.

International Agency for Research on Cancer, 1972-1981, in: *IARC Monographs on the Evaluation of the Carcinogenic Risk of Chemicals to Humans*, vols., 1-26, IARC, Lyon.

Isono, S., and Yourno, J., 1974, Non-suppressible addition frameshift in *Salmonella*, *J. Mol. Biol.*, 82: 355-360.

Latt, S.A., Schreck, R.R., Loveday, K.S., and Shuler, C.F., 1978, *In vitro* and *in vivo* analysis of sister chromatid exchange, *Pharmacol. Rev.*, 30: 501-535.

Lijinsky, W., 1974, Reaction of drugs with nitrous acid as a source of carcinogenic nitrosamines, *Cancer Res.*, 34: 255-258.

Maugh II, T.H., 1979, Cancer and environment: Higginson speaks out, *Science*, 205: 1363-1364, 1366.

McCann, J., Spingarn, N.E., Kobori, J., and Ames, B.N., 1975, Detection of carcinogens and mutagens: bacterial tester strains with R factor plasmids, *Proc. Nat. Acad. Sci. U.S.A.*, 72: 979-983.

Mirvish, S.S., 1975, Formation of N-nitroso compounds: chemistry, kinetics and *in vivo* occurrence, *Toxicol. Appl. Pharmacol.*, 31: 325-351.

Olive, P.L., and McCalla, D.R., 1975, Damage to mammalian cell DNA by nitrofurans, *Cancer Res.*, 35: 781-784.

O'Neill, J.P., Fuscoe, J.C., and Hsie, A.W., 1978, Mutagenicity of heterocyclic nitrogen mustards (ICR compounds) in cultured mammalian cells, *Cancer Res.*, 38: 506-509.

Parodi, S., Carlo, P., Martelli, A., Taningher, M., Finollo, R., Pala, M., and Giaretti, W., 1981a, A circular channel crucible oscillating viscometer: detection of DNA damage induced *in vivo* by exceedingly small doses of dimethylnitrosamine, *J. Mol. Biol.*, 147: 501-521.

Parodi, S., De Flora, S., Cavanna, M., Pino, A., Robbiano, L., Bennicelli, C., and Brambilla, G., 1981b, DNA-damaging activity *in vivo* and bacterial mutagenicity of sixteen hydrazine derivatives as related quantitatively to their carcinogenicity, *Cancer Res.*, 41: 1469-1482.

Parodi, S., Taningher, M., Pala, M., Brambilla, G., and Cavanna, M., 1980, Detection by alkaline elution of rat liver DNA damage induced by simultaneous subacute administration of nitrite and aminopyrine, *J. Toxicol. Environ. Health*, 6: 167-174.

Peck, R.M., Tan, T.K., and Peck, E.B., 1976, Pulmonary carcinogenesis by derivatives of polynuclear aromatic alkylating agents, *Cancer Res.*, 36: 2423-2427.

Peck, R.M., Tan, T.K., and Peck, E.B., 1976, Carcinogenicity of derivatives of polynuclear compounds, *J. Med. Chem.*, 19: 1422-1423.

Rao, K.P., and Rao, M.S., 1981, Effects of fluphenazine hydrochloride on the bone-marrow cells of Swiss mice, *Mutat. Res.*, 89: 237-240.

Shimkin, M.B., Weisburger, J.H., Weisburger, E.K., Gubareff, N., and Suntzeff, V., 1966, Bioassay of 29 alkylating chemicals by the pulmonary-tumor response in strain A mice, *J. Nat. Cancer Inst.*, 36: 915-934.

Smith, P.G., and Jick, H., 1977, Regular drug use and cancer, *J. Nat. Cancer Inst.*, 59: 1387-1391.

Toth, B., 1975, Synthetic and naturally occurring hydrazines as possible cancer causative agents, *Cancer Res.*, 35: 3693-3697.

Toth, B., 1980, Actual new cancer-causing hydrazines, hydrazides, and hydrazones, *J. Cancer Res. Clin. Oncol.*, 97: 97-108.

Wade, D.R., Lohman, P.H.M., Mattern, I.E., and Berends, F., 1981, The mutagenicity of isoniazid in *Salmonella* and its effects on DNA repair and synthesis in human fibroblasts, *Mutat. Res.*, 89: 9-20.

Wang, C.Y., Muraoka, K., and Bryan, G.T., 1975, Mutagenicity of nitrofurans, nitrothiophenes, nitropyrroles, nitroimidazole, aminothiophenes, and aminothiazoles in *Salmonella typhimurium*, *Cancer Res.*, 35: 3611-3617.

DISCUSSION

Dr. Farber : Is there any danger of confusing DNA replication with repair synthesis?

Dr. Cerutti : As far as I know, the amount of UDS is so much smaller than DNA replication that it is more likely that two processes overlap.

Dr. Lutz : One additional point which should be taken into account in the interpretation of UDS data is that repair but not damage is measured. It could, in principle, be possible that a DNA lesion which cannot be repaired, does not elicit UDS although such damage could be much more mutagenic than damage which is quickly repaired.

Dr. King : By use of autoradiography, we have found that UDS in rat hepatocytes elicited by N-hydroxy-2-acetylaminofluorene can be compared to adduct formation. The problem is to achieve the sensitivity desired in detecting adducts.

Dr. Lutz : We have some indication that the early eluting peak in an HPLC profile of an enzymic DNA hydrolysate does contain a high concentration of carcinogen-nucleotide adducts. After treatment of mice with ^{3}H-hexachlorocyclohexane and ^{14}TdR, we isolated liver DNA and separated the nucleosides on HPLC. The ratio of ^{3}H to ^{14}C in the first eluting peak was much higher than in whole DNA so that we concluded that there was an enrichment of bound HCH molecules per number of nucleotides. This would be in agreement with the hypothesis that enzyme degradation is hindered in the vicinity of DNA-carcinogen adducts so that the oligonucleosides have a high number of carcinogen molecules bound to them.

Dr. King : A note of caution should be made concerning the use of fluorescence for the detection of arylamine-nucleic acid adducts. Dr. Tim Peterson of the General Motors Research Labs has not been able to detect a useful spectral change of aminobiphenyl-substituted guanine derivatives by employing sensitive low-temperature techniques.These results are in direct contrast to the characteristic fluorescence of these compounds on the plates.

Dr. Lutz : Is cytotoxicity necessarily due to DNA lesions,as opposed to protein lesions?

Dr. Cerutti : Our experiments show that in rapidly dividing mouse embryofibroblasts,DNA is the major target for aflatoxin B$_1$ cytotoxicity.This result,however,cannot be generalized without great caution.

Dr. Burns : Do you believe that the so called "clastogenic intermediate"you hypothesized for TPA promotion is involved in the clastogenic action of ionizing radiation?

Dr. Cerutti : It is known that in radiation accidents patients who have been overirradiated have produced in their sera a clastogenic factor which is similar in molecular weight to the type of clastogenic factor isolated from Bloom's syndrome.It is not known if these factors are chemically identical.There is no evidence that X-ray has substantial promoter activity.The role of clastogenic factors in tumor promotion is entirely unknown.

Dr. Sarma : If we equate DNAse II-sensitive,non-sedimentable fraction of chromatin-DNA as a fraction rich in transcrible genes,as Tew et al. have shown,MNO methylates this fraction more than other fractions.Please comment on this.

Dr. Cerutti : The relationship between DNAse II sensitivity of chromosal DNA and gene activity is not entirely clear.

Dr. Friedman : Is it known why AAF adducts preferentially appear in the regulatory region of SV-40 DNA?Is this relevant for all carcinogens?

Dr. Cerutti : What we have shown and published is that with intracellular SV-40 AAF selectiviely modifies a region of DNA to the late side of the replication region.SV-40 is an extrachromosomal minichromosome.Whether replication and transcription origins of the host genome possess similar higher reactivity is not known at present.It is also not known,to my knowledge,whether actively transcribing genes possess exceptional reactivity to carcinogens.

Dr. Schulte-Hermann : I should like to stress your last point.There are many different types of promoters acting in different organs, such as saccharin,phenobarbital,estrogen,etc.,which are very different with respect to biological properties,and it seems unlikely that they all act by such a mechanism as production of active oxygen species.

Dr.Cerutti : In mouse skin system,administration of superoxide dismutase (SOD),at the same time as TPA apparently results in the quenching of the promotion effect.This may not apply to the other systems you mentioned.

Dr.Oesch : *There exists a study by Brune and Hecker on a possible correlation between skin tumor promotion and inflammatory activity;this correlation breaks down with some compounds. Can these exceptions be used as tools to determine whether the production of active oxygen is causally related to promotion or, instead,is coincidental?*

Dr.Cerutti : Dr.Troll,who is working on a similar model,gave the following satisfactory answer to this:"Superoxide production may be a necessary but not sufficient property of promoters".

Dr.Taylor : *You have shown data obtained from animals of various ages.What is the reason for this heterogeneity?I just wonder if you got different results because of the difference in the age of animals you used?*

Dr.Rajewsky : We used brain and liver of 5 week old rats to study the time course of ethylation after one pulse to the animals. There were slight different levels in liver versus brain,so I would consider the results homogeneous.We have never found any difference regarding the initial degree of ethylation by ENU, e.g.,with age or with tissue.Ethylated prenatal embryo brains had the same initial degree of 0-6 alkyl-guanine as very old rats.

Dr.Ts'O : *Concerning the accessibility of the exposure of DNA adducts in the interphase nuclei,what is the proportion of adducts that your antibodies can bind?Have you similar data on condensed chromosomes?You came up with the number 10^{-6} moles;I wonder how you computed that number.*

Dr.Rajewsky : 10^{-6} moles is that ratio of 0-6 ethyldeoxyguanosine to total guanosine if you isolate the DNA from the tissues completely,hydrolyse it and determine the molar content of 0-6 ethyldeoxyguanosine in the DNA.But you should not take this fluorescence picture as too quantitative.We are so far unable to say what the relative accessibility is.What we use here is alkali denaturated nuclei because we have about a 10-100- fold lesser affinity and recognizability by the antibodies for the products within single strand.Very recently we obtained some monoclones which have practically 1:1 recognizing potential of double versus single strand DNA in vitro.Regarding condensed chromosomes,we are studying if we can detect and distinguish chromosomes that have been carcinogen-treated,but I cannot present the results at present.

Dr.Sarma : Won't the competing nucleophiles present in the whole cells interfere with the interpretation of your results?Whole cells plus ENU should give fewer guanines alkylated while pure DNA plus ENU should give higher number of guanines alkylated.

Dr.Rajewsky : Yes,it may.

Dr.Cerutti : What is the distribution of 0-6 ethylguanine in micrococcal nuclease sensitive relative to resistant DNA?

Dr.Rajewsky : The ratio of micrococcal nuclease-sensitive to resistant DNA is about 2:1.Regarding the effect of nitrosamine on the induction of 0-6 alkylguanine-removing enzymes and of S phase cells,it was found that continuous exposure of rats to the liver carcinogen DEN,which is enzymatically activated, at constant daily dose in the drinking water at 5mg/kg body weight until tumors developed,resulted in an initial depression in ^{3}H-thymidine incorporation followed by an overshoot beginning in the 1st-2nd week treatment.This is a classical observation for carcinogens applied in a similar manner and corresponds to Dr.Montesano's necessary pretreatment time for the induction effect in the liver.Rats treated for 28 days at a constant dose level followed by ¬antoradiographic determination of the percentage of labelled cells,showed a linear relationship between dose rate of the carcinogen DEN and the increment of the fraction of labelled cells.There is no dose rate which would not produce a corresponding increment,however small,in the proportion of DNA synthesis.At low dose levels it is probable that no necrotic cells would be seen in histological sections,as any such cells would be cleared in 2-3 days in a necrotic liver.

Dr.Farber : No distinction between nodular cells and surrounding cells appears to have been made in the above experiment;regeneration often occurs in nodular cells and within 28 days would give delineated foci.

Dr.Burns : Is the increased proliferation rate associated with an increase in the total number of liver cells or is this more like regenerative reaction?

Dr..Rajewsky : It is very difficult to determine; the control labelling index in parenchymal cells is of the order of 0.1-0.2% suggesting that it is only replacement of cells,not an increase in total number.

Dr.Taylor : Is it possible to calculate a suitable dose of particular carcinogen,e.g.,DEN to cause initiation with long term development of tumors,so that one can initiate only and then use a particular promoter?

Dr.Rajewsky : There is a clear-cut dose response for carcinogenic agents where dt^n is constant,where d is dose,t is induction time constant for constant effect,e.g.,50% incidence of tumors.This was originally formulated by Druckrey for adult rats and DEN, n being equal to 2.3.Therefore,you can predict the length of daily exposure that will result in 50% death.This is an accelerated process as n is greater than one.By applying the formula,one can calculate the daily dose level for an induction time longer than the length of animals lifetive,which would probably result in initiation only.The value of n will be different for each species,age and sex and the equation was formulated with no distinction being made between initiation and promotion.

Dr.Sarma : The equation you gave must have a limited range,because in adult rat liver,a non necrogenic dose of DEN will not induce any initiation.A litle higher dose may induce initiation but not promote,where a much larger dose may not only initiate but also promote to cancer.

Dr.Montesano : In continuation of the discussion on the quantification of carcinogenic response,one thing which is of relevance is the time interval between doses in relation to tumor yield. For UV irradiation it has been shown that a total single dose is more efficient than a fractionated dose with regard to tumor yield.For chemical carcinogens a fractionated dose to the skin was more efficient in producing tumors than a single total dose.Perhaps Dr.Burns would like to comment on this and any experimental evidence in relation to split doses and chemical carcinogens and possible repair processes in DNA.

Dr.Burns : When a dose of electron radiation is split into two equal fractions given at least 24 hours apart,fewer cancers are produced than when the same dose is given in a single fraction.Such effects are probably brought about by the repair of a critical lesion involved in carcinogenesis.The identity of the repairable lesion is unknown,but a clue to its identity can be derived from the kinetics of repair.For such studies, a system must be found where cancers can be produced by a single dose of the carcinogen,a circumstance not often applicable in chemical carcinogenesis.Such is true,however,for rat skin irradiated with electrons.When the exposure was multiple the skin tolerated nearly ten times as much dose as for single doses yielding the same number of tumors.In spite of much evidence for the existence of DNA repair,nothing comparable to split dose recovery has been found for chemical carcinogens. In general,multiple doses of chemical carcinogens are more carcinogenic than single doses.

Dr.Sarma : In this context one also has to take into consideration the proliferative nature of the cell,E.g.,in adult liver,if a necrogenic dose is split into multiple non-necrogenic doses, then no initiation will be obtained.

Dr.Montesano : I would like to ask Dr.Toulme to give us a few details about his system. He has recently published a paper in Nature on a peptide which recognises apurinic sites.

Dr.Toulme : We used model peptides containing aromatic aminoacids to elucidate the origin of the specificity of recognition of DNA damage by repair enzymes. Several years ago we demonstrated that the tripeptide lys-tryp-lys exhibits and higher affinity for single strand polynucleotides than for double strand DNA. Moreover, this peptide binds very efficiently to locally destabilised regions in DNA after UV irradiation or modification by aminofluorene derivatives. The strongest sites of binding for the peptide are apurinic sites, formed by the loss of purines from the DNA. It was demostrated that amines are able to cleave the DNA backbone at apurinic sites. Incubation of the peptide with supercoiled DNA, plasmid pBR 322, in which 2 apurinic sites on average were introduced by heating, results in the relaxation of the DNA. This does not occur if DNA which does not have apurinic sites is used and is therefore due to specific breaks introduced by the peptide at apurinic sites. Therefore: a) the peptide lys-tryp-lys mimics the specificity of recognition and the activity of endonucleases specific for apurinic sites; b) this peptide can be used as a structural probe to estimate the local distortion introduced in native DNA by chemical agents and c) lys-tryp-lys can also be used for quantification of apurinic/apyrimidinic sites content of DNA.

Dr.Rueff : From what strain in the Ames' test did you compute your MPIs?

Dr.Parodi : From all the classical ones. In case of a positive result we used the most sensitive strain.

Dr.Rueff : How did you perform your DFIs? Have you done dose-response experiments?

Dr.Parodi : Actually, we did not have good information on dose-response relationship. We always administered at least two doses. After treatment at 4 and 24 hours, we utilized the most active dosage. The lack of good dose-response information increases the "noise" in the system, but in my opinion, this effect is relatively minor, in terms of reduced predictivity.

Dr.Oesch : One important limitation of the use of empirical correlations of empirical tests, is that for any unknown compound tested, one does not know whether it falls within the group of compounds which is seen correctly by the test or within that where the test produces the wrong answer. To judge this, empirical correlations do not help;instead,one needs to understand the test and to know the mechanism.

Dr.*Parodi* : We are dealing with many new compounds,and we are not able to study the metabolic activation pathways and mechanisms of action in all cases,When confronted with a large number of unknown compounds,our correlation analysis can give a preliminary estimation of the carcinogenic potency.However,I agree with you in that we must make an exhaustive investigation in the case of chemical compounds produced and used in huge amounts,for instance,in the case of vinyl chloride.

Dr.*Ts'O* : *We are now able to synthesize short DNA helixes with a known sequence.Would it be possible to make specific monoclonal antibodies against those DNA sequences?*

Dr.*Rajewsky* : Yes,it would be possible.Moreover,it would also be possible to make specific antibodies against short DNA sequences with a single modified base,i.e.,O-6-methyl-Gua.

Dr.*Ts'O* : *Would the antibodies be able to recognize those sequences with modified or unmodified bases,in native DNA?*

Dr.*Rajewsky* : Yes they would.This technique could also prove to be an important tool for investigating structural changes in DNA after exposure to alkylating agents.

Dr.*Rajewsky* : *Dr.Ts'O, how difficult is it for you to synthesize such and oligonucleotide with only one modified base by chemical means?*

Dr.*Ts'O* : It takes only about one month in our laboratory.

SECTION III

CHEMICALS AS PROMOTORS

PHENOBARBITAL AND OTHER LIVER TUMOR PROMOTERS

R. Schulte-Hermann[1], J. Schuppler[2], G. Ohde[1],

W. Bursch[1], and I. Timmermann-Trosiener[1]

[1]Institut für Toxikologie und Pharmakologie der
Philipps-Universität, Pilgrimstein 2
355 Marburg (West-Germany)

and

[2]Department Toxikologie Schering AG
Berlin-Bergkamen, Müllerstraße
1ooo Berlin 65

ABSTRACT

A number of different compounds appears to promote the
development of liver tumors from previously induced initiated
cells. These compounds include phenobarbital, hypolipidemic
drugs such as clofibrate and nafenopin, the sex steroids progesterone, cyproterone acetate, estradiol and mestranol, the
chlorinated hydrocarbons DDT, hexachlorocyclohexane, TCDD etc.
and the antioxidant butylhydroxytoluene. Studies on the mechanisms of tumor promotion by several representative prototypes of these compounds were performed in rat liver in vivo
and provided the following results:

1) All liver tumor promoters mentioned above stimulate growth
of normal liver. The growth response is due to cellular hypertrophy and/or increased rate of DNA (and cell) replication
and/or decreased rate of cell death. Some important aspects
pertinent to the control of liver growth are reviewed.

2) Hepatocytes in foci or islands of altered cells (putatively preneoplastic = pn) show higher rates of replication than
normal liver cells; various different liver tumor promoters
cause a further increase of proliferation of focal cells. The
increased proliferative activity is found in different island
phenotypes and thus seems to be a useful marker of the putative preneoplastic state. Moreover, the enhanced proliferation
of pn cells in response to promoters may provide the basis
for developing a short-term test on promotional activity. The
focal cells respond to several factors limiting proliferation
in normal liver suggesting that they are not autonomous with
respect to growth control.

3) Early pn foci grow slowly without promotion despite of
the relatively high rates of cell replication. Thus their cells
seem to have a much shorter life-time than normal hepatocytes,
or to undergo reversion to the normal phenotype ("remodelling").
Promoters seem to accelerate island enlargement by increasing
cell replication and delaying cell death or remodelling. Thus,
tumor promoters enhance the manifestation of the proliferative
advantage of the putative initiated cell population.

4) In addition promoters caused increases in the n u m b e r
of detectable islands. This can partially be explained by
enlargement of existing islands, but phenotypic changes that
would enhance the probability of detection of "remodelling"
islands, and growth of dormant initiated cells probably contribute to the apparent increase of island number.

5) Putative pn foci of unknown ("spontaneous") origin are frequent in the liver of aged Wistar rats. They are morphologically and functionally (increased proliferation) very similar to
those induced by carcinogens and are responsive to the mitogenic effect of tumor promoters. Promotion of these "spontaneous" foci may explain tumor appearance after long-term application of promoters alone. These findings imply that the long-
term carcinogenicity bioassay as currently performed does not
discriminate between initiating and promoting properties of
a test compound if the animals used develop spontaneous preneoplastic lesions in the organ affected.

INTRODUCTION

A variety of drugs and environmental pollutants has been shown to accelerate the development of liver tumors in two-stage experiments, in which an initiating carcinogen is given first, followed by long-term application of the compound itself. Examples are listed in table 1. These findings suggested tumor promoting activity of the test compounds (Peraino, 1975; Taper, 1978; Yager and Yager, 198o; Schulte-Hermann and Parzefall, 1981). However, most of the agents were hepatotumorigenic also if given without pretreatment with an initiating carcinogen (Schulte-Hermann, 1979). Observations of this type cast serious doubts on the interpretation that the agents are (pure) tumor promoters and have even prevented the general acceptance of the initiation-promotion concept in chemical (liver) carcinogenesis. In fact, we have recently shown with the α-isomer of hexachlorocyclohexane (HCH) as a model compound that discrimination between initiating and promoting properties can be impossible on the basis of the long-term carcinogenicity bioassay alone (Schulte-Hermann and Parzefall, 1981).

Obviously improved knowledge of the mechanisms of tumor promotion is required to develop methods for detection of promoting compounds which would be more reliable and more rapid than the classical long-term bioassay. Better understanding of tumor promotion would also appear to be necessary for reliable assessment of potential health risks resulting from use of promoting compounds. Below we will present a short overview on studies performed by us during the past several years on three questions pertinent to the mechanism of tumor promotion in the liver:

a) Properties of tumor promoters relevant to the promoting action?

b) Properties of the initiated cells relevant to promotion?

c) How can "pure" promoters (if they exist) lead to tumor appearance in the liver?

Tumor promotion includes as an essential component the

Table 1. Compounds believed to promote tumor development in
          rodent liver and their acute hepatic effects

class	compound	increased synthesis of	prolife- ration of	growth
Sedatives	Phenobarbital	monooxyge- nase (PB- type)	SER	+
Estrogens	Estradiol Ethinylestra- diol/Mestranol	various serum proteins		+
Progestins	Progesterone Cyproterone- acetate (=CPA)	monooxyge- nase (PCN- type)	SER	+
Hypolipi- demic drugs	Nafenopin, Clofibrate	enz. of fatty acid metab.	micro- bodies	+
Chlorinated hydrocarbons	Hexachloro- cyclohexane (=HCH), DDT, PCB's, TCDD	monooxyge- nase (PB, MC-type)	SER	+
Antioxidants	Butylhydroxy- toluene	monooxyge- nase	SER	+

PB = Phenobarbital
PCN = Pregnenolone-16α-carbonitrile
MC = 2o-Methylcholanthrene
SER = smooth endoplasmic reticulum

proliferation of the pool of initiated hepatocytes. Thus understanding the   c o n t r o l   of cell proliferation in normal
liver and its disturbance in initiated cells is of crucial
importance to the elucidation of the mechanism of tumor promotion. Therefore, some aspects of growth control in the
liver will also be considered.

It should be noted that by definition complete hepatocarcinogens and also toxic agents such as CCl_4 possess tumor-
promoting activity in the liver. Effects of these agents are
discussed by Farber (this volume) and will not be considered
in the present paper.

METHODS

Female Wistar rats (Zentralinstitut für Versuchstier-
zucht, Hannover, Germany) were used at an initial age of 4 to
8 weeks unless stated otherwise. Where indicated the animals
were adapted for three weeks to a controlled lighting rhythm
(LD 12-12) and to a daily feeding period of 5 hours. This regimen served to synchronize endogenous and mitogen-induced DNA
synthesis in the liver (Schulte-Hermann, 1977). For induction
of putative preneoplastic foci 75 or 15o mg/kg diethylnitrosamine (DENA) or 25o mg/kg N-nitrosomorpholin (NNM) were dissolved in water and administered as single oral doses.
Hepatomitogenic/promoting compounds were given as follows:
Phenobarbital (PB) orally, 1 x 5o mg/kg in aqueous solution
or daily 5o mg/kg via the food; α-hexachlorocyclohexane
(α-HCH) orally, 1 x 2oo mg/kg in oil or daily 2o mg/kg via the
food; cyproterone acetate (CPA) orally in oil, 4o or 1oo mg/kg
once or daily or 1oo mg/kg once weekly; progesterone (PRO)s.c.
5oo mg/kg once weekly. ^{3}H-thymidine (o,2 mCi/kg) was injected
i.v. to measure DNA synthesis; clock-times of injection were
scheduled to the period of maximal DNA synthesis during the
daily rhythm (Schulte-Hermann, 1977).

After decapitation specimens of liver tissue were fixed
in formalin or cold acetone, and histological sections were
prepared by standard procedures and stained with hematoxylin
and eosin or were assayed for γ-glutamyl-transferase (γ-GT)
activity (Rutenberg et al., 1968). Autoradiography was perfor-

med on the same sections to measure DNA synthesis, which was
determined by counting labelled cells ("3H-index" = percent
of hepatocytes labelled). Biochemical determination of DNA
content and of the specific activity of DNA was done as described previously (Schulte-Hermann,1977; Schulte-Hermann et
al., 198o) using the procedure of Burton (1956).

RESULTS AND DISCUSSION

1. Effects of tumor promoters in normal liver

Studies on the biological effects of tumor promoters in
n o r m a l liver should provide a clue to understanding
tumor promotion. The liver tumor promoters presently known
can be grouped into one of two categories: a) cytotoxic compounds such as acetylaminofluorene (AAF) and other complete
carcinogens; CCl_4 etc., and b) agents which increase the
functional load of the organ but without obvious hepatotoxicity as exemplified by phenobarbital. The liver may adapt to
both groups of agents by distinct patterns of responses
("adaptive strategies") consisting of changes in activity of
certain enzymes, changes in the content of organelles, and
growth (Schulte-Hermann, 1979). In the case of CCl_4, which
is activated to a toxic metabolite by the hepatic monooxygenase (Mo) system, intoxication even by small, subnecrogenic
doses results in a decrease in activity of this enzyme system,
and this serves to protect the animal from the deleterious
effects of subsequent, otherwise lethal doses. The decrease
in activity seems to be due not only to Mo destruction by
toxic metabolites but also to a temporary inability of liver
cells to respond to signals inducing Mo multiplication
(Dörffler and Schulte-Hermann, in preparation). The phenomenon
of resistance to cytotoxic effects as an adaptive response and
its implications for tumor promotion is discussed by Farber
(this volume) and will not be considered further in the present
paper.

Adaptive responses to agents (promoters) that increase
the functional load in the liver are compiled in table 1. As
seen these compounds are extremely heterogenous with respect
to chemical structures and general pharmacological or biologi-

cal effects. They share however the ability to induce in the
liver increases of specific functions and growth. Functional
changes include increased synthesis of certain serum proteins
or of enzyme families such as drug metabolizing enzymes or
enzymes of the fatty acid metabolism. These changes are frequently accompanied by multiplication of specific organelles
such as smooth endoplasmic reticulum (SER) or microbodies.
The third component of the adaptive response is the induction
of liver growth (Schulte-Hermann, 1974; Schulte-Hermann, 1979).
Indeed, stimulation of liver growth appears to be the only
known effect common to all the various tumor promoters listed
in table 1. Likewise, in various other organs compounds promoting tumor development also stimulate growth of that organ.
It therefore seemed justified to adopt the hypothesis that the
ability to induce growth is one of the critical properties of
these tumor promoters. Further evidence supporting this hypothesis will be presented below.

How is the growth response of the liver brought about?

        Some important findings will be illustrated in figs. 1
and 2, and a summary of various basic observations will be
given subsequently. Figure 1 depicts the effects of α-HCH
on the liver which was used as a model compound. The upper
part shows the increase in hepatic monooxygenase activity
(assayed by measuring the rate of aminopyrine demethylation)
and the increase in cytochrome P_{450}. The lower part of the
graph exhibits the increase of liver size and of total
hepatic DNA. The increase of DNA is mainly due to enhanced
parenchymal DNA synthesis which is followed in rat liver by
a wave of mitosis. Thus, in (adolescent) rats liver growth
appears to be produced in part by parenchymal hyperplasia.
It should be noted (fig. 1) that the increase in liver mass
relatively exceeds the increase of DNA which suggest that
a hypertrophic component is involved in the growth process.
α-HCH is slowly eliminated from the body in a matter of a
few weeks. Concomitantly, the increases in monooxygenase
and liver size regress to normal; only the enhanced DNA
content persists for a longer period but not indefinitely
(Schulte Hermann and Parzefall, 1981).

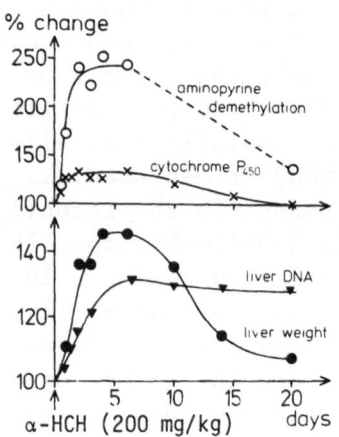

Fig.1. Effect of a single
        dose of α-HCH on
microsomal monooxygenase,
size and total DNA content
of the liver.

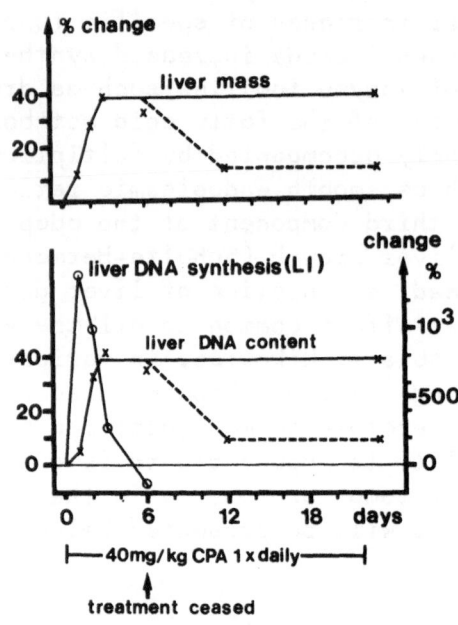

Fig. 2. Effects of cyproterone
         acetate treatment and
withdrawal on DNA content and
DNA synthesis of rat liver.
Daily dose was 4o mg/kg CPA

        Fig. 2 depicts changes seen after treatment with another
liver mitogen/tumor promoter, namely CPA. This agent has a
much shorter biological half-life than α-HCH and therefore has
to be administered daily in order to produce a sustained
effect. Concomitant with the initial phase of liver enlargement there is a steep increase of hepatic DNA synthesis which
declines again to control values even though CPA treatment is
continued. The same has been found with all other hepatomito-
gens/tumor promoters (Fig. 2) tested so far (Schulte-Hermann,
1974; Schulte-Hermann 1979; Schulte-Hermann and Schmitz,198o).
Obviously an effective feedback mechanism prevents excessive
accumulation of DNA in response to mitogenic stimuli. Fig.2
also presents another important aspect of mitogen action. It
can be seen that the increased content of DNA persists as
long as the treatment is performed. However, if the treatment
is stopped, the DNA content of the liver declines rapidly in
a matter of a few days and then more slowly until eventually

the control level will be reached. It appears that in the hyperplastic liver at least some of the cells depend on the continuous presence of the growth stimulus; its withdrawal causes rapid death of some of the cells (Fig. 2) (Schulte-Hermann et al., 1980). (Rapid elimination of liver DNA is not seen in the experiment with α-HCH (Fig. 1) possibly because of the slow elimination of this agent.)

In summary, these and other studies from several laboratories on liver enlargement produced by the agents mentioned in table 1 and by other inducers revealed the following results (Schulte-Hermann, 1974; 1979):

1) The enlargement of the organ reflects a true growth response as indicated by proportionate increases of the main cell constituents protein, RNA, lipid, glycogen, and water. Except for some "specific" enzymes (see above) which may show excessive increases the bulk of enzymes, especially those of the intermediary metabolism, seems to increase in parallel with liver size as would be expected during ordered growth.

2) Cell multiplication may contribute to the growth response as indicated by increases in the number of cells involved in DNA synthesis and mitosis. The total DNA content of the organ is enhanced.

3) The ploidy of liver cell nuclei increases. In rats treated with α-HCH or CPA there is a concomitant decrease in the percentage of binuclear cells so that total c e l l u l a r ploidy does not change significantly. In contrast, in mice higher levels of cellular ploidy may be attained. These ploidy changes do not necessarily indicate pathological processes, but appear to result from the peculiarities of cell replication in the liver of adolescent and adult rodents. Some of the ploidy changes may occur after partial hepatectomy or, less intensively, during adolescent growth (Carriere, 1969; Schulte-Hermann et al., 1980a).

4) Cellular enlargement, even without increases in ploidy, usually contributes to liver growth as shown biochemically by a decrease of DNA concentration and morphologically by a decrease in the nucleus: cytoplasm ratio. Cell enlargement is

usually most pronounced in the perivenous area of the liver
acinus and is probably largely due to the proliferation of
endoplasmic reticulum or of microbodies.

5) In summary, the growth response of the liver to mitogenic
compounds may occur with and without concomitant DNA multiplication, i.e. by an increase in genetic units and by increased expression of existing genes. Cell proliferation (the
classical hyperplasia) is a well established cause of DNA
multiplication. Growth without change in total liver DNA is
due to cell enlargement without ploidy changes. The relative
contribution of these different growth components is modified
by several factors such as properties of the inducer used,
species and age of animals, etc.

6) The hepatocyte is the predominant cell type involved in
the growth response induced by the mitogens listed in table 1.

7) The growth response is self-limited. Active liver growth
and cell multiplication are restricted to the early phase of
treatment with an inducer, and the rate of cell proliferation
returns to normal even if treatment is continued. Obviously,
the inducers shift liver size and cell content to a new steady
state at an increased level.

8) The growth response is dose-dependent. This also applies
to cell multiplication and to ploidy changes.

9) Liver enlargement is readily reversible. Part of the hyperplasia may or may not be rapidly reversible depending on the
experimental conditions; in any event there seems to be a regression of hyperplasia at least in a matter of several months
(see below and Schulte-Hermann and Parzefall, 1981).

1o) Prevention of cell death may be a mechanism by which hepatomitogens maintain cell number at an enhanced level during
prolonged treatment.

11) The competence for adaptive responses to phenobarbital or
α-HCH in rats awakes during the perinatal period. Adaptive

growth of the liver appears to be most pronounced in juvenile and young adult rats, i.e. after the mature state of differentiation has essentially been reached.

12) Increases of differentiated functions and DNA replication which seem to be mutually exclusive during developmental growth may occur simultaneously during adaptive growth. Thus, high doses of CPA induce replication of almost all paren- chymal cells; at the same time monooxygenase activity in these cells increases dramatically (Schulte-Hermann et al., 1980 a).

In conclusion, numerous studies the results of which are briefly reviewed above did not reveal signs of overt liver damage following treatment with the hepatomitogens/ promoters. Rather, in several respects the effects produced resemble those elicited by various trophic hormones in their target organs (cf. table 2).

Table 2.   Some essential characteristics of liver growth induced by single or short-term treatment with hepatomitogens/promoters

Response to functional load (e.g. drug metabolism)
Association with increase of function
Association with increase of specific organelles
No signs of overt liver damage
Self-limitation
Dose-dependency
Reversibility

It should be noted that the changes described as "adaptation" are not necessarily beneficial to the organism. Moreover, evaluation of the toxicological meaning of the growth response including its impact on liver tumor forma- tion requires knowledge of the mechanisms by which xenobiotic inducers stimulate liver growth. Up to now these mechanisms are essentially unknown.

2. <u>Mitogenic and permissive signals controlling hepatocyte proliferation</u>

Our attempts to learn more about the stimulation of liver growth by xenobiotic inducers have been focused on the control of the hyperplastic growth component. The essential events of cell replication are DNA synthesis (S) and mitosis (M), which are preceded by preparatory periods called G_1 and G_2, and these 4 phases classically constitute the replicative cycle. In the adult liver, cells do not usually proliferate and are in a quiescent state referred to as G_0. The sequence of the various stages is shown schematically in Figure 3 a.

From the G_0 state liver cells can be stimulated to enter the replicative cycle by appropriate signals such as tissue loss (partial hepatectomy, necroses) or increased functional load (Schulte-Hermann, 1974). Between the application of a stimulatory signal and the beginning of DNA synthesis cells go through a lag phase which in the liver lasts 16 to 2o hours ("prereplicative period"). Obviously during this period the cell takes the decision to enter the replicative process and prepares for DNA synthesis. If we want to understand the control of (hepatic) DNA and cell replication we must identify, at both the cellular and the molecular level, the nature and

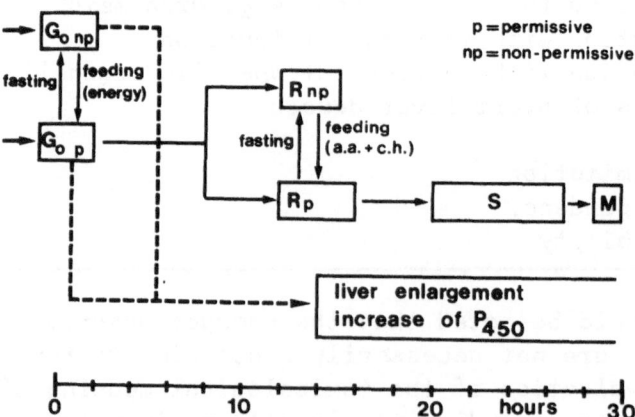

Fig. 3a. Scheme showing interactions between feeding and hepatomitogens in the control of the hepatic replicative cycle.
a.a.: amino acids; c.h.: carbohydrates

sequence of events occuring at the start and during the progression through the prereplicative period.

In the following the development of a concept will be
described which may be helpful for studies concerning growth
control in normal and preneoplastic hepatocytes. We have
found that nutrition is a permissive factor in the control of
hepatic DNA synthesis induced by α-HCH and other agents. By
using feeding schedules in which food is provided for only a
few hours per day, food consumption was shown to be required
for the eventual initiation of DNA replication at two different
stages of the prereplicative period: (1) before or at the time
of mitogen administration (G_0), and (2) 12-15 hours later,i.e.
5-8 hours before initiation of DNA synthesis, at a point called "R" (restriction) point according to Pardee (1974) ("Two-
stage control"). If food is withheld at one of these stages
hepatocytes reach a state (designated "non-permissive") in
which they are (almost) non-responsive to the mitogenic effect
of various growth stimuli (fig. 3a). Other effects of α-HCH,
i.e. organ enlargement and increase of drug-metabolizing enzyme activity, are not prevented by lack of food. The different
adaptive sponses therefore seem to be parallel rather than sequential events. Thus stimulation of liver growth cannot result from increased demands for oxygen and NADPH after multiplication of the enzymes as has been suggested by others
(Schulte-Hermann, 1977; Hoffmann and Schulte-Hermann, 1979).

These studies lead to the following conclusions:

1) Food consumption acts as an exogenous co-regulator of liver
   cell proliferation. It is not yet known whether its permissive effects are mediated directly by the postprandial
   increase of food constituents in portal blood, or indirectly via endocrine changes.

2) The prereplicative phase of parenchymal cells in the liver
   consists of at least 2 subphases separated by the R-point.
   At this point cells are already committed for replication
   but the preparatory events are still subject to exogenous
   control, which is exerted by the supply of amino acids and
   carbohydrates.

3) The non-proliferative G_0-state appears to consist of at
   least 2 sub-states: one designated G_0 p permits hepatocytes to respond to a mitogenic signal by entering the
   replicative cycle; the other sub-state designated G_0 np
   is non-permissive for induction of replication. Supply
   of nutrients to the animals induces transition from the
   G_0 np to the G_0 p state (fig. 3a).

4) Fig. 3 b shows a more complex diagram of our present concept of the control of cell number in the adult liver.
   There is evidence suggesting the existence of several
   types of signals that regulate the number of cells in the
   permissive part of the G_0-state. These may include
   nutrients, various hormones and factors involved in feedback control of hepatocyte proliferation (see above).
   Other inhibitory signals ("chalones") may stop or slow
   down the progress of hepatocytes through the replicative
   cycle by interactions shortly before initiation of S or
   during G_2 or M. The G_2-inhibitor is thought to be
   responsible for the prevention of mitosis after stimulation of DNA replication as found in mouse liver but not
   (or much less) in rat liver (Bursch and Schulte-Hermann,
   in preparation). The M-inhibitor is believed to prevent
   the completion of mitosis at telophase and to induce the
   appearance of binucleated hepatocytes (Nadal 1975).
   It is of interest to note that these inhibitory activities
   appear in the maturing organism only; monitoring ploidy
   changes during replication may thus provide a useful tool
   to indicate the state of differentiation of the liver
   (Schulte-Hermann, 1980 a). After completion of
   replication the hepatocyte may re-enter the G_0-state or
   may progress to a (hypothetical) state of terminal
   differentiation ("G_T") and may then die (fig. 3 b). The
   data shown in fig. 2 strongly suggest that also in this
   stage liver mitogens affect the control of cell number by
   preventing cell death.

In conclusion, in normal adult liver the steady state of cell proliferation and cell death is regulated by finely balanced interactions of a variety of factors acting at different stages of a cell's life cycle. As will be shown below this balance seems to be disturbed in putatively initiated cells or their progeny. Therefore, elucidation of the mechanisms controlling cell number hopefully will help to understand the nature of initiation.

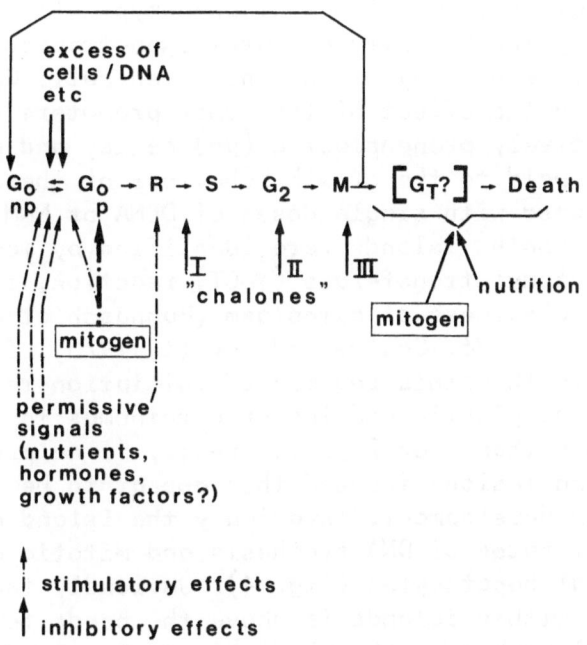

Fig. 3b.   Interactions of hepatomitogens and other factors in the control of proliferation and death of hepatocytes. The figure is explained in the text.

3. <u>Short-term effects of promoters on proliferation in foci</u>
   <u>of altered cells</u>

A question central to understanding tumor promotion
concerns identification and properties of the target cell of
promoters from which tumors eventually arise. According to
the two-stage concept this cell should be the initiated cell,
which unfortunately has not yet been identified in the liver
or other organs. There is, however, rather strong evidence
suggesting that foci or islands of phenotypically altered
cells appearing in the liver of carcinogen-treated animals
are the immediate progeny of the initiated cell. Consequently
we have studied the effect of the tumor promoters on these
altered, putatively preneoplastic (pn) cells, and particular
attention was paid to the growth behaviour of these cells.
Rats were treated with single doses of DENA or NNM, and after
3 weeks to 11 months islands were identified by means of a
positive γ-glutamyl-transferase (γ-GT) reaction, increased
basophilia or clearness of cytoplasm (Bannasch et al., 1979;
Solt and Farber, 1976; Squire and Levitt, 1975). It is important to note that this regimen of initiation results in
appearance of neoplastic nodules or carcinomas in the liver
only after more than 1 or 2 years, resp., if no promoters
are applied. Pn lesions induced thus appear to be in an early
stage of tumor development. Invariably the island cells exhibited higher rates of DNA synthesis and mitotic activity
than the normal hepatocytes (fig. 4). Obviously the rate of
proliferation within islands is above the needs for homeostasis of cell number in the whole liver. Single doses of
various types of tumor promoters resulted in a further increase of the already enhanced proliferative activity of
island cells. Obviously, islands contain a greater fraction
of cells in the G_0 p state than normal liver. The increased
proliferative activities were found in different island
phenotypes (Schulte-Hermann et al., 1981), and thus seem to
be a marker more consistently associated with the putative
pn state than the morphological and histochemical alterations
used.

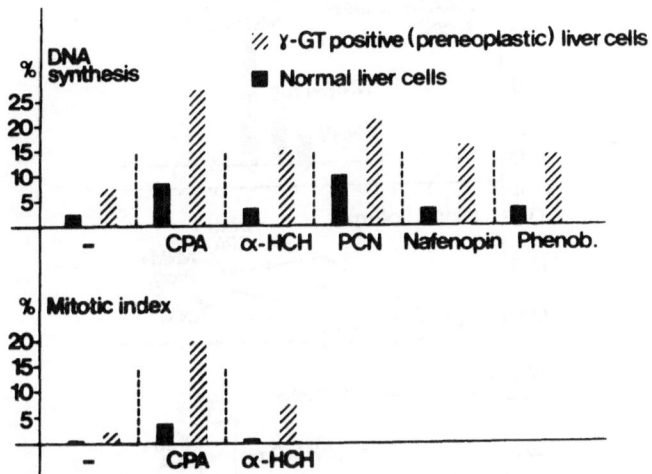

Fig. 4.   DNA synthesis and mitotic activity in foci of γ-GT
         positive cells following single doses of various
         suspected liver tumor promoters.
         PCN = pregnenolone-16α-carbonitrile, 1oo mg/kg;
         nafenopin: 1oo mg/kg; CPA: 1oo mg/kg; other doses:
              see methods

4. Long-term effects of promoters on islands of altered cells

        Islands of altered cells exhibited increased rates of
DNA synthesis at all times investigated between three weeks
and 11 months after administration of the carcinogen (figs.5
and 6). Assuming an average proliferation rate of 1,5 % per
day, islands should show rapid growth even without promotion
with a doubling time of about 45 days (fig. 6). However, the
growth rate of the average island actually found was almost
zero for several months and then increased gradually (figs.
5 and 6). Thus it appears that the altered cells have a
shorter life time than normal hepatocytes, which is several
hundred days. Alternatively, the island cells may "remodel"
to a phenotype indiscriminable from normal hepatocytes.

        Long-term effects of promoters on island development
were studied in two different experimental designs. In the
first design two suspected tumor promoters, i.e. CPA and pro-

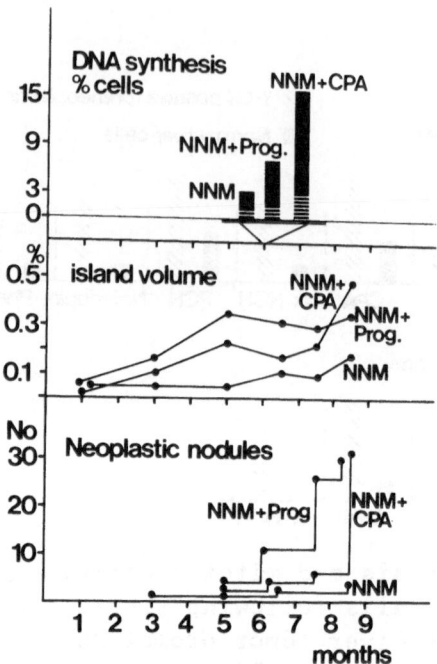

Fig. 5. Effects of intermittent treatment with cyproterone
acetate and progesterone on island growth and tumor
appearance following initiation by a single dose of
NNM. Promoter treatment was started a time "0".
Hatched columns: normal hepatocytes; black columns:
γ-GT positive island cells.

.gesterone (PRO), were given intermittently once per week, in
the other phenobarbital or α-HCH were administered continuously via the food.

Intermittent treatment with PRO or CPA caused strikingly
enhanced DNA synthesis rates in islands et each time investigated. The upper part of fig. 5 shows as an example ^{3}H-indices
found after 6 months of treatment. This effect was associated
with increases in the average island volume (fig. 5, middle
part). Island enlargement precedes the appearance of neoplastic nodules in the hormone-treated rats (fig. 5, lower part).
These findings strongly suggest that CPA and PRO promote
tumor development in rat liver and that hormone-induced increases of island cell proliferation are at least partially
responsible for island enlargement under the present condi-

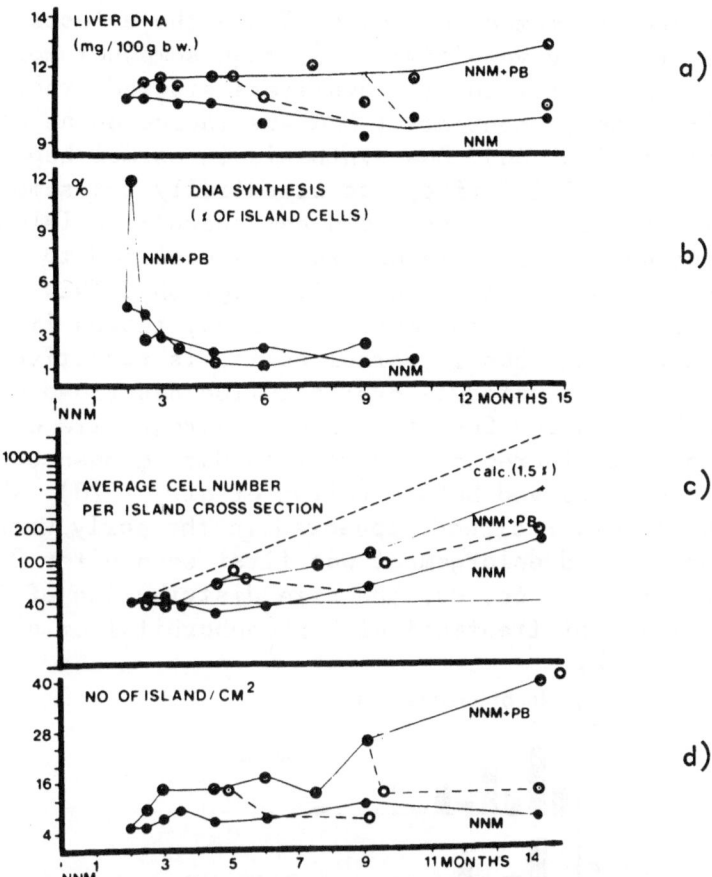

Fig. 6. Effects of continuous treatment with phenobarbital on liver DNA (a), island DNA synthesis (b), island size (c), and island number (d) following initiation by a single dose of NNM administered at time "0". PB treatment started 2 months after NNM.
    ———: theoretical island growth rate assuming cell replication of 1,5 %/day;
    - - - : changes after withdrawal of PB.

tions. Moreover, the findings are consistent with the hypothesis that island enlargement is a rate-limiting factor in liver tumorigenesis. In addition we noted an increase in the number of detectable islands (Schulte-Hermann et al., 1982).

Results obtained after continuous treatment with phenobarbital are presented in fig. 6. Since the effects of α-HCH
were qualitatively very similar (though somewhat more pronounced with respect to all parameters studied) they are not
shown. The hepatic content of DNA was increased at all times
investigated (fig. 6a). DNA synthesis in normal hepatocytes,
after a small initial rise, was essentially the same as in
untreated rats as expected (data not shown); in island cells
it was increased initially but rapidly declined to the level
found in islands of untreated rats (fig. 6b). This suggests
that DNA synthesis in the average island, though it remains
at a higher level than in normal cells, is sensitive to feedback control of hepatocyte proliferation described above
(Schulte-Hermann and Schmitz, 1980). Average size and number
of islands both increased severalfold during phenobarbital
treatment as observed before (Pitot et al., 1978). While the
increase in number already appeared in the early weeks of
promotion, island enlargement was first seen after 2 month
of promotion (fig. 6c, d). The size distribution of islands
after 28 weeks of treatment with phenobarbital or α-HCH is
shown in fig. 7.

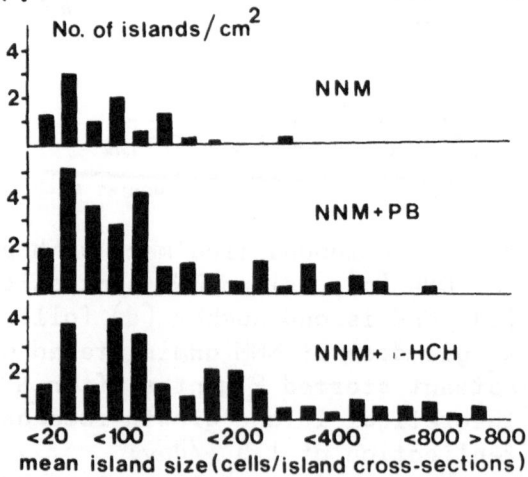

Fig. 7. Island size distribution after 28 weeks of continu-
         ous treatment with phenobarbital and α-HCH

How can these findings be explained? It appears that
increased island cell proliferation cannot be the only
factor responsible for island enlargement during
continuous exposure to α-HCH and

phenobarbital. We therefore assume that under these conditions island growth is due to a decrease in the rates of
cell death or phenotypic remodelling, either of which
appears to occur in island cells (see above). This assumption seems reasonable since prevention of cell death has
been observed to be one of the promoter effects in normal
liver (see above, fig. 2) and since promoters have already
been shown to prevent phenotypic changes in islands (Watanabe
and Williams, 1978). The increased n u m b e r of islands
should partially result from island enlargement which increases the probability of detection, and partially from
growth of mini-islands and single initiated cells to a
detectable size. This would imply that a considerable number
of initiated hepatocytes do not proliferate to form detectable islands unless a promoter is applied. In addition,
promoters may possibly lead to phenotypic changes within
existing but undetectable islands in a non-promoted liver
in such a way that they are more clearly demarcated from the
surrounding normal tissue.

     These considerations are supported by findings ob-
tained after withdrawal of PB (fig. 6). The total DNA content
of the liver returned to the control level although more
slowly than in the experiment presented in fig. 2. In
parallel number and average size of islands returned to the
levels found in non-promoted animals (fig. 6c, d). Some of
the residual islands exhibited signs of phenotypic reversion
to a more normal appearance, such as partial loss of γ-GT.
Thus both remodelling of island cells to the normal phenotype and island cell death (suggested by the loss of liver
DNA) may have contributed to the decreases of island size
and number. In any event part of the island cells found
after a period of promotion seem to be promoter-dependent
for survival or specific phenotypic appearance. These results are compatible with the assumption that PB induces
growth of a subpopulation of promoter-dependent islands.
The basic defect in this subpopulation would be a persisting
imbalance of cell proliferation vs. cell death/remodelling
during prolonged promoter treatment when the normal liver
has reached a new steady state of cell number (see above).
This property seems to be different from another feature of
putative initiated cells, i.e. resistance which is thought

responsible for island growth during promotion with AAF (Solt
and Farber 1976; Farber 1980; Farber: this volume).

The regression of islands after promoter withdrawal is
of considerable interest from a practical toxicological
point of view, since it confirms previous findings made with
skin tumors suggesting that the action of a promoter is reversible within certain limits.

We conclude that the ability to induce liver growth or
the hormone-like effect is an essential, though not necessarily the only critical property of the tumor promoters. Island
cells have a proliferation advantage over normal hepatocytes;
tumor promoters seem to enhance the manifestation of this advantage. Properties of promoters and of putative preneoplastic
islands relevant for tumor promotion and also of possible help
for identification of both are listed in tables 3 and 4.

Table 3. Properties of liver tumor promoters

---

1) Induction of growth and functional changes in the liver
   (hormon-like effect)
2) Enhanced proliferation of putative preneoplastic cells
3) Accelerated growth of putative preneoplastic islands
4) Histochemical/morphological changes in putative preneoplastic islands
5) Accelerated appearance of tumors

---

5. Growth control in foci of altered cells

Despite of their increased proliferative activity island cells are not autonomous with respect to growth control.
First, their proliferation rate although higher than in normal liver cells is still much lower than in liver lesions
further advanced towards the malignant state. Second, island
cells appear to respond to feedback inhibition of DNA synthesis during prolonged promoter treatment (fig. 6) as do
normal liver cells (see above and fig. 2). Third, island
cells seem to depend as normal cells on permissive signals

Table 4. Properties of cells in islands of altered (ini-
        tiated) hepatocytes which are relevant to island
        growth

---

1) Proliferation rate in excess of homeostatic need of the
   whole liver
2) Decrease of life-span or reversion to normal phenotype
3) Response to liver tumor promoters:
   - Increase of proliferation rate
   - Increase of life-span and/or prevention of pheno-
     typic reversion
4) Sensitive to feedback-inhibition of cell proliferation
5) Dependence on permissive signals exerted by food consumption

---

released by consumption of food:

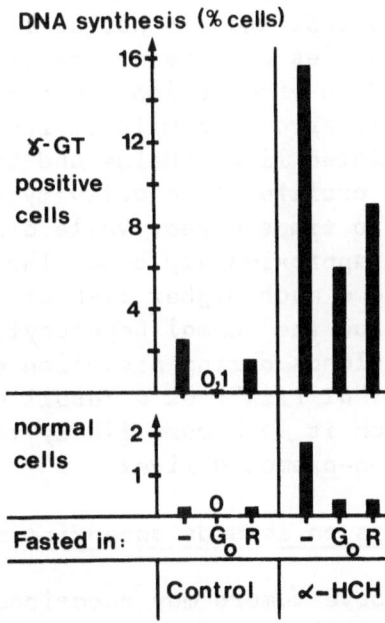

Fig. 8. Effect of fasting during the G_0 and R-phase of the
        replicative cycle on DNA synthesis in foci of altered
        hepatocytes

As shown in fig. 8 fasting in either the G_0 or R-state partially suppresses DNA synthesis in foci of altered cells similar as in the normal liver cells. In conclusion, with respect to their proliferative behaviour island cells do not show autonomy but depend on the presence of permissive and promoting factors.

6. Progression

If some or all of the foci of altered cells are potential intermediates on the pathway to cancer, progression to more malignant phenotypes should occasionally occur within islands. This has been observed by others (Farber, 198o) and also in the present study. Progression may be due to a (rare) event similar to that causing initiation (Farber, 198o). On the basis of our findings we propose the hypothesis that the relatively high replicative activity of island cells may be responsible for progression. Since cell replication seems necessary to fix any damage potentially leading to initiation (or progression) the chances of fixation of critical damage are much higher in islands than in normal liver. Moreover, replication itself carries a certain risk of errors which occasionally may lead to progression. In the adult rat, the frequency of abnormal, erroneous mitoses reportedly is high even in the non-initiated liver (Heine and Stöcker, 197o). Due to the increased proliferative activity each island cell may replicate about 1o times a year while a normal liver cell would replicate approximately once. Thus the average island cell should have a much higher risk of initiation-like phenotypic changes than the normal hepatocyte. Multiplication and enlargement of islands during promotion dramatically expands the population "at risk"; as a result a rare event leading to progression is much more likely to occur at an early time than in non-promoted liver.

7. Effect of promoters on islands appearing spontaneously

As mentioned above tumors may occasionally develop after sole treatment with a promoter without initiating pretreatment. This finding has similarly been made with the promoters par excellence, i.e. the phorbol esters, in studies on skin tumorigenesis and has supported doubts expressed by

several workers on the validity of the promotion concept. The
defenders of the concept explained the formation of tumors by
promoters alone by assuming promotion of s p o n t a -
n e o u s initiated cells, but to our knowledge this claim
has not yet found much experimental support.

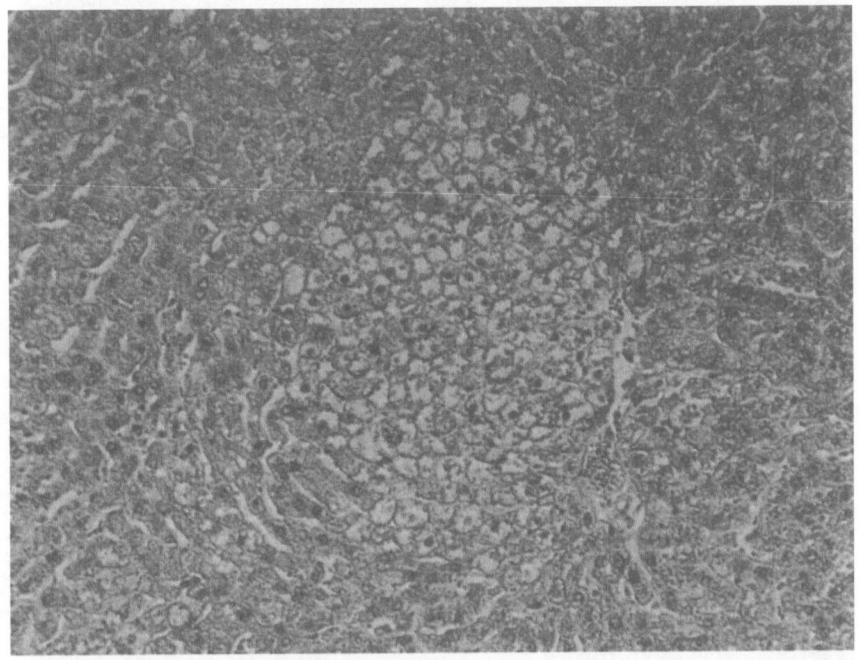

Fig. 9.   Island of altered cells in the liver of an untreated
(9 a)   2 years old Wistar rat.
          Scale: a) 25 x;   b) 18o x
          Note the presence of numerous island cells labelled
          with silver grains indicating DNA replication

       We have searched for putatively initiated cells in the
liver of two years old Wistar rats, using for identification
the proliferative characteristics of carcinogen-induced island cells (see above), in addition to the usual morphological and histochemical markers. Although the Wistar substrain
used has a low background of spontaneous hepatoma (2 %), all
of 41 animals studied had in the liver islands of altered
cells which on the basis of histochemical, morphological and
functional criteria (increased cell proliferation) were very

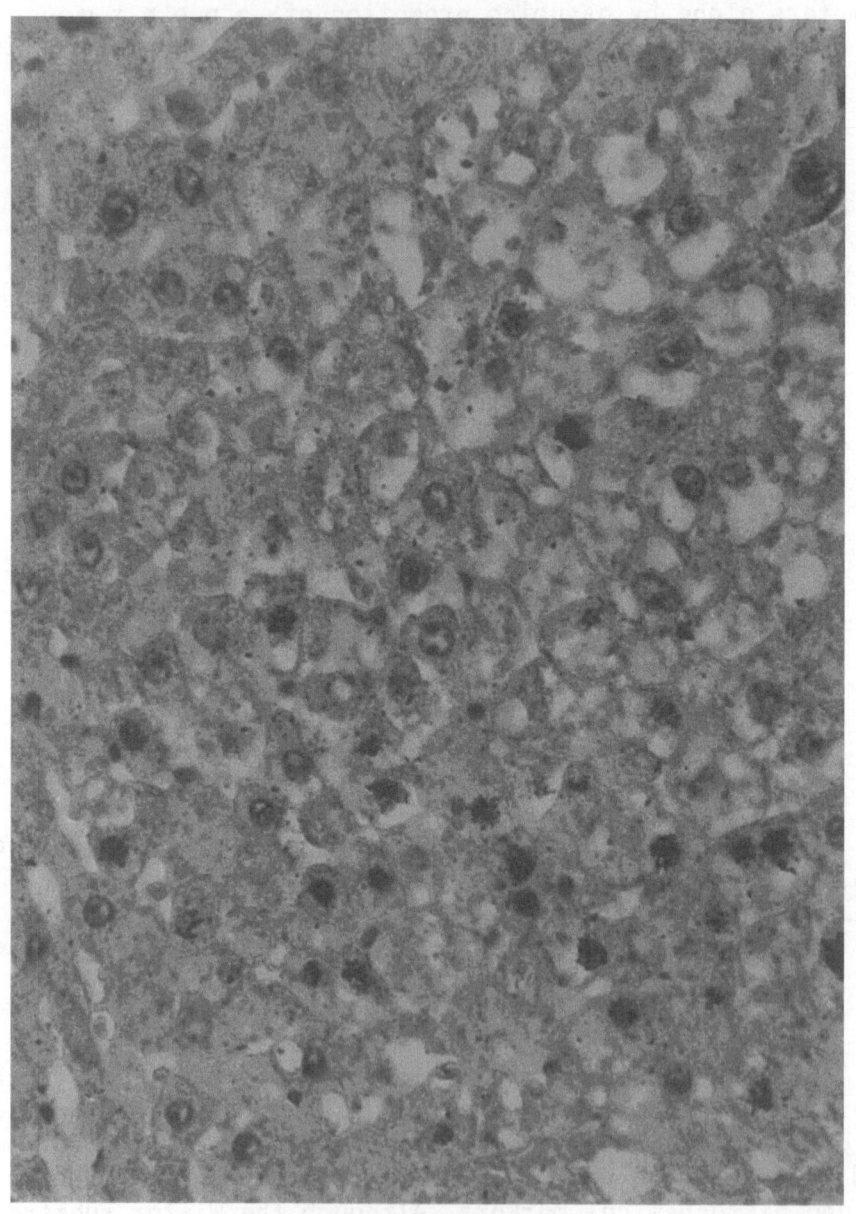

Fig. 9 b.   Scale 180 x

similar if not identical to those produced in young animals by application of hepatocarcinogens (fig. 9). As shown in fig. 1o these "spontaneous" islands exhibit an increased rate of DNA synthesis over that of normal hepatocytes. Most importantly various different liver tumor promoters cause a further increase of the DNA replication rate; this shows that the "spontaneous" islands are responsive to the mitogenic effects of the tumor promoters. Prolonged application of the promoters therefore should result in rapid island growth and eventually in tumor formation.

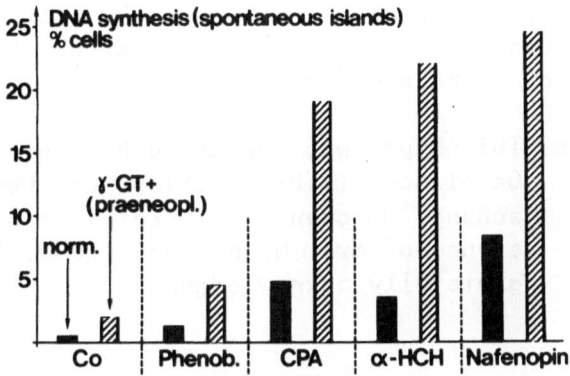

Fig. 10.   DNA synthesis in "spontaneous" foci of altered
           cells
           Treatment: see methods and fig. 3
           Columns: Black: normal cells;
                         Cross-hatched: γ-GT positive islands

     This finding implies that long-term carcinogenicity bioassays of chemical agents do not discriminate between initiating and promoting properties of a test compound, if preneoplastic lesions develop spontaneously in the affected organ. Obviously additional tests are required for reliable interpretation of data and risk assessment. The properties of tumor promoters listed in table 3 would appear to provide useful parameters for the detection of promoting agents. In particular the observed enhancement of proliferation of island cells in response to tumor promoters might provide a useful and reliable short-term test in vivo. This possibility should be checked in further studies.

In view of the ubiquitous presence of a vast number of carcinogenic factors in our environment the formation of initiated cells may be a frequent event in the liver and in other organs of animals and humans. According to some current evaluations of long-term carcinogenicity studies a number of drugs and other chemicals including various natural and synthetic hormones have been classified as (initiating) carcinogens. However, several of these agents induce growth and promote tumor development in their target organs. On the basis of the present results it is tempting to consider the possibility that promotion of spontaneous initiated cells may explain the development of cancer by non-mutagenic drugs and hormones in various organs of animals and humans.

Acknowledgement: This study was supported by a grant from the Gesellschaft für Strahlen- und Umweltforschung, München. The careful technical assistance of Mrs. G. Barthel and J. Sprenger is gratefully acknowledged.

REFERENCES

Bannasch, P., Hacker, H.-J., and Mayer, D., 1979, Early biological markers during liver carcinogenesis. Arch. Toxicol. Suppl. 2: 145.
Boutwell, R.K., Sivak, A., 1974, The function and mechanism of promoters of carcinogenesis, Crit.Rev.Toxicol.2: 419.
Burton, K., 1956, A study of the conditions and mechanism of the diphenylamine reaction of the colorimetric estimation of deoxyribonucleic acid, Biochem. J. 62: 315.
Carriere, R., 1969, The growth of liver parenchymal nuclei and its endocrine regulation, Int. Rev. Cytol. 35: 2o1.
Farber, E., 198o, The sequential analysis of liver cancer induction, Biochim. Biophys. Acta 6o5: 149.
Heine, W., Stöcker, E., 197o, Der Proliferationsmodus der Leber seniler Ratten nach Teilhepatektomie, Verh.Dtsch. Ges. Pathol. 54: 55o.
Hoffmann, V., and Schulte-Hermann, R.,1979, The regulative

role of food consumption in the induction of rat liver
cell proliferation by drugs and environmental pollutants,
Arch. Toxicol. Suppl. 2: 457.

Nadal, C., 1975, Inhibition of rat hepatocyte multiplication
by serum factors. Physiological significance, Virchows
Arch. B Cell Pathol. 18: 273.

Pardee, A.B., 1974, A restriction point for control of normal
animal cell proliferation, Proc.Nat.Acad.Sci.71: 1286.

Peraino, C., Fry, R.J.M., Staffeldt, E., and Christopher, J.P.,
1975, Comparative enhancing effects of phenobarbital,
amobarbital, diphenylhydantoin, and dichlorodiphenyl-
trichloroethane on 2-acetylaminofluorene-induced hepatic
tumorigenesis in the rat, Cancer Res. 35: 2884.

Pitot, H.C., Barsness, L., Goldsworthy, T., and Kitagawa, T.,
1978, Biochemical characterisation of stages of hepatocarcinogenesis after a single dose of diethylnitrosamine,
Nature 271: 456.

Rutenberg, A.M., Kim, H., Fischbein, J., Hauker, J.S.,
Wasserkrug, H.C., and Seligman, R., 1968, Histochemical
and ultrastructural demonstration of γ-glutamyl trans-
peptidase activity, J. Histochem. Cytochem. 17: 517.

Schulte-Hermann, R., 1974, Induction of liver growth by xenobiotic compounds and other stimuli, Crit. Rev. Toxicol.
3: 97.

Schulte-Hermann, R., 1977, Two-stage control of cell proliferation induced in rat liver by α-hexachlorocyclohexane,
Cancer Res. 37: 166.

Schulte-Hermann, R., 1979, Reactions of the liver to injury:
Adaptation, Farber/Fisher (Eds.): Toxic Injury of the
liver (Marcel Dekker) New York, Chapter 9: 385.

Schulte-Hermann, R., and Schmitz, E., 1980, Feedback inhibition of hepatic DNA synthesis, Cell Tiss. Kinet. 13: 371.

Schulte-Hermann, R., Hoffmann, V., Parzefall, W., Kallenbach,
M., Gerhardt, A., and Schuppler, J., 1980, Adaptive
responses of rat liver to the gestagen and anti-androgen
cyproterone acetate and other inducers. II. Induction of
growth, Chem.-Biol. Interact. 31: 287.

Schulte-Hermann, R., Hoffmann, V., and Landgraf, H., 1980 a,
Adaptive responses of rat liver to the gestagen and
anti-androgen cyproterone acetate and other inducers.
III. Cytological changes, Chem.-Biol. Interact. 31: 3o1.

Schulte-Hermann, R., and Parzefall, W., 1981, Failure to dis-
    criminate initiation from promotion of liver tumors in
    a long-term study with the phenobarbital-type inducer
    α-hexachlorocyclohexane and the role of sustained stimu-
    lation of hepatic growth and monooxygenases, Cancer Res.
    41: 4140

Schulte-Hermann, R., Ohde, G., Schuppler, J., and Timmermann-
    Trosiener, I., 1981, Enhanced proliferation of putative
    preneoplastic cells in rat liver following treatment
    with the tumor promoters phenobarbital, hexachlorocyc-
    lohexane, steroid compounds, and nafenopin, Cancer Res.
    41: 2556.

Schulte-Hermann, R., Schuppler, J., Ohde, G., and Timmermann-
    Trosiener, I., 1982, Effect of tumor promoters on pro-
    liferation of putative preneoplastic cells in rat liver,
    Carcinogenesis 7: 99.

Solt, D., and Farber, E., 1976, New principle for the analy-
    sis of chemical carcinogenesis, Nature (Lond.) 263: 7ol.

Squire, R.A., and Levitt, M.H., 1975, Report of a workshop on
    classification of specific hepatocellular lesions in rats.
    Cancer Res. 35: 3214.

Taper, H.S., 1978, The effect of estradiol-17-phenylpropriona-
    te and estradiol benzoate on N-nitrosomorpholine-induced
    liver carcinogenesis in ovariectomized female rats,
    Cancer (Phila.) 42: 462.

Watanabe, K., and Williams, G.M., 1978, Enhancement of rat
    hepatocellular-altered foci by the liver tumor promoter
    phenobarbital: Evidence that foci are precursors of neo-
    plasms and that the promoter acts on carcinogen-induced
    lesions, J. Natl. Cancer Inst. 61: 1311.

Yager, J.D., and Yager, R., 1980, Oral contraceptive steroids
    as promoters of hepatocarcinogenesis in female Sprague-
    Dawley rats, Cancer Res. 40: 3680.

MOLECULAR MECHANISMS

OF MULTISTAGE CARCINOGENESIS

I. Bernard Weinstein

Division of Environmental Sciences and
Cancer Center/Institute of Cancer Research
Columbia University College of Physicians and Surgeons
New York, New York 10032

INTRODUCTION

The subject of chemical carcinogenesis is an exciting one for at least three reasons. One, it deals with a disease of major magnitude. Cancer is the second leading cause of death in the United States and the Western World. Two, it probes some of the most fundamental questions in contemporary biology, i.e. questions related to DNA structure, chromatin and the control of gene expression, membrane structure and function, the very basic problem of growth control and the specificity and stability of cellular differentiation. Three, it brings together investigators from such diverse disciplines as epidemiology, toxicology, cell biology and molecular genetics.

Epidemiologic studies have provided persuasive evidence that a major fraction of human cancer is due to environmental (i.e. exogenous) rather than endogenous factors (1). This is an optimistic message since it means that if we could identify the exogenous causative factors we could hope to prevent a major fraction of human cancer, either by reducing human exposure or somehow protecting the host. Significant progress has already been made through the identification of cigarette smoking as the major cause of lung cancer. In addition, over 20 chemicals or chemical processes have been implicated in various forms of human cancer (2). However, the specific causes of other major cancers (i.e. cancers of the large bowel and breast) have not been identified with certainty. In addition, several important general questions remain unresolved. These include the current controversies concerning the extent to which human cancers are due to naturally occuring versus man-made chemicals, the relative contribution of initiators and promoters, the roles of chemical versus viral agents, the role of general nutritional factors (i.e. fat, fiber and vitamins) and the role of multifactor interactions. This chapter will briefly review what I believe are the major known facts and unanswered questions related to the mechanism of action of chemical carcinogens.

THE ACTION OF INITIATING AGENTS; METABOLISM AND COVALENT BINDING TO MACROMOLECULES

The principle that many carcinogens undergo metabolic activation to electrophiles that bind covalently to DNA, as well as RNA and protein, has become an axiom in our field (3,4). There is some, but not conclusive, evidence that the covalent binding to DNA is a critical event in the carcinogenic process (4). Thus factors that limit or inhibit DNA excision repair appear to enhance carcinogenesis. The evidence is, however, indirect and certainly does not exclude the possibility that RNA and protein binding are also critical events in the action of some carcinogens.

At the present time we know very little about what determines carcinogen potency, organ specificity and species specificity. In some cases differences in metabolic activation or detoxification, or differential rates of repair of specific DNA adducts (i.e. O^6 methylguanine), have been demonstrated and associated with organ and species specificity (1,4). However, detailed comparative biochemistry and the actual mechanisms underlying these differences are poorly understood at the present time. In addition, I believe that other mechanisms, such as those related to tumor promotion and progression and cofactor interactions, are also major factors in determining carcinogen potency and specificity.

With several carcinogens the chemistry and steric aspects of their interactions with nucleic acids are now understood in considerable detail. (3-10). Different carcinogens can attack different sites on the DNA, and even a single carcinogen can form multiple types of adducts. This complicates attempts to formulate a unified or simple theory relating specific types of DNA damage to the mechanism of carcinogenesis. Although several chemical carcinogens form specific covalent adducts with DNA it is likely that other carcinogenic agents (ionizing radiation, free radicals, activated oxygen, etc.) produce their effects by a "hit and run" attack on the DNA. The detection and quantification of these effects is much more difficult, but is obviously an important area for further research.

An additional complexity is the emerging evidence that although the B DNA helix of Watson and Crick is the predominant conformation of DNA, alternative conformations can exist (11).

Sage and Leng (15), and our group in collaboration with A. Rich (12,13), have obtained evidence that the modification of poly (dG.dC), (dG.dC) by AAF induces it to flip from the conventional right-handed B helix to the left handed Z DNA. If similar events occur in vivo, then unusual base sequences of DNA might be preferential targets and/or undergo specific conformational changes in response to carcinogen modification. This could be particularly important when one considers the likelihood that in the chromatin structure regions of the DNA might be held in specific conformations because of their association with proteins.

Most of the studies on carcinogen-DNA interactions have focused on nuclear DNA. We have found, however, that when cell cultures are exposed to either radioactive BP or BPDE there is also very extensive modification of mitochondrial DNA (mtDNA) (14). Allen and Coombs (15) have also seen this with a variety of PAH carcinogens. Extensive modification of mtDNA by alkylating agents has also been seen in vivo (16). The functional significance of carcinogen attack on mtDNA is not known. This could of course cause disturbance in energy metabolism, although we favor the possibility that perturbations of mitochondrial ion flux, particularly intracellular Ca^{2+} homeostasis, might be more important, and thus contribute to alterations in growth control in carcinogen-exposed cells.

A multiplicity of DNA excision repair mechanisms exist (17), but much less is known about the consequences of persistent lesions with respect to DNA replication and gene transcription, particularly in eukaryotes. The in vitro modification of DNA, RNA and synthetic nucleic acids by carcinogens impairs their template activities during in vitro replication, transcription and translation (4,6,8). Although in some cases mispairing errors can be demonstrated, I am struck by the fact that the most predominant effects are usually inhibition of template function and often arrest of synthesis at the site of carcinogen modification. It is possible, therefore, that complex host responses to the latter events, analogous to the "SOS" response in bacteria, might be more important in carcinogenesis than simple errors in base pairing (18).

Table 1 lists several possible mechanisms by which covalent modification of DNA by carcinogens might initiate the carcinogenic process. I have argued elsewhere (4,19) that it is unlikely that the process involves random point mutations. Evidence against this includes: 1) the above described effects on template function, 2) the fact that the in vitro transformation of rodent cells by chemical carcinogens and radiation can occur with a much higher efficiency than random mutation (for review see ref. 19), 3) the fact that although human and rodent cell cultures are equally susceptible to mutagenesis human cells appear to be much more

Table 1. Possible Molecular Mechanisms of Initiation
          of the Carcinogenesis Process

<u>A</u>. <u>With Permanent Changes in DNA Sequence</u>:

   1. Random point mutation
      a. Direct: base substitution, frame shift,
         deletion in structural or regulatory
         gene.

      b. Indirect: induction of "SOS-type" error-
         prone DNA synthesis.

<u>B</u>. <u>Without Permanent Changes in DNA Sequence</u>:

   Altered chromatin structure, altered feedback loops,
   DNA methylation, etc.

For a detailed discussion see text and ref. 19.

resistant to cell transformation, 4) the long lag between carcinogen exposure and tumor formation, and 5) the striking parallels
between differentiation and carcinogenesis (19,21). Of the possible mechanisms listed in Table 1, I believe that the induction of
gene rearrangements and/or alterations in the state of methylation
of specific genes are likely to be the key events in carcinogenesis. The latter mechanism is of considerable interest because
of the increasing evidence that activation of gene expression is
often associated with a decrease in 5 methylcytidine content of
the expressed gene, although other factors must also play an important role (22). Later I shall return to the possible role of
gene rearrangements in carcinogenesis.

TUMOR PROMOTION & MULTIFACTOR INTERACTIONS

Two Stage Skin Carcinogenesis

There is increasing appreciation of the fact that in the intact animal carcinogenesis is a multistage process than can
proceed over a considerable fraction of the lifespan of the individual, and that the evolution of a fully malignant tumor is subject to a variety of promoting as well as inhibitory factors
(19,23). These basic phenomenae are also becoming apparent during
the transformation of cells in culture, whether the process is induced by chemical carcinogens or certain oncogenic viruses
(19,24). Indeed, it seems likely that a full understanding of the

molecular mechanisms of the initial events in the carcinogenic process will also require an understanding of the later events.

The most powerful paradigm for understanding these complex phenomanae has been the model of two stage carcinogenesis on mouse skin, where at least two stages, initiation and promotion have been clearly defined (23,25). Each of these stages is elicited or inhibited by different types of agents, and the two stages have different biologic properties. As stressed elsewhere (19,26), the major difference is that whereas initiation appears to involve DNA damage, this is not the case for promotion. The two stage mouse skin carcinogenesis system has also served as a paradigm for studies on the multistage aspects of carcinogenesis in several other tissues and species. Evidence that hepatocellular cancer, bladder cancer, colon cancer and breast cancer also proceed via processes analogous to initiation and promotion has been reviewed elsewhere (23,27). The concept of promotion appears to be particularly relevant to the causation of human breast cancer (27).

Whereas just a few years ago there were very few specific cellular or biochemical markers for the action of tumor promoters, exciting advances have recently been made through studies on the biochemical effects of the phorbol esters in cell culture systems and on mouse skin (for review see refs. 19,23,28). Indeed, there has been such a plethora of findings that it will now require a considerable scientific effort to determine which of them are relevant to the mechanism of tumor promotion, and which are epiphenomonae. It will be important, for example, to distinguish effects peculiar to the particular specialized cells examined (i.e. macrophages or lymphocytes), or in vitro toxic effects, from those that actually occur during tumor promotion on mouse skin.

In an attempt to rationalize the numerous effects elicited by the phorbol ester tumor promoters I have classified them into three categories (19,26), all of which conveniently begin with the letter "M": 1) Mimicry of transformation, 2) Modulation of differentiation, and 3) Membrane effects. Perhaps the most intriguing capacity of the potent tumor promoter 12-0-tetra-decanoyl-phorbol-13-acetate (TPA), and related phorbol esters, are their abilities to induce in normal cells the expression of several phenotypic traits characteristic of tumor cells, and to enhance the further expression of some of these traits in cells that are already transformed (19,26,28). These findings provide a clear demonstration of a recurring theme in cancer biology, i.e. that the phenotypic properties of tumor cells pre-exist but lie dormant in the normal tissue of origin. The phorbol esters provide potent pharmacologic agents for studying the cellular mechanisms that control the expression of these genes.

Since it is likely that carcinogenesis involves major disturbances in differentiation, it is of interest that TPA is a highly
potent inhibitor or inducer of differentiation in a variety of
cell systems (19,26,28). The examples include a variety of programs of differentiation and cells from such diverse species as
avian, rodent, human and even echinoderm. The ability of tumor
promoters to inhibit terminal differentiation may be central to
their action as tumor promoters (19,26). The basal cells in the
adult epidermis are continually dividing, yet the tissue is in a
state of balanced growth because of asymmetric division of stem
cells. One daughter cell remains a stem cell and the other is
committed to keratinize and terminally differentiate, thus, irreversibly losing its growth potential. If an "initiated" stem
cell were restrained to this mode of division, it could not increase its proportion in the stem cell pool. If this mode of tissue renewal was interrupted by a tumor promoter, the initiated
cell could undergo exponential division this yielding a clone of
similar cells. Since TPA can also induce phenotypic changes in
cells that mimic those of transformed cells, the microenvironment
of a clone of such cells might itself enhance their further outgrowth and development into a tumor. In addition, clonal expansion of the population of intiated cells would provide a larger
population from which variants that have undergone progression to
later stages of neoplasia might emerge. I assume that in those
tissues in which TPA induces rather than inhibits terminal differentiation it would not be a tumor promoter. This could provide
one explanation for the tissue specificity of the phorbol esters
as tumor promoters. It might be possible to design phorbol analo-
gues that induce the terminal differentiation of certain neoplastic cells yet lack significant tumor promoting activity. Such
compounds would offer a novel approach to cancer chemotherapy.

Phorboid Receptors

Our studies on the cell culture effects of the phorbol ester
tumor promoters led us to suggest that they act by binding to and
usurping the function of membrane-associated receptors that are
normally utilized by an endogenous growth factor (19). Indirect
evidence for this hypothesis includes: (a) the fact that these
compounds act in a concentration range similar to that of several
hormones and growth factors (i,e. $\sim 10^{-8}$ 10^{-10}M),(b) the fact that
these compounds display very similar structure-function requirements on cells from diverse species and tissues, and (c) the fact
that like known hormones they induce highly pleiotropic effects
which vary considerably depending upon the target cell. Since the
earliest cellular responses to these agents occur at the cell surface membrane (26), we suggested that the putative receptors were
associated with the plasma membrane (19,26).

By utilizing ^{3}H-phorbol dibutyrate (PDBu), which is much less hydrophobic than TPA, to overcome the problem of non-specific binding, Blumberg et al have obtained direct evidence for specific high affinity saturable receptors in crude membrane preparations of chick embryo fibroblasts (29) and mouse epidermis (30). Our laboratory and others (32-34) have extended this approach to studies on phorboid receptors in intact cells. A Scatchard analysis of ^{3}H-PDBu binding to intact ray embryo fibroblasts suggests that there are at least two classes of specific binding sites, a high affinity class with K_D of about 8nM, and 1.6 x 10[5] sites per cell, and a low affinity class with a K_D of 710 nM, and about 2 x 10[6] sites per cell (31). Specific high affinity phorbol ester receptors have been detected in a variety of both normal and transformed cell cultures and in a variety of normal tissues, with the exception of mature red blood cells (29-34). With prolonged exposure cell cultures display what appears to be down-regulation of the phorboid receptors, a phenomenon characteristic of several other membrane-associated receptors. This aspect could play a role in dose-schedule and tissue specific effects of TPA.

In general, the abilities of a series of TPA analogs to compete with ^{3}H-PDBu for binding to cell surface receptors correlates with their known potencies in cell culture and with their activities as tumor promoters on mouse skin (29-34). These results provide evidence that the ^{3}H-PDBu receptors mediate the biologic action of the phorbol esters. In collaborative studies we have found that the indole alkaloid teleocidin B is also a potent inhibitor of ^{3}H-PDBu binding (35). This result is of particular interest since, although this compound is structurally unrelated to the phorbol esters (Figure 1), Sugimura and his colleagues have found that it shares with these compounds a number of similar cell culture effects, and is also as potent as TPA as a tumor promoter on mouse skin (36).

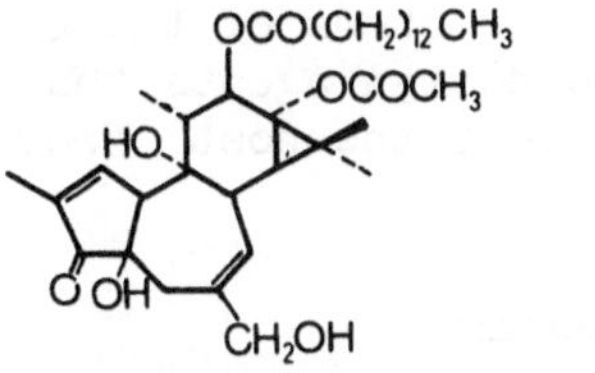

TPA 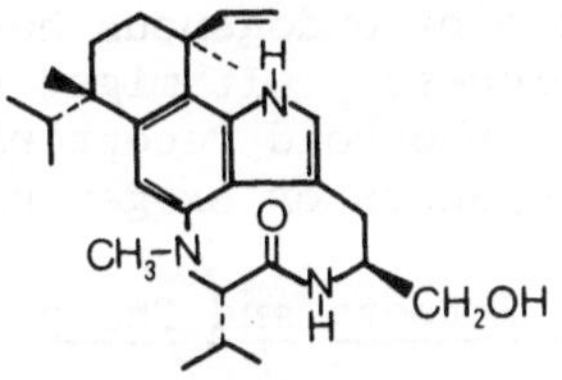   TELEOCIDIN

Figure 1

We have also found that, like TPA, nanomolar concentrations of
teleocidin B and dihydroteleocidin induce a rapid increase in
2-deoxyglucose uptake, induce arachidonic acid release and prostaglandin synthesis, and inhibit EGF receptor binding(36). The
results obtained with the teleocidins suggest that the phorboid
receptors mediate the effects of both the phorbol esters and the
teleocidin tumor promoters, thus explaining their similar, if not
identical, effects on cells. Despite their dissimilar chemical
structures, model building studies suggest that TPA and teleocidin
share similar three-dimensional features and this may explain
their apparent affinities for the same set of receptors (Horowitz,
A., Jeffrey, A. and Weinstein, I.B., unpublished studies).

A number of polypetide growth factors and various hormones
fail to inhibit ^{3}H-PDBu-receptor binding (29-32). We have found
that sera from a variety of species, amniotic fluid and various
tissue extracts do inhibit specific ^{3}H-PDBu binding, and this factor has been partially purified from human serum (31). Studies
are in progress to determine whether this substance merely inhibits binding or whether it binds directly to the phorboid receptors and serves as an endogenous agonist or antagonist.

What might be the normal function of phorboid receptors and
their putative endogenous ligand? We postulate that this effector
system could play a role during embryogenesis by enhancing the
outgrowth of new stem cell populations. In the adult this same
system might enhance expansion of stem cell populations during hyperplasia, wound healing and regeneration. In all of these situations it might be necessary to transiently inhibit terminal differentiation so as to expand the proliferative population, and
then at a later time turn off this effector system to allow terminal differentiation to proceed and to return to a stable state of
tissue renewal. During tumor promotion aberrant stem cells (generated during initiation) might undergo preferential clonal expansion as a result of excessive stimulation of the phorboid receptor
system. This model has obvious implications in terms of the possible role of endogenous host factors as promoters of the carcinogenic process. It might be possible to design agents that would
block the phorboid receptors and thus protect the host from certain endogenous or exogenous promoters.

Membrane Effects and Phospholipid Metabolism.

The earliest responses of cells to the phorbol ester tumor
promoters involve alterations in membrane function (19,26) (Table
2). This also appears to be the case with teleocidin (35). Some
of these membrane effects occur within minutes and are not blocked
by inhibitors of protein or RNA synthesis. Therefore, they are
mediated directly at the level of the cell membrane presumably
through the activation of pre-existent enzymes or other membrane

associated proteins. It is not clear whether the primary effect of these tumor promoters is due to alterations in ion flux (37-39) or activation of proteases (40), esterases (41), protein kinases, phospholipases, etc.

Table 2. Effects of TPA on Cell Surfaces and
Membranes in Cell Culture

Altered Na/K ATPase
Increased Uptake 2-DG, ^{32}P, ^{86}Rb
Increased Membrane Lipid "Fluidity"
Increased Phospholipid Synthesis
Increased Release Arachidonic Acid, Prostaglandins
Altered Morphology and Cell-Cell Orientation
Altered Cell Adhesion
Increased Pinocytosis
Altered Fucose-Glycopeptides
Decreased LETS Protein
"Uncoupling" of β-Adrenergic Receptors
Inhibition of Binding of EGF to Receptors
Decrease in Acetylcholine Receptors
Synergistic Interaction with Growth Factors
Inhibition of Metabolic Cooperation

For specific refs. see refs. 19,26.

Exposure of cells to the phorbol ester tumor promoters causes a rapid increase in membrane phospholipid turnover. TPA stimulates the incorporation of p^{32} and choline into membrane phospholipids; it also induces deacylation of phospholipids with release of arachidonic acid and an increase in prostaglandin synthesis (for review see refs 19,26). Recently, we discovered that within 5 min. TPA induces the release of choline from the phosphatidyl choline fraction of C3H 10T1/2 cells (19,41). Figure 2 presents a hypothetical scheme of the effects of TPA and other compounds on phospholipid metabolism. Our results (19,26) suggest that TPA-induced choline release from membrane phospholipids is due to activation of an endogenous phospholipase C or D. This would result in the accumulation of diacylglycerol. TPA-induced arachidonic acid release and prostaglandin synthesis may be due to the subsequent action of a diacylglycerol lipase. Alternatively, TPA could have an independent effect on phospholipase A_2. These events might then be followed by compensatory resynthesis of phosphatidyl choline via CDP choline transferase (Figure 2).

Several questions remain unresolved with respect to the effects of the phorbol esters on phospholipid metabolism. Are these effects due to perturbation in the phospholipid substrate or to activation of membrane-associated phospholipases? Since phospholipases are activated by Ca^{2+}, does TPA produce its effects on phospholipid metabolism by altering Ca^{2+} flux or intracellular distribution? Does the phorbol ester-induced degradation of phosphatidyl choline generate metabolites that mediate subsequent events in this cascade. These mediators could include: arachidonic acid metabolites (cyclooxygenase or lipoxygenase products), lysophospholipids, phosphatidic acid, or diacylglycerol. Do the effects of the phorbol esters on phospholipid metabolism produce a generalized change in the physical properties of the lipid matrix of cell membranes, for example increased fluidity (19,26), which then alters the activities of a number of membrane-associated proteins and functions? We have suggested that the role of dietary lipid in enhancing colon and breast cancer might be mediated by changes in membrane lipids in the target tissue, changes that are similar to those produced by tumor promoters (27). Thus, much more work is required to clarify the role of lipid metabolism in tumor promotion.

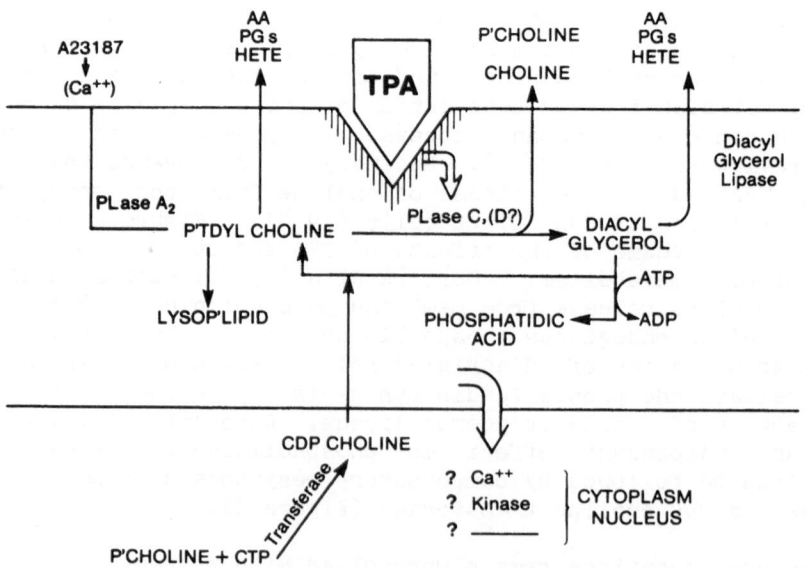

Figure 2. Effects of TPA on Phospholipid Metabolism
(for details see ref. 19,42)

In view of current evidence that the viral "sarc" genes are protein kinases(43), an attractive mechanism to explain the mimicry of transformation by tumor promoters is that they might activate endogenous protein kinases. Direct tests of this hypothesis with respect to the avian pp60 sarc protein kinases have been negative (44,45), but because of the complexities of the "sarc" gene system these results do not rule out the general hypothesis. The search for novel protein kinase activities in cells treated with tumor promoters and various growth factors will, no doubt, be an intensive area of future research.

Tumor Promoting Activity of Polycyclic Aromatic Hydrocarbons

Although the application of a single low dose of BP or other PAH carcinogens to mouse skin does not induce skin tumors unless this is followed by repeated applications of a tumor promoter, repeated applications of a PAH carcinogen will induce skin tumors (25). This suggests that PAHs can have tumor promoting activity. Therefore, we have recently studied the possibility that PAH carcinogens might induce cell membrane changes that are similar to those induced by the phorbol ester tumor promoters. We have indeed found that the exposure of C3H 10T1/2 cells to BP and certain other PAHs leads to a loss of EGF-receptor binding (46,47). These and other results have led us to propose that binding of certain compounds to the cytosolic "Ah" receptor induces a pleiotropic program that includes not only increases in certain drug metabolizing enzymes, but also changes in membrane structure and function (46,47). Thus certain PAHs might be complete carcinogens because they not only are they converted to metabolites that bind covalently to cellular DNA, but they also induce membrane changes that alter growth and differentiation. Other classes of compounds might also be complete carcinogens because they have both genotoxic and membrane effects. We have presented evidence that glucocorticoids may inhibit carcinogenesis by inducing membrane effects that are reciprocal to those induced by PAHs and tumor promoters (47).

Chromosomal Effects and Activated Oxygen

It has been suggested that tumor promoters act by inducing a heterozygous recessive mutation (established by the initiator) to be expressed (48). A few studies have shown that TPA can induce sister chromatid exchange (SCE) as well as various chromosomal aberrations (48,49,50). These effects have not, however, been highly reproducible between laboratories, often require high concentrations of the TPA, sometimes are seen only with certain batches of TPA (raising the question of a contaminant) and do not occur with all cell types. Moreover, we know that when a population of cells is exposed to TPA the entire population responds within minutes or hours and the effects are usually reversible when the agent is removed (19). In addition, the papillomas on mouse skin often regress when application of the tumor promoters is stopped (25). Thus, chromosome aberrations or segregation could not account for the early effects of tumor promoters. The malignant tumors that appear much later on mouse skin are auto-nomous and often show chromosomal abnormalities. Thus if the in vitro chromosomal effects of TPA have any significance I suggest that they relate more to late stages in the process such as tumor progression rather than to tumor promotion.

TPA and teleocidin induce oxygen radicals and peroxides in polymorphonuclear leukocytes (40). The stimulation of arachidonic acid metabolism and lipid turnover by tumor promoters could gen-erate highly reactive forms of activated oxygen (51) that could lead to lipid peroxidation and other toxic effects, including chromosomal damage. It is essential to determine whether or not such effects are confined to only certain cell types, whether they occur only under conditions of toxicity, and whether they can ac-tually be associated with tumor promotion or progression on mouse skin.

Chemical-Viral Interactions

There are several examples in which initiating carcinogens, tumor promoters or other chemical and physical agents interact synergistically with viruses in the carcinogenic process, both in vivo and in cell culture (for review see refs. 24,52). Indeed, it seems likely that certain human cancers may be due to interactions between chemical agents and types of viruses which alone would have little or no oncogenic potential. This appears to be the case for liver cancer in Africa, nasopharyngeal cancer in Asia and Burkitt's lymphoma (27,52).

We discovered that the transformation of rat embryo (RE) cells by an adenovirus is enhanced when the infected cells are grown in the presence of phorbol ester tumor promoters; EGF and melittin also enhanced adenovirus transformation (52). TPA and EGF also induce the growth in agar of morphologically altered adenovirus-transformed RE cells (52), which may provide a useful in vitro model for studying the process of tumor progression. Subsequent studies have revealed that TPA also enhances cell transformation induced by EBV virus (53), polyoma virus (54) and SV40 virus (55). In addition, it accelerates the replication and cytopathic effects of adenovirus in human cells (56), enhances EBV replication and antigen expression in lymphoblast cell lines (53), and enhances the replication of mouse mammary tumor virus (57), and an endogenous murine xenotropic type-C retrovirus (58). TPA also enhances the expression of markers of transformation in chick embryo fibroblasts transformed by RSV (44,45). It is unfortunate that in the past cancer research has been polarized into two camps, those in search of viruses as causes of human cancer and those in search of human chemical carcinogens. I suspect that much greater progress will be made if one takes the view that certain human cancers result from complex interactions between viruses and chemicals.

A UNIFIED THEORY OF INITIATION AND PROMOTION

I would now like to return to the question of the mechanism of initiation and describe a unified theory of initiation and promotion. This theory attempts to explain carcinogenesis within the framework of normal development and differentiation and also provides a bridge to current theories about the origin and mechanism of action of certain tumor viruses.

Earlier in this paper I presented several reasons why I think that initiation of carcinogenesis does not involve simple random point mutation resulting from errors in replication at the sites of DNA damage. It should be stressed that several laboratories have found that the frequency of transformation of rodent cell cultures induced by radiation or carcinogens can be ten to several hundred times that obtained for the induction of mutations to specific markers such as drug resistance, even when both types of phenomenae are scored in the same cell culture system (for review see ref. 19). This discrepancy is even greater when one considers the likelihood that cell transformation occurs via a multistep process which is limited, therefore, by the joint probabilities of each of the successive steps. Thus the initial step induced by the carcinogen may occur with even a greater frequency than the net transformation frequency. Indeed, there is evidence that when exposure to chemical carcinogens (59) or radiation (60) occurs at low cell densities almost 100% of the exposed cells are capable of giving rise to progeny that are transformed. This result provides evidence against random mutation, which usually occurs with a frequency in the range of 10^{-4} 10^{-6}).

We have previously postulated that the establishment of normal populations of stem cells involves gene rearrangements (for review of gene rearrangements see refs. 61,62) and that DNA damage by initiating carcinogens might induce with high frequency aberrant stem cells (19). The cassette model for the control of mating type in yeast (62) is a particularly attractive model for thinking about how gene rearrangements might be involved in differentiation and carcinogenesis. Some of the evidence favoring gene rearrangements rather than random mutations in the action of initiating carcinogens is summarized in Table 3.

Table 3.   Mechanism of Action of Initiating Carcinogens:
Evidence Against Random Mutation and
Favoring Gene Rearrangements

A.   High efficiency of cell transformation in vitro speaks
against random mutation:

1.   With chemicals or x-ray; in 10T1/2 or hamster
embryo cultures.
2.   Transformation frequency >> random mutation.
3.   "Initiation" of transformation can approach
100% efficiency.

B.   Characteristic of gene tranposition

1.   Occurs in prokaryotes and eukaryotes (i.e. cassette
model in yeast, immunoglobulin synthesis)
2.   High specificity and efficiency

C.   Models suggested from the action of retroviruses:

1.   Multiple sarc genes exist in normal vertebrate cells
2.   Transformation by retroviruses resembles gene
transposition

For details related to points A) and B) see text and ref. 19.
For reviews on gene transposition, sarc genes and retroviruses
see refs. 19,61,62,43.

The subsequent role of tumor promoters could be to enhance
the outgrowth of these aberrant stem cells, as well as to "switch
on" their abnormal programs of differentiation, just as endogenous
growth factors are apparently required to induce normal stem cells
to grow and express their specialized functions.   As discussed
above, presumably the phorbol ester tumor promoters accomplish
this by binding to and usurping the function of receptors normally
occupied by endogenous factors that control stem cell replication
and differentiation. Following repeated exposure of initiated
cells to a tumor promoter, a neoplastic population might eventually emerge which grows autonomously in the absence of the promoter,
perhaps due to further changes in genome structure. It is also
possible that the mechanism by which the transformed phenotype is
eventually "locked in" with respect to constitutive expression occurs by mechanisms (yet to be discovered) similar to those that
provide stability to normal states of differentiation. Cairns
(63) has also proposed that carcinogenesis involves gene rearrangements, although he arrived at this conclusion on the basis of
somewhat different evidence.

A major challenge to future research in carcinogenesis is to identify the specific host genes involved in the transformation of cells by chemical and physical agents and to utilize recombinant DNA techniques to analyze the state of integration and/or expression of these genes in normal and carcinogen-transformed cells. Recent studies (64,65) suggest that the techniques of DNA transfection may prove to be extremely useful for such studies. Studies of the RNA sarcoma viruses have led to the concept that they arose by the recombination of retroviruses with specific "onc" genes (also called sarc genes or proto-oncogenes) endogenous to normal vertebrate species (46). It is possible, therefore, that the same "onc" genes are involved in the transformation of cells by chemical carcinogens, but that in this case DNA damage triggers rearrangement and/or switch-on of these genes in the absence of a virus vector. Our research group is currently testing this hypothesis in carcinogen-transformed rodent cells (66,67).

REFERENCES

1. H. H. Hiatt and J. D. Watson (eds): "Origins of Human Cancer, Cold Spring Harbor Conferences on Cell Proliferation," Cold Spring Labs, Cold Spring Harbor, New York (1977).
2. IARC Monographs, Supplement 1 "Chemicals and Industrial Processes Associated with Cancer in Humans," International Agency for Research on Cancer, Lyon, France (1979).
3. E. Miller, Cancer Res. 38:1479 (1978).
4. I. B. Weinstein, in: S. Crooke and A. Prestayko (eds), "Cancer and Chemotherapy Vol. 1, Introduction to Neoplasia and Anti-Neoplastic Chemotherapy," pp. 169-196, Academic Press, New York (1980).
5. H. Gelboin and P.O.P. Ts'o (eds), "Polycylic Hydrocarbons and Cancer, Vol. 1 and 2," Academic Press, New York (1978).
6. B. Singer and B. Kroger, Prog. in Nucleic Acid Res. and Mol. Biol. 23:151 (1979).
7. D. Grunberger and I. B. Weinstein, in: P. L. Grover (ed), "Chemical Carcinogens and DNA," p. 59, CRC Press, Boca Raton, Florida (1979).
8. D. Grunberger and I. B. Weinstein, in: W. Cohen (ed), Prog. in Nucleic Acid Res. and Mol. Biol, Vol 23, pp 105-149, Academic Press, New York (1979).
9. I. B. Weinstein, R. A. Mufson, L. S. Lee, P. B. Fisher, J. Laskin, A. Horowitz and V. Ivanovic, in: B. Pullman, P.O.P. Ts'o and H. Gelboin (eds), "Carcinogenesis: Fundamental Mechanisms and Environmental Effects," pp 543-563, R. Reidel Pub. Co., Amsterdam, Holland (1980).
10. A. M. Jeffrey, T. Kinoshita, R. M. Santella, D. Grunberger, L. Katz and I. B. Weinstein, in: B. Pullman, P.O.P. Ts'o and H. Gelboin (eds), "Carcinogenesis: Fundamental Mechanisms and Environmental Effects," pp 565-579, R. Reidel Pub. Co., Am-

sterdam, Holland (1980).

11. A. H. Wang, G. J. Quigley, F. J. Kolpak, J. L. Cranford, J. A. Van Boom, G. Vander Macel and A. Rich, Nature, 282:680 (1979).

12. E. Sage and M. Leng, Proc. Natl. Acad. Sci. USA 77:4597 (1980).

13. R. Santella, D. Grunberger, I. B. Weinstein and A. Rich, Proc. Natl. Acad. Sci. USA 78:1451 (1981).

14. J. Backer and I. B. Weinstein, Science 209:297 (1980).

15. J. A. Allen and M. M. Coombs, Nature 287:244 (1980).

16. V. Wunderlich, I. Tetzlaff and A. Graffi, Chemical-Biological Interactions 4:81 (1971/72).

17. P. C. Hanawalt, E. C. Friedberg and C. F. Fox (eds), "DNA Repair Mechanisms," Academic Press, New York (1978).

18. V. Ivanovic and I. B. Weinstein, Cancer Res. 40:3508 (1980).

19. I. B. Weinstein, R. A. Mufson, L. S. Lee, P. B. Laskin, A. Horowitz and V. Ivanovic, in: B. Pullman, P. O. P. Ts´o and H. Gelboin (eds), "Carcinogenesis: Fundamental Mechanisms and Environmental Effects," pp 543-563, R. Reidel Pub. Co., Amsterdam, Holland (1980).

20. G. B. Pierce, R. Shikes and L. M. Fink, "Cancer: A Problem in Developmental Biology," Prentice-Hall, Inc., Englewood Cliffs, New Jersey (1978).

21. A. C. Braun, An Epigenetic Model for the Origin of Cancer, Quart. Rev. Biol. 56:33 (1981).

22. A. Razin and A. D. Riggs, Science 210:604 (1980).

23. T. J. Slaga, A. Sivak and R. K. Boutwell (eds), "Mechanisms of Tumor Promotion and Cocarcinogenesis, Vol. 2," Raven Press, New York (1978).

24. P. B. Fisher, N. I. Goldstein and I. B. Weinstein, Cancer Res. 39:3051 (1979).

25. I. Berenblum, in: F. F. Becker (ed), "Cancer," p. 323, Plenum Press, New York (1975).

26. I. B. Weinstein, L. S. Lee, P. B. Fisher, A. Mufson and H. Yamasaki, J. of Supramolecular Struct. 12:195 (1979).

27. I. B. Weinstein, in: C. McGrath, M. J. Brennan and M. A. Rich (eds), "Cell Biology of Breast Cancer," Academic Press, New York (1981).

28. L. Diamond, T. G. O´Brien and G. Rovera, Life Sci. 23:1979 (1978).

29. P. E. Driedger and P. M. Blumberg, Proc. Natl. Acad. Sci. USA 77:567 (1980).

30. K. B. Delclos, D. S. Nagle and P. M. Blumberg, Cell 19:1025 (1980).

31. A. D. Horowitz, E. Greenebaum and I. B. Weinstein, Proc. Natl. Acad. Sci. USA 78:2315 (1981).

32. M. Shoyab and G. J. Todaro, Nature 288:451 (1980).

33. V. Solanki and T. J. Slaga, Proc. Natl. Acad. Sci. USA 78:2549 (1981).

34. C. L. Ashendel and R. K. Boutwell, Biochem. Biophys. Res.

Commun. 99:543 (1981).

35. K. Umezawa, I. B. Weinstein, A. D. Horowitz, H. Fujiki, T. Matsushima and T. Sugimura, Nature 290:411 (1981).
36. H. Fujiki, M. Mori, M. Nakayasu, M. Terada, T. Sugimura and R. Moore, Proc. Natl. Acad. Sci. 78:3872 (1981).
37. C. Wenner, J. Hackney, H. Kimellog and E. Mayhew, Cancer Res. 34:1731 (1978).
38. E. Rozengurt, Annals of the New York Academy of Sciences 339:175 (1980).
39. P. B. Fisher and I. B. Weinstein, Carcinogenesis 2:89 (1981).
40. W. Troll, G. Witz, B. Goldstein, D. Stone and T. Sugimura, in: E. Hecker (ed), "Cocarcinogens and Biological Effects," Raven Press, (in press) (1981).
41. P. W. Wertz and G. C. Mueller, Proc. Amer. Assoc. Cancer Res. 21:128 (1980).
42. R. A. Mufson, E. Okin and I. B. Weinstein, Carcinogenesis, (in press) (1981).
43. "Cold Spring Harbor Symp. Quant. Biol, Vol. 44: Viral Oncogenesis (1981).
44. A. R. Goldberg, K. B. Delclos and P. M. Blumberg, Science 208:191 (1980).
45. C. Pietrapaolo, J. Laskin and I. B. Weinstein, Cancer Res. 41:1565 (1981).
46. V. Ivanovic and I. B. Weinstein, J. Supramolec. Struct. Suppl. 5 (Abstr.) 232 (1981).
47. V. Ivanovic and I. B. Weinstein, Nature 392:404 (1981).
48. A. R. Kinsella and M. Radman, Proc. Natl. Acad. Sci. 75:6149 (1978).
49. H. Nagasawa and J. B. Little, Proc. Natl. Acad. Sci. 76:1943 (1979).
50. I. Emerit and P. A. Cerutti, Nature 293:144 (1981).
51. I. Fridovich, Science 201:875 (1978).
52. P. B. Fisher and I. B. Weinstein, in: R. Montesano, H. Bartsch and L. Tomatis (eds), "Molecular and Cellular Aspects of Carcinogen Screening Tests," pp. 113-131, Intl. Agency Research on Cancer, Lyon, France (1980).
53. N. Yamamota and H. Zur Hausen, Nature 280:244 (1979).
54. R. Seif, J. Virol. 36:421 (1980).
55. R. G. Martin, V. P. Setlow, C. A. Edwards and D. Vembu, Cell 17:635 (1979).
56. P. B. Fisher, C. S. H. Young and I. B. Weinstein, and T. H. Carter, Molecular and Cellular Biology 1:370 (1981).
57. S. K. Arya, Nature 284:71 (1980).
58. K. Hellman, A. Hellman, Int. J. Cancer 27:95 (1981).
59. S. Mondal and C. Heidelberg, Proc. Natl. Acad. Sci. USA 65:219 (1970).
60. A. R. Kennedy, M. Fox, J. Murray and J. B. Little, Proc. Natl. Acad. Sci. USA 77:7262 (1980).
61. R. McKay, Nature 287:188 (1980).
62. I. Herskowitz, L. Blair, D. Forbes, J. Hicks, Y. Kassir, P.

Kushner, J. Rine, G. Sprague and J. Strathern, in: T. Leighton and W. F. Loomis (eds), "Molecular Genetics of Development," Academic Press, New York, (1980).

63. J. Cairns, Nature 289:353 (1981).

64. C. Shih, L. C. Padhy, M. Murray and R. A. Weinberg, Nature 290:261 (1981).

65. T. G. Krantiris and G. M. Cooper, Proc. Natl. Acad. Sci. USA 78:1181 (1981).

66. S. Gattoni, P. Kirschmeier, I. B. Weinstein, J. Escobedo and D. Dina, Molecular and Cellular Biology, (in press) (1981).

67. P. Kirschmeier, S. Gattoni, D. Dina and I. B. Weinstein, (manuscript submitted for publication) (1981).

ALTERATIONS OF LIVER ARCHITECTURE IN MICE TREATED WITH ANABOLIC
ANDROGENS AND DIETHYLNITROSAMINE

W. Taylor[*], S. Snowball, C.M. Dickson[**] and
Milena Lesna[***]

Department of Physiological Sciences, The Animal Unit[**]
The Medical School, The University, Newcastle upon Tyne
NE1 7RU and Department of Pathology[***], Royal Victoria
Hospital, Shelley Road, Bournemouth, BH1 4JG; England

INTRODUCTION

It has been recognised for decades that there is a relationship
between endogenous steroid sex hormones and cancers of organs and
tissues which are target organs of these steroids. The most extensively studied cancers are those of the breast, uterus and prostate
gland. However, it is still a matter of debate as to whether or
not the steroids themselves (or activated metabolites) are implicated in the start of the process(es) which cause the tissues to
develop malignant tumours. That is, are endogenous steroid
hormones initiators of carcinogenesis? Many other factors have
been implicated in the development and progress of hormone-related
cancers in man; family history, parity, ethnic origins, oncongenic
viruses, etc. Thus it seems that many complex and interacting
processes are involved in the incidence and development of many
human cancers (see Review by Taylor, 1981a).

With the development of steroidal oral contraceptives and the
increasing use of diverse types of anabolic androgens in human
therapeutics a further dimension was added to the possible carcinogenic activity of natural steroids and their pharmacological anal-
ogues. This applies particularly to benign and malignant tumours
of the liver (Evans, 1978; Sherlock, 1978). Another matter of
current concern is the possible hazard to the human population of
residues of anabolic agents in meat products from farm animals
treated with such agents (Taylor, 1981b).

*To whom all correspondence should be addressed.

The relationship between alterations in liver architecture caused by oral contraceptives and anabolic androgens became confused for two main reasons.   Firstly, it was considered by some that the steroidal structure itself would produce the same type of liver lesions and disturbances of hepatic function, since it was not realised that a close similarity in chemical structure is not necessarily related to a similar physiological (or pathological) response.   Thus, components of oral contraceptives produce, amongst other effects, marked changes in biliary lipids leading to an increased tendency to develop cholesterol gallstones (e.g. Anderson et al., 1980), whereas in some animals anabolic androgens have little if any effect on biliary lipids (Dickson et al., 1979). Secondly, as pointed out in the authoritative Review of Ishak (1979), there was, and to a certain extent still is, considerable confusion in the literature about the nomenclature used by pathologists to describe the same or even different types of hepatic lesions, especially those caused by oral contraceptives or anabolic androgens.

The purpose of the present investigation was to compare the effect of a 17α-alkylated anabolic steroid, methyltestosterone (MeT) with a commonly used anabolic androgen without a 17α-alkyl substituent, 17β-hydroxy-19-nor-4-androsten-3-ene-17β-n-decanoate (Decadurabolin*) (DecaD) on liver architecture in Balb/C mice, a strain with little or no tendency to develop hepatic or mammary tumours spontaneously.   The route of administration and the doses used approximated to those used in man in terms of mg/kg.   The second part of the work was concerned with the possible role of diethylnitrosamine (DEN) as an initiator of hepatic cancer and of DecaD as a promoter.

EXPERIMENTAL

Experiment A

Sixty male and 60 female Balb/C mice, aged 3 months, were fed a commercial diet containing MeT such that the daily oral dose of the steroid was 150μg per day.   The same numbers of age-matched controls received diet only.   Similarly, 60 mice of each sex were given 125μg of DecaD in 0.1 ml of arachis oil by subcutaneous injection once weekly.   Age-matched control animals received arachis oil only by the same route.

Experiment B

Sixty male and 60 female mice, 3 months old, were given 160μg of DEN in 0.2 ml of water by stomach tube every 3 days for 8 weeks.

The DEN solution was made up immediately before use.   After an
interval of 8 weeks the DEN-treated animals were divided into 2
groups of 30 (A and B below) and 3 groups of 30 age-matched
untreated animals were introduced (Groups C-E below).   Group A
received weekly injections of 50μg of DecaD in 0.1 ml of arachis
oil (i.e. DEN plus DecaD); Group B were injected once weekly with
0.1 ml of arachis oil (i.e. DEN plus arachis oil); Group C (no
previous treatment) were given 50μg of DecaD in 0.1 ml of arachis
oil once weekly (DecaD only); Group D (not previously treated)
were given 0.1 ml of arachis oil once weekly (i.e. arachis oil
only); Group E received no treatment.   Treatment extended over 8
weeks.   During this time some animals in all groups died of non-
specific causes.   All animals were killed 3 months after the last
treatment.   Livers, lungs and kidneys were removed and placed in
10% buffered formol-saline.

RESULTS

Experiment A.   The livers from MeT-treated mice were more thoroughly studied, although the results of DecaD-treatment were the same
in most respects.   Livers of all male animals killed 12 weeks
after treatment showed hyperplasia, especially in mid-zonal areas,
and numerous binucleated forms were found.   Female mice were only
slightly affected.   No true neoplasms or peliosis were observed in
animals of either sex.

The remaining animals were killed 10 months after the end of
treatment.   Hyperplastic changes were present in all mid-zonal and
centrizonal areas of livers of animals in both sexes.   Multiple
dysplastic areas with various nuclear abnormalities were present:
these included nuclear enlargement and hyperchromatism, lobulation,
multinucleated forms, coarse patterns of nuclear chromatin and
occasional intranuclear eosinophilic inclusions usually in the
largest nuclei.   The areas of large dysplastic liver cells altern-
ated with zones of smaller uniform hepatocytes and many were found
close to the capsule or hilum.

There appears to be a sex difference in response to MeT treatment since 22/35 (63%) male mice but only 13/33 (39%) female mice
developed areas of dysplasia.   Non-parametric analysis of these
results by a 2 x 2 Chi-squared test gave $Chi^2 = 3.743$, which is
barely significant at the 5 per cent level for which $Chi^2 = 3.84$ is
required.   Experiments with larger groups of animals are required
to confirm whether or not there is a true sex difference in response
to MeT.   Small tumours, about 2 mm in diameter, were found in two
mouse livers, one of each sex (Fig. 1-3).

The effects of DecaD were very similar to those exerted by MeT,

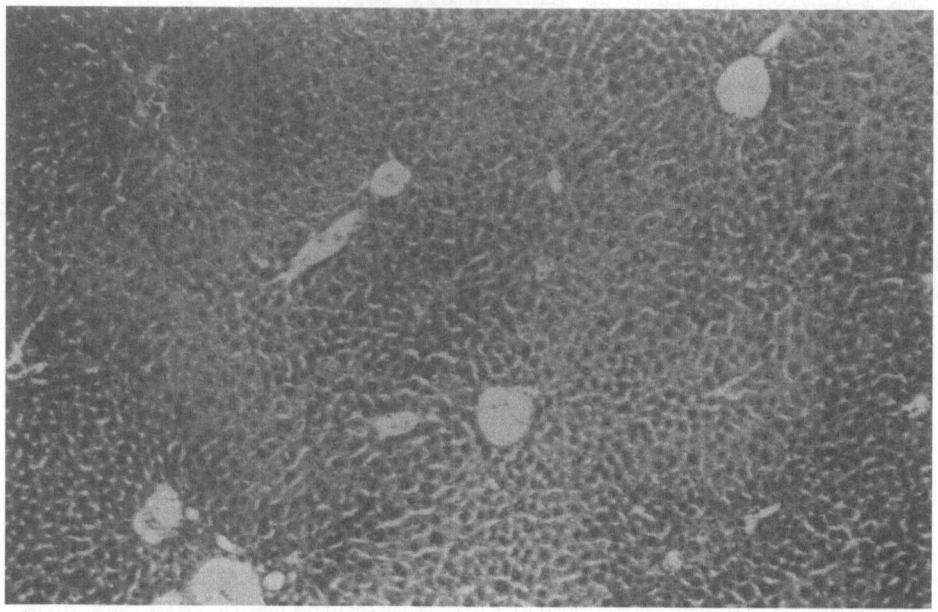

Fig. 1.   Liver from male mouse treated with methyltestosterone for
          10 months showing random distribution of hyperplasia
          (low power).

but more benign hepatocytic nodules were found in the livers: 3 in
25 males and 4 in 23 females.   Although no statistical significance
can be placed on these values, the results indicate that DecaD is as
hepatotoxic and carcinogenic as MeT (Fig. 4).

Experiment B. Marked anatomical differences were observed in the
livers and lungs of animals subjected to the different treatments.
The combined DEN plus DecaD treatment produced grossly enlarged and
malformed livers, in most of which no parenchymal tissue could be
seen.   An extreme example is shown in Figure 5(A).   DEN treatment
alone also caused marked anatomical changes, some of which were as
large as those found in the livers of animals on the combined treatment.   Figure 5(B) shows a more typical response to DEN, character-
ised by the presence of small, pale yellow cysts mainly distributed
along the periphery of the large liver lobes.   Livers from animals
treated with DecaD (Fig. 5C) or arachis oil (Fig. 5D) showed no
marked gross abnormalities or differences.

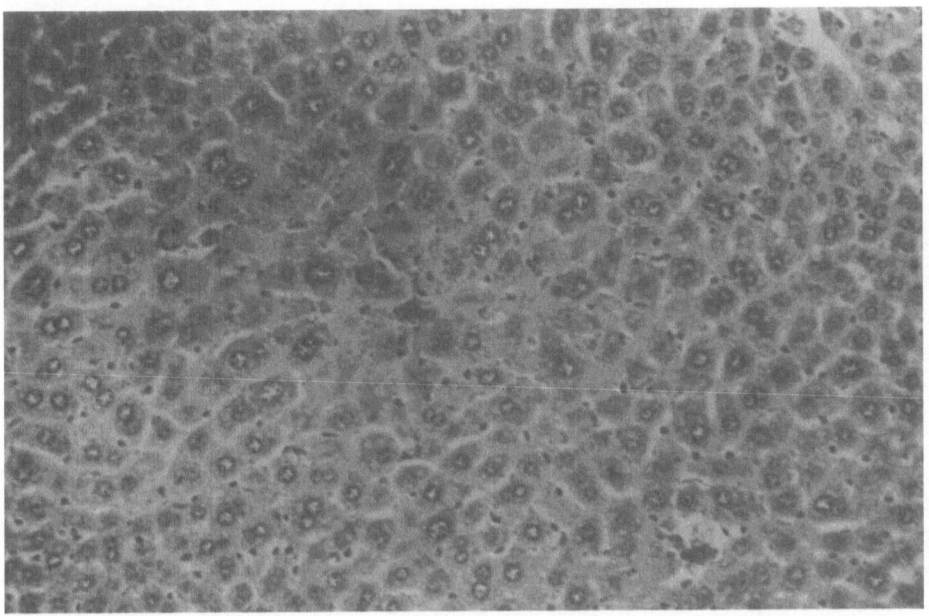

Fig. 2.   Higher power illustration of hyperplasia in methyltestost-
          erone-treated male mouse.

        Histological examination showed that the livers of animals
treated with DEN alone or with DEN plus DecaD, regardless of sex,
showed multiple tumours of variable histological patterns, many with
extensive degeneration, sinusoidal dilatation or peliotic-like
changes within the tumour masses.   The scanty adjacent liver
parenchyma showed virtually overall diffuse dysplasia.   The many
cystic structures seen macroscopically are cystadenomas derived
from bile ducts.   In some livers a full spectrum of changes from
small basophilic hepatocytic adenomas with peripheral proliferation
of bile ducts to a large cytologically "malignant" variant of hepatocellular tumours was seen.   There were no obvious differences due
to either sex or DecaD.

        All the animals treated with DEN, with or without DecaD, had
multiple papillary adenocarcinomas of the lungs which could not be
attributed to metastases from the liver tumours.

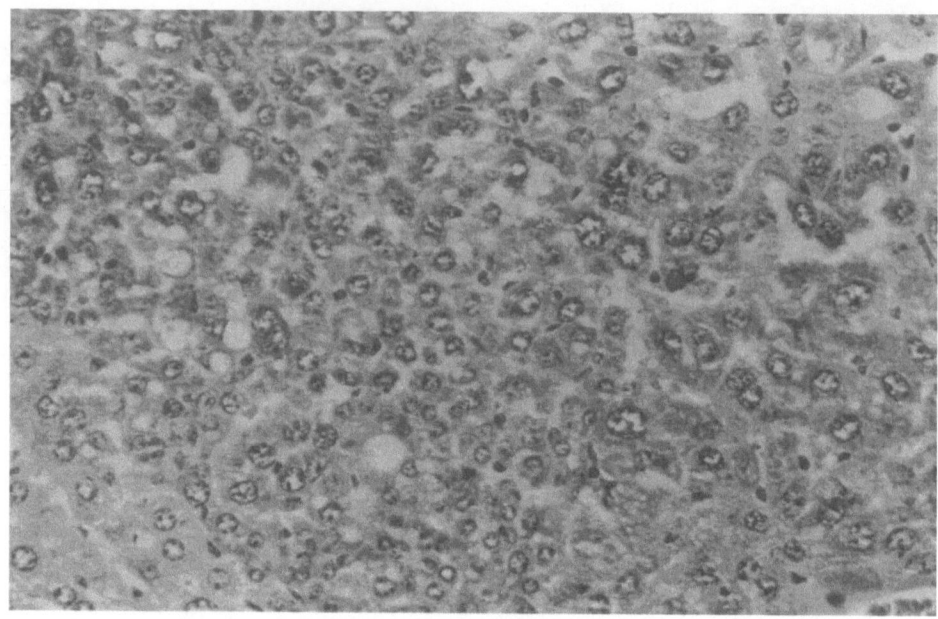

Fig. 3. Liver tumour in male mouse treated for 10 months with
methyltestosterone. Note the small dark cells contrast-
ing with the pale dysplastic parenchyme in the bottom
left-hand corner where there is no clearly defined margin.
(High power).

DISCUSSION

     Evidence is accumulating that benign and malignant hepatic
tumours occur in some human subjects following long-term treatment
with anabolic androgens. Paridinas et al. (1977) and Ishak (1979)
have listed the cases of androgen-associated neoplasms reported
between 1952 and 1976. However, the present paper appears to be
the first report of production of hepatic tumours by administration
of anabolic androgens alone to experimental animals. Hepatocytic
hyperplasia and increase in liver weight after anabolic androgen
treatment are well-known phenomena, but prior to the present work
the production of hepatic tumours has only been reported when those
agents were used in conjunction with known carcinogens with or
without orchidectomy (Firminger et al., 1961; Reuber, 1974). The
incidence of hepatic neoplasms induced by N-2-fluorenyldiacetamide
in rats was lowest after bilateral orchidectomy (Reuber, 1976).
This finding may be related to our results in Experiment A which

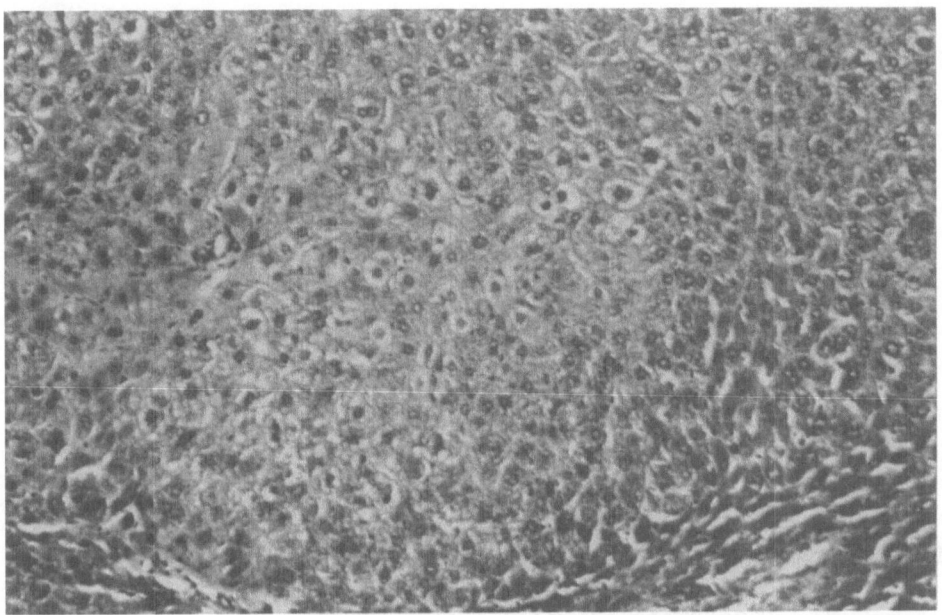

Fig. 4.   Liver tumour in female mouse treated with Decadurabolin*
          for 10 months with narrow rim of normal liver.

showed that male mice are more responsive to the anabolic androgens
than are female mice.

However, in spite of the absence of such lesions from age-
matched control animals, it cannot be stated with any certainty
that the anabolic steroids used in our experiments can act as
initiators of carcinogenesis, particularly as the steroids were
administered for a considerable part of the life span of the
animals.   Nevertheless, at dose levels comparable to those used in
human therapeutics dysplasia was observed in livers of most of the
livers and tumours were found in these animals.   It is also of
interest that male mice appear to be more susceptible to the action
of the androgen than are female mice.   This finding is worthy of
further study, since most investigators do not seem to consider
that such a sex difference is a possible factor in carcinogenesis.

The results of Experiment B are open to the interpretation
that the DEN acted as an initiator of tumorigenesis and DecaD as a
promoter (Farber, 1980).   However, under the experimental conditions used the dose of DEN alone produced a wide spectrum of

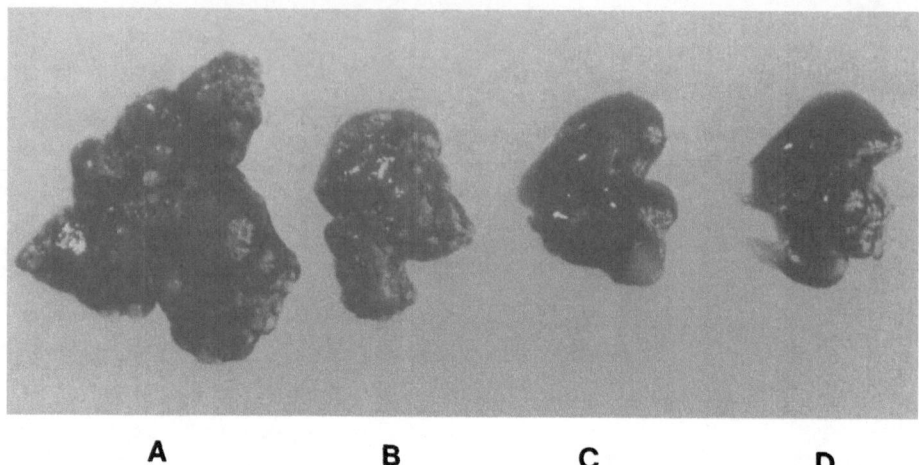

A   B   C   D

Fig. 5.   Livers of mice treated with (A) diethylnitrosamine
          followed by Decadurabolin*; (B) diethylnitrosamine alone;
          (C) Decadurabolin* alone; (D) arachis oil only.   Note
          the cysts on the surface and periphery of the lobes of
          A and B.   These are cystadenomas derived from bile ducts.

neoplastic changes barely distinguishable from those produced when
DecaD was also given.   Therefore in this Experiment DEN acted as
both iniator and promotor of the carcinogenic process, and the
DecaD may have exaggerated the response because of its ability to
produce liver hyperplasia.   Further experiments with different
doses and times of exposure to DEN and DecaD are required to
resolve this problem.

     DEN is usually considered to be a fairly specific hepato-
carcinogen.   However, in Experiment 2 all animals treated with
this agent developed tumours in their lungs.   This may be due to
the administration of the DEN by mouth, although great care was
exercised during the feeding to ensure that no fluid could enter
the bronchial tree.   The nature and extent of the tumours lead
us to believe that they were not secondary tumours metastasing
from the liver.   No spontaneous tumours of the lung were found in
animals not dosed with DEN.

The experiments described provide no information about the mechanism of action of the agents used, and, indeed, were not designed to provide such information, which will be derived from further and more elaborate studies.

SUMMARY

Male and female Balb/C mice were treated for 10 months with methyltestosterone (a 17α-alkylated steroid) or Decadurabolin* (which has no 17α-alkyl substituent) at dose levels and by routes normally used in human patients. Hyperplasia and dysplasia was found in the livers of most animals, but males were more affected than females. Contrary to expectations, Decadurabolin* was found to be at least as hepatotoxic and carcinogenic as methyltestosterone. Tumours were found in the livers of a few mice treated with these agents.

In a second experiment oral pretreatment of mice with diethylnitrosamine followed by no treatment or dosing with Decadurabolin* caused massive changes in liver architecture and induced multiple hepatic tumours. Although the livers of mice treated with the two agents seemed to be more affected, the distribution and multiplicity of the tumours was similar to those animals treated with diethylnitrosamine only.

Animals treated with diethylnitrosamine alone or with Decadurabolin* also developed massive papillary tumours in their lungs.

We conclude that, under the experimental conditions used, anabolic androgens alone are weak carcinogens which can initiate and promote preneoplastic and tumour growth. The evidence does not suggest that anabolic androgens are obligatory promoters for hepatocytic tumours induced by administration of diethylnitrosamine.

ACKNOWLEDGEMENTS

We are grateful to the Smith Kline and French Foundation for financial assistance to W.T., and to the Dorset Area Health Authority for financial support for M.L. S. Snowball is a Luccock Research Student of this Medical School.

REFERENCES

Anderson, A., James, O.F.W., MacDonald, H.S., Snowball, S., and
        Taylor, W., 1980, The effects of ethynyl oestradiol on
        biliary lipid composition in young men, Eur. J. Clin.
        Invest., 10:77-80.
Dickson, C.M., Lesna, M., and Taylor, W., 1979, The effects of
        anabolic androgens on gall-bladder bile acids and cholest-
        erol in mice, J. Steroid Biochem., 11:1567-1571.
Evans, D.J., 1978, Liver tumours elicited by specific factors:
        synthetic androgens and anabolic steroids, in: "Primary
        Liver Tumours", H. Remmer, H.M. Bolt, P. Bannasch, and
        H. Popper, ed., MTP Press, Lancaster, England, pp.213-216.
Farber, E., 1980, The sequential analysis of liver cancer induction,
        Biochim. Biophys. Acta, 605:149-166.
Firminger, H.I., and Reuber, M.D., 1961, Influence of adrenocort-
        ical, androgenic and anabolic hormones on the development of
        carcinoma and cirrhosis of the liver in A X C rats fed
        N-2-fluorenyldiacetamide, J. Natl. Cancer Inst., 27:559-570.
Ishak, K.G., 1979, Hepatic neoplasms associated with contraceptive
        and anabolic steroids, in: "Carcinogenic Hormones",
        C.H. Ligeman, ed., Springer-Verlag, Berlin, pp.73-128.
Paradinas, F.J., Bull, T.B., Westaby, D., and Murray-Lion, I.M.,
        1977, Hyperplasia and prolapse of hepatocytes into hepatic
        veins during long-term methyltestosterone therapy: possible
        relationships of these changes to the development of
        peliosis hepatis and liver tumours, Histopathology, 1:
        225-238.
Reuber, M.D., 1974, The importance of the testes in the induction
        of hyperplastic nodules, carcinomas and cirrhosis of the
        liver in A X C strain male rats ingesting 0.025 per cent
        N-2-fluorenyldiacetamide, J. Natl. Cancer Inst., 53:883-891.
Reuber, M.D., 1976, Effect of age and testosterone on the induction
        of hyperplastic nodules, carcinomas and cirrhosis of the
        liver in rats ingesting N-2-fluorenyldiacetamide, Eur. J.
        Cancer, 12:137-145.
Sherlock, S., 1978, Hepatic tumours and sex hormones, in: "Primary
        Liver Tumours", H. Remmer, H.M. Bolt, P. Bannasch, and
        H. Popper, ed., MTP Press, Lancaster, England, pp.201-212.
Taylor, W., 1981a, Toxicology and carcinogenicity of anabolic
        agents in human subjects, in: "Anabolic Agents in Beef and
        Veal Production", Proc. Workshop, Brussels, under auspices
        of the European Communities Directorate General for Agric-
        ulture, B. Hoffman and J.F. Roche., ed., Agricultural
        University, Dublin, Ireland, pp.113-138.
Taylor, W., 1981b, The relationship between steroids and cancer in
        man, and its relevance to the use of steroidal anabolic
        agents in farm animals, in: "Steroids in Animal Production",
        H. Jasiorowski, ed., Warsaw Agricultural University, Warsaw,
        Poland, pp.235-247.

DISCUSSION

Dr.Friedman : Can you explain what is known about the mechanism of carcinogenesis by a high level of carcinogen compared to the effect of a low dose of carcinogen plus promoter?

Dr.Weinstein : Using a very high doses or repeated doses of initiating carcinogens,for instance B(a)P,we do not need a promoter, so what is going on?There are two possibilities:one is that B(a)P itself can serve as a promoter,the second one is that carcinogenesis proceeds through some entirely different mechanism. We tested the first theory,that if you only use B(a)P it must have effects similar to those of promoters.So we added B(a)P to cells in culture and measured EGF receptors and indeed,we saw a progressive loss of EGF receptors.We also looked at a series of PAH;all the PAH which are complete carcinogens for the mouse skin had the same effect as B(a)P.So our model is that B(a)P enters the cell,binds to the AHH receptor,is translocated to the nucleus and may in some way interact with chromatin and induce some enzymes.We can extend this model by saying that when this occurs there are also biochemical functions which are induced that alter membrane structure and function and actually mimc the action of phorbol esters.B(a)P is also very good in the induction of arachidonic acid release and in changing phospholipid metabolism.So if you look at B(a)P carefully,it also changes membranes in a way very similar to phorbol esters.Thus, we would say that a complete carcinogen not only damage DNA but also induces changes in the membrane.This is only a theory but I think that there is good evidence to support it.

Dr.Burns : Can you explain your concept of promotion as inhibition of terminal differentiation(keratinization of epidermis) in light of the powerful stimulation of cell proliferation caused by TPA on mouse skin?It seems to me that the new equilibrium,hyperplasia, hyperkeratinization,etc.,represents more differentiation not less.

Dr.Weinstein : Yes,we recently published a study in "Cell" in which we exposed mouse skin to TPA or various control compounds.We took fragments of epidermis,incubated them for short periods of

time with ^{35}S-labelled methionine,extracted the proteins and did
two-dimentional gels.We found a cluster of spots which range
from about 42,000 to 65,000 daltons which are keratins.What
is very striking is that within 3 to 6 hours after exposure
to TPA,there is a marked inhibition of incorporation of labeled
methionine into these keratins.We found that TPA shifts the keratin
profile to a mature one as you move to the lower layers.So I think
that this is consistent with an inhibition of the terminal differ-
entiation.In terms of why there are more basal cells,I think there
are two alternatives.One is that cell cycle of basal cells is
shorter after treatment with TPA.I do not know of any evidence
for that.The second one is that basal cells that were dormant were
recruited into the cell cycle.One third possibility is that the
same number of basal cells are in cycle but the daughter cells
also remain in cycle.So,when you remove TPA,you have a larger
population which starts to defferentiate and which should be
keratinized.

*Dr.Dragsted : Can you elicit a graded response to TPA so that only
certain membrane effects correspond to certain dose levels
of TPA? Can you correlate those levels to the threshold dose
of tumor promotion in vivo?*

Dr.Weinstein : The changes that I described are concentration
dependent.The concentrations which are required are in the range
of about 10^{-9}M which is in the range of mitogenic effects and
approximate concentrations used on mouse skin.Some of these
effects have also been seen on mouse skin,like induction of
arachidonic acid release,etc.So I think that there is a correlation between the two in terms of concentration dependence.

*Dr.Dragsted : Have you tried to isolate the membrane receptor
for TPA by trying chemical reactions between TPA and the receptor,
for istance with UV light or by chemical means?*

*Dr.Weinstein :*We have not been successful and I do not know of any
reports on the successful solubilization of the receptor.So far
the receptor binding is done either with intact monolayers or
with the whole membrane preparations and our attempts so far
to solubilize the receptor in an active form have not been
successful,but we are trying as are a number of other laboratories.
One approach is to have,as you suggested,derivatives of the
phorbol esters that might be covalently linked to the receptor,
e.g.,some photoactivatable group,but the synthesis of such
derivatives is not easy and there are a number of groups working
on this.At present time,the receptor has not been isolated,
therefore,whether it is a distinct protein or some other chemical component of the membrane is not known.

Dr.Hubert-Habart : Does any complete carcinogen compound inhibit phorboldibutyrate binding?

Dr.Weinstein : No.If we just add B(a)P or DMBA,they do not compete directly for phorbol ester binding.Therefore,we invoke the mechanism that they can nevertheless alter the membrane function but through a more indirect mechanism.

Dr.Arus : In your lecture you mentioned chalones.Have you any information whether chalones compete for this binding site or these receptors on the membrane?

Dr.Weinstein : We have not tested any chalones,I do not have any available.We have found a serum factor (a 60,000 dalton protein) which has been partially purified,present in normal serum and which inhibits the binding of the labelled phorbol ester to the receptor.It is present in high concentration in female serum and in even higher concentration in pregnant women.We have also found it in rodent serum and amniotic fluid but not in urine or spinal fluid.We do find,however,a similar activity in a variety of tissue extracts.The factor inhibits binding at 4°C and in membrane preparations,pointing to a direct physical effect not requiring cell metabolism.We are a bit disappointed because the factor itself does not induce the effects that TPA induces on cells,e.g.,it does not induce phospholipid turnover or alter the binding of other receptors.It is not a mitogen and we have not tested it as a promoter on mouse skin,but I am skeptical that it will work.So the most trivial explanation is that this serum factor may itself bind the phorbol ester, trap it,so that phorbol ester is not available for the membrane receptor.We have tested this explanation and found no evidence that it binds phorbol ester,so we have to asuume that it binds to the membrane either on the receptor (but not the active site of the receptor),or it binds adjacent to the receptor and interferes with the function of the receptor.However,it does not activate the receptor,it is not an agonist.I remind you that the concentration of this factor is in the physiological range, it is equivalent to about 10% serum,so if you grow cells in 10% serum you always have a significant level of the serum factor and are always partially inhibiting binding.Actually,this is how we discovered it.We found that there was better binding if we left serum out of the binding assay.So if this has any in vivo significance,it might really inhibit the function of the phorbol ester receptor and in that sense serve as an antipromoter or anti-proliferative agent.We do not know if this factor is a chalone,but it does raise the possibility that there are host factors which might protect the host against external factors that might enhance promotion,but this is very speculative.

Dr.Dogliotti : Cerutti spoke last week about the mechanism of action of TPA via active oxygen species. What do you think about this model of action of TPA?

Dr.Weinstein : Well,frankly I am very skeptical about that.There is no doubt that if you add TPA to poymorphonuclear leukocytes, to granulocytes,to lymphocytes or to macrophages you can activate the production of activated oxygen.But I think that is the expression of a specialized function of these cells,that is,e.g., whenever macrophages are activated with TPA,what you see is the induction of its normal functions,namely,phagocytosis, chemotaxis,release of cathepsins and of activated oxygen.So, if the specialized program of the cell,when activated,is to release superoxide,then TPA can induce that.The release of activated oxygen has not been demonstrated for fibroblasts. This may be due to limitations of detection of the method and there is a small release which may be important,but I would tend to think that this is a specialized function.This is a general problem in interpreting the findings with TPA because on different cells it does different things and which ones are relevant to tumor promotion is difficult to tell. Cerutti has seen chromosomal abnormalities in lymphocytes treated with TPA but others have treated fibroblasts and seen at best borderline effects.No major abnormalities have been seen,perhaps a small increase in SCE.The results,however,seem to vary from one laboratory to another depending on the concentrations of TPA used and the source of the TPA.The concentrations are much higher than those required to saturate the receptor or produce the effects that I described in my talk.So I think that the release of superoxide and the chromosome damaging effects of TPA are toxic manifestations and unrelated to tumor promotion.

Dr.Sarma : Does promotion represent simple amplification of initiated cells or do promoters contribute to or modify initiated cells?

Dr.Weinstein : I think they probably do both.First of all,promotion itself is also a multistep process;it has been demonstrated in vivo and in culture.E.g.,rat fibroblasts infected with adenovirus look morphologically altered clones of these cells do not give tumors in mice or grow in soft agar:in summary they are partially transformed.Passage of these cells in the presence of TPA leads to progression and development of tumorigenicity,demonstrating a multistage process.But if you add TPA to normal rat fibroblasts not infected with adenovirus it does not cause them to grow in soft agar and it does not make them tumorigenic. I think of initiation as acting to set up a cell population which responds preferentially or responds in a qualitatively different manner to the phorbol esters than normal cells do . The same is true if we initiate cells in culture with chemicals: these cells are altered in their response and we call this an enhancement. One possibility to explain this is that the initiated cell or the partially transformed cell might have acquired more receptors and so is more responsive,but we do not find more receptors in these cells. So there must be other reprogramming, perhaps at the chromatin level.

Dr. *Farber : Is there any hormone you know which does what TPA does in terms of diversivity of effects?*

Dr. *Weinstein :* Well,epidermal growth factor in cell culture has these highly diverse effects.It does almost the same things as TPA.Also other polypeptide growth factors have very pleiotropic effects on a variety of tissues.

Dr. *Taylor :* It is important to bear in mind that some substances are cholestatic,some are choleretic and some have little effect on bile flow.Since a very important function of the liver is biliary excretion of compounds,the effect on bile flow may be important.For example,estrogens are cholestatics and disturb biliary lipid composition in a particular way which tends to lead to gallstone formation.However,anabolic androgens do not have this effect,whereas progesterones tend to have effects almost the opposite of those of estrogens,etc.

Dr. *Schulte-Hermann :* We are,of course,at a very early stage of investigation and I am fully aware that there are numerous complicating factors which may modify the results and promoting effects.

Dr. *Burns : I was surprised at the large increase in total DNA during promoter treatment and the equally large decrease after cessation of promotion in comparison to the relatively small changes in proliferation rate. Could there be infiltration by other cells, e.g.,inflammatory cells,as a result of the promotion?*

Dr. *Schulte-Hermann :* No.We have not seen any evidence of such type of response.There are no more inflammatory cells than there are in normal parenchyma.I think that there are really two processes which balance each other: the multiplication of parenchymal cells and the loss of parenchymal cells.However,the finding you refer to is a very early finding of ours. We repeated the experiments to be sure that it really occurs.Of course,the process that you mentioned may be really important in the regulation of growth in normal tissue and in tumors.

Dr. *Dragsted : I can supplement your slides on the different kinds of induction from different promoters.BHT shows the same pattern of cyt.P 450 induction as phenobarbital in mouse liver as opposed to the kind of induction caused by 3-methylcholanthrene.As it is known that low doses of BHT may induce cyt.P 450 and some liver enlargement without increase in total DNA,can you correlate this graded response to BHT to its threshold dose as a tumor promoter?*

Dr.Schulte-Hermann : So far we have not done studies on the promotion efficiency of BHT.As far as the threshold doses for monooxygenase induction and induction of liver growth are concerned
I think it depends on the compound.With phenobarbital,it is
probably true that it is more active at lower doses as an inducer
of monooxygenase than for liver growth,as is BHT.But it may not
be true for all compounds,e.g.,CPA.

Dr.Lutz : *Is it possible to override the arrest of cells in R due
to feeding schedule with any agent,e.g.,hormones?*

Dr.Schulte-Hermann : I assume that at least part of these fasting
effects are mediated by changes in the hormone "milieu".
As far as the early feeding/fasting effects are concerned,I think
they are endocrinologically mediated.

SECTION IV

CARCINOGENESIS AS MULTISTEP PROCESS

SOME CRITICAL CONSIDERATION CONCERNING

SEQUENTIAL ANALYSIS OF CARCINOGENESIS WITH CHEMICALS

Emmanuel Farber

Department of Pathology and Professor of Biochemistry
University of Toronto, 100 College Street
Toronto, Ontario M5G 1L5

Cancer development with chemicals can begin with a brief exposure (a few hours or days) to an activated form of a carcinogen
and the chemical need not be present as such ever again, as far as
can be determined. This is valid not only in the skin, which was
the first tissue in which this was demonstrated clearly but also
in liver, colon, mammary gland, urinary bladder, kidney, brain and
other organs or tissues[2,3,6,7]. The brief exposure to the chemical induces neither a cancer cell nor a neoplastic cell but
rather some cell that can be differentially stimulated to produce
a focal proliferation. By neoplastic is meant a cell that can proliferate without the need for an added or known stimulus for growth,
i.e., a cell that has acquired some degree of autonomy.

The existence of an initiated state cannot be detected per se
but makes itself evident only when some promoting or selecting environment is created, i.e., by the occurrence of subsequent focal
proliferation. Thus, the concept of initiation is intricately
bound up with the subsequent appearance of discreet proliferative
lesions.

The separation of this first sequence, initiation - promotion,
is justified because of the dependence of each of its steps on the
environment for their appearance. With a single exposure to an
initiating dose of a carcinogen, the further history is closely
dependent upon the imposition of a suitable promoting environment.
This can be created by a "pure" promoter or by further exposure to
a carcinogen. In the former case, repeated exposure over a relatively long period (weeks to months in rats or mice) is usually
required. In the latter case, a briefer exposure to an active
carcinogen may suffice.

This first sequence generates a new cell population that is at risk for a second "rare event" from which a second new population can develop. The occurrence of this new focal change in a rare cell and its amplification by selection or differential growth seems to be no longer environment dependent but appears to be self-generating. Because of this relative autonomy, at least with respect to added exogeneous agents, we consider this second rare event as the beginning of "neoplasia" and everything preceding this change as "preneoplasia". The subsequent steps are poorly understood and are discussed below.

INITIATORS

Until fairly recently, one of the most puzzling and confusing aspects of chemical carcinogenesis was the diversity in chemical structure of carcinogens. This problem has now been largely resolved by the discovery of metabolic conversion of many carcinogens to highly reactive metabolites[4]. Although the principle was quite well established by the late 1960's, the many details concerning the specific forms of the metabolites are only now being clarified. The best known form of reactive moieties, generated from several different types of carcinogens, is the "electrophilic reactant", a positively charged molecule that reacts well with sites of electron densities in many different cellular components including DNA, RNA, protein, glutathione and probably also polysaccharides[4]. A minority of chemical carcinogens such as some nitrosamides (e.g., alkyl nitrosoureas), bis-chlormethyl ether and nitrogen mustard, are active per se and do not seem to require any metabolic conversion to more reactive metabolites.

Activation and Metabolism of Procarcinogens

The first major type of metabolic activation discovered was the conversion of an aromatic amine, 2-acetylaminofluorene (2-AAF) by N-hydroxylation to an N-OH derivative[4]. This reactive product may in turn be esterified to a more reactive form, an N-O-ester, which is believed to be the ultimate type of carcinogen for some aromatice amines. The human bladder carcinogen 2-naphthylamine (β-nathylamine) is a type of aromatic amine.

More recently, much effort has been placed on the clarification of the activation of benzo(a)pyrene (B(a)P) and other polycyclic aromatic hydrocarbons (PAH). Many of those easily generated by burning (pyrolysis), are widely distributed, therefore, in our environment and are thought to be responsible, in part at least, for the carcinogenicity of coal tar products, oils, tars, etc. These compounds undergo epoxidation to form reactive epoxides, some forms of which are considered to be ultimate carcinogens[8]. In the case of B(a)P and probably other PAH, the initial site of epoxidation may undergo hydration to form a dihydrodiol, a reaction catalyzed by epoxide hydrolase. This inactive derivative in turn can be converted to another epoxide at a second site to form a dihydrodiol epoxide. These are considered to be the most likely ultimate carcinogens for at least some polycyclic aromatic hydrocarbons. Another potentially important carcinogen for humans that is subject to activation via epoxidation is aflatoxin B_1[4]. This undergoes oxidation at its 2,3-position and this derivative, the 2,3-oxide, appears to be one form of ultimate carcinogen of this mycotoxin. Vinyl chloride is also activated via epoxidation[4].

Very likely, these reactions with B(a)P, aflatoxin B_1 and vinyl chloride are illustrative of the probable activation of many other aliphatic, aromatic or heterocyclic compounds, both carcinogenic and non-carcinogenic (e.g., bromobenzene).

Other types of metabolic conversions also are considered to be important in carcinogenesis[4]. Nitrosamines are converted to highly reactive alkylating moieties, probably through oxidation. Aromatic or heterocyclic nitro compounds, such as nitrofurans and 4-nitroquinoline-N-oxide (4NQO) probably undergo initial reduction to hydroxyamino-derivatives. In the case of 4NHQ, this form is considered to be an ultimate carcinogen.

Thus, several types of metabolic conversions to ultimate carcinogens are now known and offer interesting problems for detailed analysis of the chemistry, enzymology, modulation and control.

For the majority of known conversions, the system most active in the cell is the "mixed function oxygenase" system (MFO) consisting of several cytochromes P450, NADPH cytochrome C reductase and lipid[9]. This inducible system is located predominantly in the microsomal fraction of the cell, (endoplasmic reticulum,ER) although recent work increasinbly points to a second comparable system in the nucleus[10]. In addition to these oxidative systems, reducing systems also exist for some precarcinogens, such as the aromatic or heterocyclic nitro compounds. Diaphorase or other NADPH or NADH reductases are widely distributed among different cells and are effective in reducing the nitro group to the amino or hydroxyamine derivative.

The liver is by far the most active and most versatile organ in the metabolism of precarcinogens and of xenobiotic agents generally. It and other organs show an ability to detoxify as well as activate potential carcinogens and the ultimate fate of a chemical depends largely upon the balance between activation and inactivation, a balance that is easily modulated in major ways by drugs and other chemicals, age, nutrition and hormones as well as genetics[11-16]

For example, the carcinogenicity of several aromatic amines for the liver can be completely prevented by simultaneous exposure to phenobarbital or 3-methylcholanthrene, agents that induce many liver enzymes [11,16-17] This phenomenon of resistance of the induced liver to some carcinogens may be of great importance to humans. Virtually all humans in the western world have levels of several xenobiotic agents, such as DDT, dieldrin, aldrin, PCB's (polychlorinated biphenyls) and dioxins in their adipose tissues. These agents as a group are very effective enzyme inducers in the liver. Also, many drugs induce various microsomal or other enzymes in liver or other tissues. Are these inducers making tissues more or less susceptible to the carcinogenic effect of other environmental agents?

It is considered probable that the organ or tissue distribution of the carcinogen-metabolizing enzymes may play a role in the organotropism of carcinogens. Since there is an almost certain obligatory requirement of activation and since the metabolic patterns affecting carcinogens and other xenobiotic agents are so variable from cell to cell or from organ to organ, the absolute activities of the various enzymes and especially their relative balance may play key roles in determing which organ, if any, may be a target for a particular carcinogen. An interesting example of modulation at this level is the liver-kidney axis with dimethylnitrosamine. This potent carcinogen normally induces liver cancer when taken in via the gastrointestinal tract. However, if the animal is placed on low protein diet, the hepatic activation and metabolism falls off. This allows more carcinogen to be available for action on the kidney and changes the dominant cancer pattern from liver to kidney [18].

A puzzling phenomenon relating to the metabolic activation of many carcinogens is its possible physiological role. A reasonable interpretation of the major importance of "drug-metabolizing" enzymes is in the genesis of derivatives that can be excreted as such or that can be conjugated to facilitate excretion. These types of conversions occur with chemical carcinogens as well as with many other xenobiotics. What is the survival value for the host, if any, of metabolic activities that lead to highly reactive more "toxic" derivatives, not less toxic. Are there naturally occuring substrates for these metabolic reactions which require "activation" for the performance of their metabolic roles?

POSSIBLE MOLECULAR TARGETS FOR ULTIMATE CARCINOGENS

The molecular targets for the electrophilic reactants are many. To date, the bulk of the effort has been concentrated on DNA with some interest in RNA and protein. In principle, many other molecular targets exist at the macromolecular and "micromolecular" levels. Because of the relative ease of relating change in DNA to

a permanent change in biological behaviour of cells, DNA has received the lion's share of attention.   Since the first discovery of
the chemical nature of an adduct of a carcinogen with nucleic acids
in a target organ in vivo [19], there has been an increasing interest
in establishing the chemical nature and site of interaction with
several different carcinogens[5] . Virtually every potential site
for interaction with DNA bases (as well as with phosphates) reacts
with one or more carcinogens.   In order to narrow down the possibilities for relevance to cancer, sites more likely to be involved
in hydrogen-bonding between bases (purines-pyrimidines) in DNA and
thus to be involved in possible miscoding are often considered to
be most relevant.   This presupposes that the major or only biochemical lesion in DNA that is relevant to cancer initiation is a
miscoding one.   This judgement may not be justified, since the
evidence is circumstantial and inconclusive.   Conceivably, other
types of alterations in DNA, besides miscoding, such as recombina-
tions, gaps, translocation, etc. may be important to the early
events in cancer development[5,20-23].   In fact, Cairns has suggested
that mutagenesis may be of only minor importance in the initial
events in chemical carcinogenesis and that genetic transposition
involving relatively large segments of the genome might be more
relevant to the process[23] .   The application of this newer technology to appropriate "clean" cell populations during the development
of cancer is to be awaited with interest.

Another important aspect is the site of interaction of the ultimate carcinogen within the long DNA molecules.   With the use of
several different approaches such as susceptibility to nucleases,
separation of transcriptionally active from inactive DNA or isolation of linker and nucleosome regions in chromatin, some of the
interactions of carcinogens with DNA have been found to be non-
random. However, to date, no single region of hig affinity has
been found [5] .   This interesting aspect of DNA as a probable target
for carcinogens must await the further advances in DNA functional
segmental fractionation, such as through the use of appropriate
restriction enzymes and DNA cloning for specific genes in biologically well defined preneoplastic and early neoplastic cell populations. Included in this will be the possible roles of histones
and of the non-histone chromosomal proteins in favouring certain
regions over others.

DNA REPAIR

In view of the essentially irreversible nature of initiation
with chemicals, and the apparent focal nature of the initiation
process (see below), major emphasis at the molecular level is given
the DNA as a probable target in initiation.   However, the evidence
is largely circumstantial.

Great indirect support comes from the well known high incidence of skin cancer in patients with xeroderma pigmentosum (XP). The vast majority of these patients have some degree of interference with repair of DNA damaged by ultraviolet light. The latter is the major if not sole carcinogenic stimulus in these patients and patients can be protected from skin cancer by careful avoidance of exposure to ultraviolet light[24]. Fibroblast cultures from patients with XP show increased sensitivity not only to ultraviolet light but also to some chemical carcinogens and mutagens[25]. Other human disease, e.g., ataxio telangiectasia and Fanconi's anemia, also show repair deficiencies in DNA as well as increased risk for neoplasia [26].

Thus, the bulk of evidence implicating DNA as a major target for initiation of cancer development comes from studies on humans implicating ultraviolet light as the etiological agent, This is buttressed by a large amount of less definitive data on experimental chemical carcinogenesis and a general feeling that DNA repair may be a critical component in the development of cancer with chemicals. For example, there is a correlation under some conditions between the formation of O^6-methylguanine (O^6-MeG) in brain, persistence of this lesion and the ultimate occurrence of gliomas[27]. This type of correlation is also prosent in liver and kidney under some conditions[28]. Another interesting example relates to the carcinogen 1,2-dimethylhydrazine (DMH). This compound is most active in inducing colon cancer and is not generally effective as an hepatocarcinogen. However, it does induce angiosarcoma of the liver. It has been found recently that the vascular lining cells of the liver are much less effective in the removal of O^6-methylguanine from their DNA than are the hepatocytes, an observation that correlates well with the "organotropism" of DMH[29].

Yet, other studies indicate that the genesis and persistence of O^6-MeG may be important but insufficient for cancer production with some nitrosamines or nitrosamides[30]. Also, in the liver, with some carcinogens such as 1,2-dimethylhydrazine and using a very early step in carcinogenesis as the end point, only DNA lesions removed within about 48 hours seem to be of major importance and the persistent ones much less so if at all[31].

It is often theorized that our major protection against cancer resides in the efficiency with which we repair the DNA damaged by the many carcinogens and mutagens in our environment. As pointed out by German[26] and by Cairns[23], since fibroblasts from patients with xeroderma pigmentosum show a defect in the repair of DNA damage by some chemicals [25] as well as by ultraviolet light, such patients should show an elevated risk for cancer development in organs or tissues other than the skin if chemical carcinogens are playing important roles in the genesis of many forms of cancer.

Yet, the available data show no apparent increased risk in patients with XP for cancer other than in the skin[23]. Patients with Bloom's syndrome do show such an elevated risk. Such observations are interpreted as evidence against a role for the many environmental chemical hazards in the etiology of human cancers generally, except in well established instances such as respiratory cancer in smokers and in occupational exposures[23]. However, an alternate hypothesis must be entertained, namely that the role of repair may be quite different in the dynamics of cancer induction with chemicals as compared to ultraviolet light.

The past ten years has seen a large expansion of studies on DNA repair, largely in _in vitro_ systems. These studies should lead to a much clearer delineation of the types of repair that _might_ be occuring in carcinogenesis. What _does_ happen remains poorly understood. Repair by basic excision, by "long versus short patch" removal, by possible recombination or other forms of "postreplication" repair, by removing interstrand cross-links or other more complex forms of damage or by other mechanisms are slowly being studied in many different systems _in vitro_ and to a much less degree _in vivo_[5,25]. The enzymology, although difficult, is also slowly becoming clarified. In the case of methylating carcinogens, an interesting recent finding is the discovery of an enzyme in bacteria that removes the methyl group from the O^6-positive of guanine in DNA by transmethylation with its transfer to a S-containing moiety in protein[32]. This raises the question whether some of the enzymes involved in repair of DNA damage perform physiological functions that subserve normal cellular requirements, other than repair.

An obvious failing in much of the attempts to correlate patterns of repair of DNA with carcinogenicity is the wide gap between the relatively advanced state of the chemistry on the one hand and the primitive state of the art in identifying and quantitating discreet biological steps in the carcinogenic process on the other hand.

CARCINOGEN METABOLISM IN HUMAN TISSUES

A gratifying aspect of recent studies on the early chemical and biochemical events in carcinogenesis is the overall similarity in patterns of activation and types of adducts seen in human tissues as compared to the experimental animal tissues. Studies with some nitrosamines, benzo(a)pyrene, aflatoxin B_1 and other carcinogens (e.g.[33-39]) have shown that human tissues in general resemble one or more animal tissues in their patterns of activation and in the type of carcinogen-DNA adducts formed. Since the metabolism of any single carcinogen, including the quantitative aspects of adduct formation, varies in detail with the source and form of the activating system, such as whole cell versus microsomes or microsomes-supernatant, it is not yet possible to attempt a highly detailed analysis of the biological significance of the similarities and differences.

An interesting development that may help to clarify some aspects of this important phase of activation is the use of radioimmunoassays for specific adducts in DNA, especially with highly sensitive new approaches to radioimmunoassay[40-42]. Such detection of minute quantities of carcinogen-induced adducts in DNA opens up the possibility of studying the exposure patterns of individuals to carcinogens. This coupled with adequate medical examination and appropriate epidemiological studies might well offer new approaches to the ultimate problem of risk assessment. Although it is far too early to discuss such possibilities in other than general terms, it is important to emphasize that adduct formation is an index of exposure,not initiation, and that persistence of a chemical lesion in DNA is by no means synonomous with cancer development. As discussed below, initiation of the carcinogenic process is not an inevitable consequence of adduct formation. Nevertheless, the possibilities that seem imminent in this area of chemical carcinogenesis may allow the study of human carcinogenesis to enter a new phase of sensitivity with a new perspective.

INITIATION

In the "classical" system of skin carcinogenesis in mice and rabbits, a single or brief exposure to a carcinogen induces some change in the tissues called initiation, such that focal proliferations called "papillomas", can be made to appear by application of croton oil or other agents called promoting agents, which by themselves are non-carcinogenic or only weakly so. This phenomenon was more recently found also in several other organs such as liver, brain, mammary gland, colon and urinary bladder[1-3]. Such focal proliferations (papillomas,polyps, hyperplastic nodules) in turn, are sites for further evolution to"neoplasia". Thus, initiation can only be defined so far in terms of subsequent event in response to exposure to a promoting or selecting environment, i.e., in biological terms, not in chemical or biochemical. Initiation of skin, liver, mammary gland and probably at most sites is largely permanent. Although some loss of intensity may occur with time, the general experience is that this biological "event" probably persists for the lifetime of the animal.

These observations are most easily interpreted as reflecting some permanent change in the DNA in the rare cell affected during initiation in vivo. Whether the change is a mutation in a structural or regulatory segment of DNA[43-45] or involves more complex rearrangements of larger segments of DNA such as in transpositions[23] remains unknown. Pertinent are the observations on transformation initiated with x-rays or with polycyclic aromatic hydrocarbons in

which some change or changes other than a mutation in a rare cell
appears to be involved as an early step in initiation in vitro
with a highly selected cell type[79,80]. Until concrete evidence
in support of one or another proposed mechanism becomes available,
and until the molecular nature of the focal irreversible steps in
normal development and differentiation is understood, it is pre-
ferable to denote the initiation and other rare focal changes
during carcinogenesis as "rare events".

One cannot equate activation of carcinogens leading to DNA-
adduct formation with initiation. For example, many carcinogens
such as B(a)P and 7,12-dimethyl benzo(a)anthracene (DMBA) can be
activated by liver to form adducts without initiating or inducing
liver cancer in adult animals. However, if coupled with one round
of cell proliferation, many can initiate[46-48] and can induce liver
cancer [49]. In vitro, with different cell systems, cell proliferation early in the carcinogenic process has been shown to be required
for transformation with x-rays[50], some viruses and some chemicals
Although suspected for in vivo carcinogenesis as well[3,49] it has
only been established for liver cancer formation[49] and very recently
for liver cancer initiation[46,48]. Thus, initiation is at least a
two-step process, a biochemical step that is reparable followed by
a round of cell proliferation that "fixes" some change so as to
make it essentially permanent. The cell proliferation can be
generated by some primary mitogenic stimulus such as partial hepatectomy or by a chemical mitogen[46] or as a response to a cell
death[53].

The mechanistic role of cell proliferation in initiation is
not understood. The commonest hypothesis involves DNA synthesis
or replication as somehow "fixing" damage in a daughter strand.
While attractive, one must be aware of other possibilities related
to the cell cycle such as variations in activation or inactivation,
unsual availability of susceptible regions of DNA or alterations
in the repair processes at different times. With at least two
models of liver carcinogenesis[31,54] cell proliferation to be effective must occur within one to three days after the administration of the carcinogen.

The lack of a major degree of reversibility of the initiated
state indicates that the very early carcinogen-induced altered
cells are not recognized by the host in a manner that leads to
their destruction. This raises serious doubts about the validity
of the concept of immune surveillance at an early stage in chemical
carcinogenesis [55], as it has been proposed for the host control
of cancer development[56].

If the initiation process in the liver or elsewhere involves
an occasional single or rare target cell, as is probable[72,77,78],

such isolated cells have yet to be characterized as to phenotype
or genotype, since they have not been seen. Although many markers
appear after the proliferation of the initated cells, it is not
known what role the cell proliferation plays in their appearance.

The probable requirement for cell proliferation for initiation
has important implications for cancer development in many sites in
humans. In the tissues showing continual proliferation (skin, bone
marrow, gastrointestinal tract, etc.), initiation of carcinogenesis
with chemicals could be dependent largely on the metabolic patterns
of activation and repair, providing initiated cells are retained.
However, in the non-proliferating tissues, such as pancreas, sali-
vary gland, liver, kidney, urinary bladder and brain, an important
rate limiting step for beginning the carcinogenic process may be
cell proliferation. Thus, concommitant cell necrosis induced by
viruses, toxic agents, parasites, dietary deficiencies etc., fol-
lowered by cell regeneration,could be a major determinant for cancer initiation in many sites. In addition, the presence of many
proliferating cells is probably one basis for the susceptibility
of the fetus and neonate to many chemical carcinogens [57] and could
account for the peak in cancer incidence in the first decade. Some
conterbalance for this could be the relatively poor development of
the metabolic activating systems for some types of carcinogens in
some species[58-59]. It is noteworthy and perhaps significant that
the human fetus, unlike the fetus in rodents, acquires the capability of activation of some carcinogens early in development[58] and
thus may be at greater risk than some experimental animals for cancer development with chemicals.

Essential Nature of Initiated Cells

A most important question for initiation concerns the essential biological nature of the initiated cells. What properties have
they acquired that enables them, as a group, to be precursors for
the ultimate development of cancer? What property or properties
confer on these relatively few cells the ability to be stimulated
to form a focal area of proliferation? The available evidence is
against any conclusion that the initiated cells have acquired any
autonomy of growth[1,3]. Without appropriate promotion by non-carcinogenic or carcinogenic agents, few if any post-initiation focal
proliferations are seen in the systems so far studied.

In most systems, the properties critical to initiation remain
unknown. In two continuously proliferating tissues, the skin[60] and
the colon [61] an early property of carcinogen-altered cells appears
to be some disturbance in the programming or control such that the
cells do not show the normal progression of differentiated properties. Whether these are "inherent" properties of the altered
cells or a reflection of some change in the local environment has
not been established.

In the liver, three properties of initiated cells have been observed. The first, the appearance of enzyme deficiencies or excess or other biochemical changes, has been used to identify putative preneoplastic hepatocytes[48,62,69]. However, so far no hypothesis has appeared implicating any one or more of such changes in mechanisms of carcinogenesis. The second property, resistance to the inhibitory effects of carcinogens on cell proliferation, has been shown to be one type of initiated cell in which a mechanism for focal proliferation can be formulated (differential inhibition)[63]. An assay for the quantative assessment of such resistant hepatocytes has been used to study a variety of properties of initiation and initiated cells [63]. A third functional property has been proposed - retention of a response to mitogens by initiated cells and loss of such response by the majority of surrounding cells on repeated stimulation[64]. This approach also can be used as a model for a mechanism of promotion (differential stimulation)[65].

In this context, it is attractive to consider that many different types of initiated cells may be induced by exposure to an active carcinogen and that the nature of the cells selected or "promoted" may be a property of the promoting or selecting environment. Conceivably, each target organ or tissue for a carcinogen might well have a spectrum of types of potentially initiated cells selected or promoted which may reflect the mechanism of promotion appropriate for that particular tissue or organ. Since a round of cell proliferation seems to be an essential step for initiation, the only cells that are targets for the initiating effects of a carcinogen would be those that are cycling or those that enter the cycle before repair of the critical molecular lesions is complete.

Thus, initiation of chemical and some other forms of carcinogenesis can be viewed as the induction of altered cells that can be selected by an environment appropriate for those cells and for the tissue or organ in which they are induced.

Whether some or all initiated cells have, in addition to a "handle" for selection, properties that relate directly or intimately to cancer remains to date unknown. At one extreme is the hypothesis that the initiation process does nothing relevant to cancer other than allow a rare cell or group of cells to develop into a focal proliferative lesion and that all subsequent steps related to cancer are acquired at later times. At the other extreme is the hypothesis that the initiating dose of a carcinogen imparts some more direct cancer-related property or properties to the initiated cells and it is such properties that play a role in determining which of the many preneoplastic lesion progress to cancer. The obvious challenge to the cancer research is to devise experimental approaches to test these hypotheses.

Prehn[82] and others have periodically suggested that a carcinogen or carcinogenic stimulus might not <u>induce</u> an altered cell
during initiation but rather might encourage the selection of a
preformed cell already present in the target tissue. Since promoting agents or environments for the skin or liver often do not lead
to the appearance of preneoplastic or neoplastic lesions in the
absence of an initiating exposure to a carcinogen, it does not appear likely that initiated or later cells exist preformed in most
models of carcinogenesis. In the many studies on skin and in the
increasing number on liver, exposure to a carcinogen under "initiating conditions" is a prerequisite for carcinogenesis except in
a rare strain of susceptible animals (see[67-72]). However, the
unusual susceptibility of a rare preformed cell to the inducing or
initiating effects of carcinogens cannot be ruled in or out with
the currently available methods of cell analysis in tissues. A
negative conclusion concerning the selection of a preformed altered
cell by a carcinogen <u>in vitro</u> has been reached by Heidelberger[73].

Thus, in several different systems, it appears that exposure
to a carcinogen under initiating conditions <u>induces</u> rather than
<u>selects</u> altered target cells, although an unusual or rare suscep-
tibility of some preformed cells to such an inducing effect has not
been ruled out. If, as seems probable, many different types of
initiated cells may be induced by exposure to an activated carcinogen, the existence of a small population of preformed cells that
are peculiarly programmed for susceptibility becomes much less
likely.

In the liver, the initiated resistant cell that can be selected in the Solt-Farber model appears to be randomly distributed
without any apparent predilection for one or other zones of the
liver acinus[72]. This plus other considerations[3] make it highly unlikely that the target cell in the liver for carcinogenesis is a
hypothetical stem cell. Whether such hypothetical stem cells exist
and are targets in many other tissues remains unknown. In those
tissues in which a reserve of proliferating cells are considered to
be stem cells (e.g., bone marrow, skin?), it is unknown whether
such cells are peculiarly susceptible to the initiating effects of
a carcinogen. Naturally in such tissues, if a round of cell proliferation is obligatory for initiation, as is very probable, the replicating cells would be the exclusive targets in carcinogenesis.
However, in the skin at least, situations exist in which cell division appears in supra-basal layers of the epidermis. These cells
recruited for proliferation also might well be susceptible to initiation of carcinogenesis.

Although the majority of chemical carcinogens fall well within
the current paradigm of initiating effects being related to some
form of DNA damage, there are known carcinogens that appear to be
exceptions. A growing list of hypolipidemic agents[74], several pesticides, herbicides and other xenobiotics[75] and at least one drug,

methapyrelene [76] have so far not been shown to generate mutagenic or other DNA-damaging effects. Is this merely a reflection of deficiencies in our technology or are there pathways to cancer that do not involve DNA damage of exogenous origin as essential early steps in the process?

REFERENCES

1.   Foulds L: Neoplastic Development. 1969, 1975. New York: Academic Press, Vols. 1 and 2

2.   Pitot HC: Biological and Enzymatic Events in Chemical Carcinogenesis. Ann Rev Med. 30: 25 - 39, 1979

3.   Farber E, Cameron R: The Sequential Analysis of Cancer Development. Adv Cancer Res. 31: 125-226, 1980.

4.   Miller EC: Some Current Perspectives on Chemical Carcinogenesis in Humans and Experimental Animals: Presidential Address. Cancer Res 38: 1479-1496, 1978.

5.   Rajalakshmi S, Rao PM, Sarma DSR: Chemical Carcinogenesis: Interactions of Carcinogens with Nucleic Acids. In: Becker FF, ed. Cancer: A Comprehensive Treatise. 2nd ed. New York: Plenum Press in press.

6.   Berenblum I: Sequential Aspects of Chemical Carcinogenesis. In: Becker FF. ed. Cancer: A Comprehensive Treatise. New York: Plenum Press 1: 323-244, 1975.

7.   Scribner JD, Suss R: Tumour Initiation and Promotion. Int Rev Exp Pathol 18: 137-198, 1978

8.   Gelboin HV, Ts'o POP, eds: Polycyclic Hydrocarbons and Cancer. Vols 1 and 2. New York: Academic Press 1978.

9.   Lu AYH, West SB: Multiplicity of Mammalian Microsomal Cytochromes P-450. Pharmacol Rev 31: 277-295, 1979.

10. Bresnick E: Nuclear Metabolism of Polycyclic Hydrocarbons and Interaction of Polycyclic Hydrocarbons with Nuclear Components. Adv Enzyme Regulation 16: 345-361, 1978.

11. Wattenberg LW: Inhibitors of Chemical Carcinogenesis. Adv Cancer Res 26: 197-226, 1978.

12. Weisberger JH, Williams GM: Metabolism of Chemical Carcinogens. In: Becker FF, ed. Cancer: A Comprehensive Treatise. New York: Plenum Publ Corp 1: 185 - 234, 1975.

13. Levin W, Lu AYH, Ryan D, et al: Properties of Liver Microsomal Monoxygenase System and Epoxide Hydrase: Factors Influencing the Metabolism and Mutagenicity of Benzo(a)pyrene. In: Hiatt HH, Watson JD, Winsten JA, eds. Origins of Human Cancer. New York: Cold Spring Harbor Laboratory 659-682, 1977.

14. Bentley P, Oesch F: Enzymes Involved in Activation and
     Inactivation of Carcinogens and Mutagens. In: Remmer H,
     Bolt HM, Bannasch P, Popper H, eds. Primary Liver Tumours.
     Lancast, MTP Press 239-252, 1978.

15. Schulte-Hermann R: Reactions of the Liver to Injury:
     Adaptation. In: Farber E, Fisher MM, eds.   Toxic Liver
     Injury. New York: Marcel Dekker 285-444, 1979.

16. Farber E: Toxicological Significance of Liver Hypertrophy
     Produced by Inducers of Drug-metabolizing Enzymes. In:
     Environmental Chemicals, Enzyme Function and Human Disease.
     CIBA Foundation Symposium 76. Amsterdam: Excerpta Medica
     261-274, 1980.

17. Environmental Chemicals, Enzyme Function and Human Disease.
     CIBA Foundation Symposium 76. Amsterdam: Excerpta Medica
     1980.

18. McLean AEM, Magee PN: Increased Renal Carcinogenesis by
     Dimethylnitrosamine in Protein Deficient Rats. Br J Exp
     Pathol 51: 587-590, 1970.

19. Magee PN, Farber E: Toxic Liver Injury and Carcinogenesis.
     Methylation of Liver Nucleic Acids by Demylnitrosamine In
     Vivo. Biochem J 83: 114-124, 1962.

20. Singer B: N-nitrosoalkylating Agents: Formation and Per-
     sistence of Alkyl Derivatives in Mammalian Nucleic Acid as
     Contributing Factors in Carcinogenesis. J Natl Cancer Inst
     62: 1329-1339, 1979.

21. Lawley PD: Approaches to Chemical Dosimetry in Mutagenesis
     and Carcinogenesis: the Relevance of Reactions of Chemical
     Mutagens and Carcinogens with DNA. In: Grover PL, ed.
     Chemical Carcinogens and DNA. Boca Raton, Florida: CRC
     Press 1: 1-36, 1978.

22. Marquardt H: DNA - The Critical Cellular Target in Chemical
     Carcinogenesis? In: Grover PL, ed. Chemical Carcinogens and
     DNA. Boca Raton, Florida: CRC Press, 2: 159-179, 1978.

23. Cairns J: The Origin of Human Cancers. Nature 289:
     353-357, 1981.

24. Takebe H: Genetic Complementation Tests for Japanese Xero-
     derma Pigmentosum Patients and Their Skin Cancers and DNA
     Repair Characteristics. In: Magee PN, Takayama S, Sugimura
     T, Matsushima T, eds. Fundamentals in Cancer Prevention.
     7th Int Symp of Princess Takamatsu Cancer Res Fund, Tokyo:
     Univer Tokyo Press 383-395, 1975.

25. Maher VM, McCormick JJ: DNA Repair and Carcinogenesis.
    In: Grover PL, ed.   Chemical Carcinogens and DNA.
    Boca Raton, Florida, CRC Press 2:   133-158, 1978.

26. German J, ed: Chromosomes and Cancer. New York: Wiley
    and Sons, 1974.

27. Goth R, Rajewsky MF: Persistence of O^6-ethylguanine in Rat
    Brain DNA: Correlation with Nervous System Specific Car-
    cinogenesis by Ehtylnitrosourea. Proc Natl Acad Sci.
    USA 71: 639-643, 1974.

28. Magee PN, Swann PF, Mohr U, Resnik G, Green U: Possible
    Repair of Carcinogenesis by Nitroso Compounds. In:
    Magee PN, Takayama S, Sugimura T, Matsushima T, eds.
    Fundamentals in Cancer Prevention. Tokyo: University of
    Tokyo Press 281-289, 1976.

29. Lewis JG, Swenberg JA: Differential Repair of O^6-methylgua-
    nine in DNA of Rat Hepatocytes and Non-parenchymal Cells.
    Nature 288: 185-188, 1980.

30. Buechler J, Kleihues P: Excision of O^6-methylguanine from
    DNA of Various Mouse Tissues Following a Single Injection of
    N-methyl-N-nitrosourea. Chem Biol Interact 16: 325-333,
    1977.

31. Ying TS: Studies on Acute Cell Injury, Cell Replication and
    DNA Repair during Initiation of Liver Carcinogenesis.
    Ph.D. Thesis, University of Toronto 1980.

32. Olsson M, Lindahl T: Repair of Alkylated DNA in Escherichia
    Coli. Methyl Group Transfer from O^6-methylguanine to a
    Protein Cysteine Residue. J. Biol Chem 255: 10569-10571,
    1980.

33. Conney AH, Levin W: Carcinogen Metabolism in Experimental
    Animals and Man. In: Montesano R, Tomatis L, Davis W,
    eds. Chemical Carcinogenesis Essays. Lyon: Int Agency
    for Res on Cancer Publ 10 3-22, 1974.

34. Montesano R, Magee PN: Comparative Metabolism In Vitro of
    Nitrosamines in Various Animal Species including Man. In:
    Montesano R, Tomatis L, Davis W, eds. Chemical Carcino-
    genesis Essays. Lyon: Int Agency for Res on Cancer Publ
    10 39-56, 1974.

35. Shinohara K, Cerutti P: Formation of Benzo(a)pyrene - DNA
    adducts in Peripheral Human Lung Tissue. Cancer Lett 3:
    303-310,1977.

36. Prough RA, Patrizi VW, Okta RT, Masters BSS, Jakobsson SW:
     Characteristics of Benzo(a)pyrene Metabolism by Kidney,
     Liver and Lung Microsomal Fractions from Rodents and Humans.
     Cancer Res 39: 1199-1206, 1979.

37. Autrup H, Schwartz RD, Essigman JM, Smith L, Trump BF,
     Harris CC: Metabolism of Aflatoxin B_1, Benzo(a)pyrene and
     1,2-dimethylhydrazine by Cultured Rat and Human Colon.
     Teratogenesis, Carcinogenesis and Mutagenesis 1: 3-13, 1980.

38. Autrup H, Jeffery AM, Harris CC: Metabolism of Benzo(a)pyrene
     in Cultured Human Bronchus, Trachea, Colon and Esophagus.
     In: Bjørseth A, Dennis AJ, eds. Polynuclear Aromatic Hydro-
     carbons. New York: Raven Press 4: 89-105, 1980.

39. Mass MJ, Rodgers NT, Kaufman DG: Benzo(a)pyrene Metabolism
     in Organ Cultures of Human Endometrium. Chem Biol Int 33:
     195-205, 1981.

40. Hsu IC, Poirier MC, Yuspa SH, Yolken RH, Harris CC: Ultra-
     sensitive-enzymatic Radioimmunoassay (USERIA) Detects
     Femtomoles of Acetylaminofluroene-DNA adducts. Carcinogenesis
     1: 455-458, 1981.

41. Poirier MC, Dubin MA, Yuspa SH: Formation and Removal of
     Specific Acetylaminofluorene-DNA adducts in Mouse and Human
     Cells Measured by Radioimmunoassay. Cancer Res 39: 1377 -
     1381, 1979.

42. Hsu IC, Poirier MC, Yuspa SH, Grunberger D, et al: Measure-
     ment of Benzo(a)pyrene-DNA adducts by Enzyme Immunoassays
     and Radioimmunoassay. Cancer Res 41: 1091-1095, 1981.

43. Cairns J: Mutation, Selection and the Natural History of
     Cancer. Nature 255: 197-200, 1975.

44. Nowell PC: The Clonal Evolution of Tumour Cell Populations.
     Science 194: 23-28, 1976.

45. Burnet FM: Cancer: Somatic-genetic Considerations. Adv
     Cancer Res 28: 1-29, 1978.

46. Cayama E, Tsuda H, Sarma DSR, Farber E: Initiation of
     Chemical Carcinogenesis Requires Cell Proliferation.
     Nature 275: 60-62, 1978.

47. Tsuda H, Lee G, Farber E. Induction of Resistant Hepatocytes
     as a New Principle for a Possible Short-term In Vivo Test for
     Carcinogens. Cancer Res 40: 1157-1164, 1980.

48. Emmelot P, Scherer E: The First Relevant Cell Stage in Rat
     Liver Carcinogenesis. A Quantitative approach. Biochem
     Biophys Acta 605: 247-304, 1980.

49. Craddock, VM: Cell Proliferation and Experimental Liver Cancer. In: Cameron HM, Linsell DA, Warwick GP, eds. Liver Cell Cancer. Amsterdam: Elservier-North Holland Blomed Press 153-201, 1976.

50. Borek C.Sachs L: In Vitro Cell Transformation by X-irradiation. Nature 210: 276-278, 1966.

51. Tooze J: The Molecular Biology of Tumour Viruses. New York: Cold Spring Harbour Laboratory, 1973.

52. Kakunaga T: Requirement for Cell Replication in the Fixation and Expression of the Transformed State in Mouse Cells treated with 4-nitro-quinolin-1-oxide. Int J Cancer 14: 736-42, 1974.

53. Ying TS, Sarma DSR, Farber E: Role of Acture Hepatic Necrosis in the Induction of Early Steps in Liver Carcinogenesis by Diethylnitrosamine. Cancer Res 41: 2096-2101, 1981.

54. Columbano A, Rajalakshmi S, Sarma DSR: Requirement of Cell Proliferation for the Initiation of Liver Carcinogenesis as Assayed by Three Different Procedures. Cancer Res 41: 2079-2083, 1981.

55. Stutman O: Immunodepression and Malignancy. Adv Cancer Res 22: 261-422, 1975.

56. Thomas L: Discussion. In: Lawrence HS, ed. Cellular and Humoral Aspects of Hypersensitivity. New York: Harper and Row 529: 532, 1959.

57. Rice JM. ed. Perinatal Carcinogenesis. Natl Cancer Inst Monograph 51, 1979.

58. Neubert D, Merker H-J, Nau H, Langman J, eds. Role of Pharmacokinetics in Pernatal and Perinatal Toxicology. Stuttgart: G. Thieme Publ, 1978.

59. Pelkonen O: Environmental Influences on Human Foetal and Placental Xenobiotic Metabolism. Eur J Clin Pharmacol 18: 17-24, 1980.

60. Berenblum I: Speculative Review: Probable Nature of Promoting Action and its Significance in Understanding of Mechanism of Carcinogenesis. Cancer Res 14: 471-477, 1954.

61. Lipkin M, Deschner E: Early Proliferative Chances in Intestinal Cells. Cancer Res 36: 2665-2668, 1976.

62. Pitot HC, Sirica AE: The Stages of Initiation and Promotion in Hepatocarcinogenesis. Biochem Biophys Acta 605: 191-215, 1980.

63. Farber E: The Sequential Analysis of Liver Cancer Induction.

Biochem Biophys Acta 605: 149-166, 1980.

64. Ohde G, Schuppler J, Schulte-Hermann R, Keiger H: Prolifera-
     tion of Rat Liver Cells in Perneoplastic Nodules after
     Stimulation of Liver Growth by Xenobiotic Inducers. Arch
     Toxicol Suppl 2 451-455, 1979.

65. Farber E: Sequential Events in Chemical Carcinogenesis.
     In: Becker FF, ed. Cancer: A Comprehensive Treatise.
     2nd Edition. New York: Plenum Press Corp, in press, 1981.

66. Boutwell RK: Some Biological Aspects of Skin Carcinogenesis.
     Prog Exp Tumour Res 4: 207-250, 1964.

67. Boutwell RK: The Function and Mechanism of Promoters of
     Carcinogenesis. CRC Crit Rev Toxicol 2: 419-443, 1974.

68. Peraino C, Fry RJM, Grube DD: Drug-induced Enhancement of
     Hepatic Tumourigenesis. In: Slaga TJ, Sivak A, Boutwell
     RK, eds. Carcinogenesis: Mechanisms of Tumour Promotion and
     Cocarcinogenesis. Raven Press, New York 2: 421-432, 1978.

69. Pitot HC, Barsness L, Kitagawa T: Stages in the Process of
     Hepatocarcinogenesis in Rat Liver. In: Slaga TJ, Sivak A,
     Boutwell RK, eds. Carcinogenesis: Mechanisms of Tumour
     Promotion and Carcinogenesis, Raven Press, New York 2:
     433-442, 1978.

70. Scherer E, Emmelot P: Kinetics of Induction and Growth of
     Enzyme-deficient Islands Involved in Hepatocarcinogenesis.
     Cancer Res 36: 2544-25, 1976.

71. Solt DB, Farber E: A New Principle for the Analysis of
     Chemical Carcinogenesis. Nature 263: 701-703, 1976.

72. Solt DB, Medline A. Farber E: Rapid Emergence of Carcino-
     gen-induced Hyperplastic Lesions in a New Model for the
     Sequential Analysis of Liver Carcinogenesis. Am J Pathol
     88: 595-618, 1977.

73. Heidelberger C: Mammalian Cell Transformation and Mammalian
     Cell Mutagenesis In Vitro. J Environmental Pathol Toxicol
     3: 69-87, 1980.

74. Reddy JK, Azarnoff DL, Hignite CE: Hypolipidaemic Hepatic
     Peroxisome Proliferators Form a Novel Class of Chemical
     Carcinogens. Nature 283: 397-398, 1980.

75. Rinkus SJ, Legator MS: Chemical Characterization of 465
     Known or Suspected Carcinogens and Their Correlation with
     Mutagenic Activity in the Salmonella Typhimurium System.
     Cancer Res 39: 3289-3318, 1979.

76. Lijinsky W, Reuber MD, Blackwell BN: Liver Tumours Induced in Rats by Oral Administration of the Antihistaminic Methapyrilene Hydrochloride. Science: 209: 817-819, 1980.

77. Scherer E, Hoffmann M: Probable Clonal Genesis of Cellular Islands Induced in Rat Liver by Diethylnitrosamine. Eur J Cancer 7: 369-371, 1971.

78. Iannaconne PM, Gardner RL, Harris H: The Cellular Origin of Chemi-ally Induced Tumour. J Cell Sci 29: 249-269, 1978.

79. Kennedy AR, Fox M, Murphy G, Little JB: Relationship Between X-ray Exposure and Malignant Transformation in C3H10T1/2 cells. Proc Natl Acad Sci USA 77: 7262-7266, 1980.

80. Mondal S, Heidelberger C: In Vitro Malignant Transformation by Methylcholanthrene of the Progeny of Single Cells Derived from C3H Mouse Prostate. Proc Natl Acad Sci 65: 219-225, 1970.

81. German J: Carriers in Chromosome-breakage Syndromes. Proc 6th Int Congress Radiation Res: 496-505, 1979.

82. Prehn RT: Tumor progression and homeostasis. Adv Cancer Res 23: 203-236, 1976.

BENIGN AND MALIGNANT TUMOR INDUCTION IN MOUSE SKIN

Fredric J. Burns, Roy E. Albert and Bernard Altshuler

NYU Institute of Environmental Medicine
550 First Avenue
New York, New York

INTRODUCTION

Carcinogenesis has often been assumed to be a multistage disease where a single cell progresses from normal to cancer in discrete sequential stages[1,2,3]. There is statistical support for the existence of such stages in the shape of functions that describe the dependence of cancer yield on dose and time. Biological evidence in favor of the multistage theory is derived from chromosomally marked clones seen in exacerbations of myeloid leukemia and in the progressive acquisition of automony seen in certain types of tumors, especially, hormone dependent tumors[4,5].

In an attempt to explain mouse skin tumor data in terms of multistage progression, we have formulated a cell generation hypothesis. In this formulation, the initial event in carcinogenesis is assumed to be an interaction between the carcinogen and the cell (probably the DNA of the cell) that changes the cell in such a way that it is identifiable as initiated, i.e., it forms a benign clonal growth, known as a papilloma, when exposed to a promoter, such as, 12-0-tetradecanoyl-13-phorbolacetate (TPA)[6,7]. Furthermore, it is assumed that the original initiated cell and all of its progency are unstable in the sense that they are subject at each cell division to the risk of additional changes leading to progressive acquisition of cancerous properties[8].

Papillomas that are dependent on continued promotion, i.e., those that would regress if the promotion were stopped, may acquire autonomy[6]. The cells in automomous papillomas continue to be at risk of progression to cancer whether or nor promotion is continued. Probably many changes not produced directly by the

315

carcinogen are needed to convert an initiated cell into a cancer
cell. These additional changes or transitions are an indirect
result of initiation and are assumed to be distributed in a
stochastic manner in time subsequent to initiation.

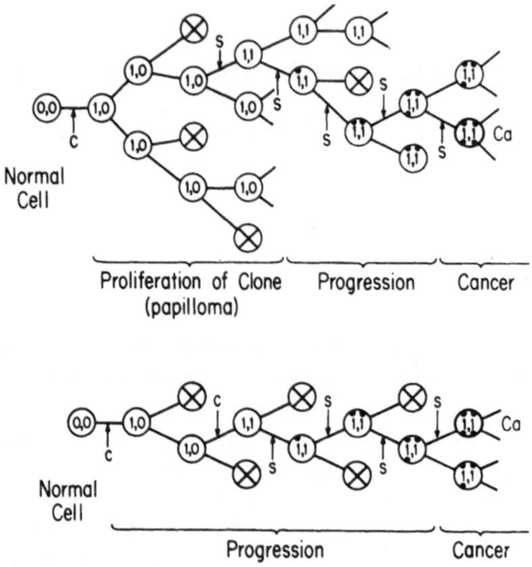

Figure 1. A schematic diagram of the multistage-multi-generational
hypothesis. The initial event is depicted as being produced by a
carcinogen (arrow with a C). In the upper panel the cell (1,0)
with one event multiplies into a clone, and at a subsequent cell
division suffers a spontaneous event (arrow with S) to become
a cell that is equivalent to one having suffered two carcinogen
induced (without clonal multiplication) events as depicted in the
lower panel. The further progression of 1,1 cells is depicted as
requiring 4 additional events. As discussed in the text, this
number is somewhat uncertain, because it depends on the amount of
clonal multiplication assumed for intermediate stages.

     We propose a cell generation hypothesis where the acquisition
of each of the various properties necessary for a cancer cell
proceeds in a sequential manner as a direct result of instability,
probably in the chromosomes, caused by the carcinogen having
interacted with the cell (Figure 1).

Multistage theory holds that the value of the exponent of the
function of tumor rate versus time equals the number of stages in
carcinogenesis. Accordingly, that exponent ought to be constant,
but there are many examples where it varies. This can be handled
by invoking clonal expansion as an important determinant of the
temporal function whenever promotion, intrinsic or extrinsic, is
present[9]. Thus, there are two routes a cell may take as it
progresses to cancer. The first route involves one carcinogen
induced alteration (initiation) followed by additional alterations
that are observable only because of the multiplication of probability implicit in clonal growth. The second route involves 2 or
3 carcinogen-induced alterations that presumably damage the cell
so severely that additional alterations are probable even without
substantial clonal growth.

To make these ideas more concrete, we can formulate them into
a mathematical framework. First let it be assumed that cancer
requires n stages. These stages correspond to transitions that
can be described by transition probabilities (for the ith transition) of the form:

$$K_i = a_i + b_i \, d \tag{1}$$

where a_i is the spontaneous transition rate, b_i is the dose
coefficient of the ith transition and d is the dose of the
carcinogen[2].

If a_i and b_i are constants and the dose rate is constant, the
cumulative probability of the ith transition is given by $K_i t$
where t is elapsed time. Accordingly, the cumulative probability
per unit time of cancer occurrence, often referred to as the
cumulative hazard function $H(t,d)$ can be written:

$$H(t,d) = \prod_{i=1}^{n} K_i \, t^n. \tag{2}$$

For any transition where the spontaneous rate is neglibible in
comparison to the carcinogen induced rate, i.e., $a_i \ll b_i d$, the
transition probability can be written as $b_i d$. If there are m
such transitions, the cumulative hazard becomes:

$$H(t,d) = \prod_{i=1}^{m} b_i \prod_{m}^{n} K \, d^m t^n. \tag{3}$$

Since the tumors are assumed to be randomly distributed among the
animals, the proportion with tumors, $P(t,d)$, is related to the
cumulative hazard, $H(t,d)$, by the equation:

$$P(t,d) = 1 - e^{-H(t,d)}. \tag{4}$$

It follows that 50% of any given group of animals will have at least one tumor when $H = 0.693$[10]. If the time when 50% have developed at least one tumor is designated t_{50}, it follows from equations 3 and 4 that:

$$d \, t_{50}^{n/m} = constant. \hspace{3cm} (5)$$

The above equation can be considered to be a dose—response function where m is the number of dose-dependent transitions and n is the total number of transition in carcinogenesis.

Equation 5 was originally found empirically by Druckrey to apply to liver carcinogenesis when either AAF or DEN were given in the diet, and the value of n/m was estimated to be about 2.3[11]. Values of n/m were derived from the epidemiological data on lung cancer in cigarette smokers and found to be 2.6[12]. The multistage theory seems generally to fit the experimental and epidemiological data quite well for situations where the carcinogen exposure is prolonged, and the dose rate is constant.

The principle defect of the multistage theory is that the stages are not identifiable and their order or sequence is unknown. Peto concluded that the carcinogen-dependent stages were probably early in the sequence because older mice, that presumably had accumulated many of the non-carcinogen related stages, showed no greater response to topical application of a carcinogen, benzo(a)pyrene, than younger mice[13]. The stages themselves are purely speculative entities but certainly can encompass the concept of carcinogenic progression as it is currently understood. Cancer cells may need to acquire a number of specific properties, such as the ability to stimulate host blood vessels by means of angiogenesis factor, the ability to dissolve connective tissue proteins by secreting proteases, the ability to block the immune defenses of the host by producing blocking factor. The acquisition of each of these properties occurring sequentially in a given period of time could be considered to represent transitions between stages in the multistage model. Of course, there are many other properties of cancer cells that might represent stages and certainly more biological studies are needed to refine our understanding of stages and the transitions between them.

The mouse skin is an ideal model system to test these ideas and to study dose and time related aspects of benign and malignant tumor formation. A series of experiments were performed in an attempt to answer certain specific questions related to these ideas.

The first and most important question was what shape to assume for
the dose-response function of benign and malignant tumors.
Carcinogens and promoters were applied topically in 0.2 ml acetone
by pipette onto the dorsal skin of mice. In one experiment the
following amounts of benzo(a)pyrene (B(a)P) were applied as
single initiating doses: 0 µg, 4 µg, 8 µg, 16 µg, 32 µg, 64 µg and
128 µg followed by a standard protocol of promotion consisting of
5 µg of 12-0-tetradecanoyl-13-acetate three times weekly. The
second experiment involved giving multiple initiating doses of
B(a)P once per week. The total amount of B(a)P along with the
number of fractions were as follows: 4 µg (4, 8, 32 fractions;
8 µg (2, 8, 32 fractions); 16 µg (4, 8, 16, 32 fractions); 32 µg
(2, 8, 32 fractions); 64 µg (4, 8, 16, 32 fractions) and 128 µg
(8, 32 fractions). Each treatment group contained 20 or 25 animals.
In the latter experiment, promotion was begun one week after the
last dose of initiator. A third experiment involved total doses
of 4 µg, 16 µg, 32 µg and 128 µg in 8 weekly fractions followed by
promotion one week after the last initiating dose.

Animals were observed every other week and the progress of
individual tumors was charted. Regression of tumors and progression
of benign lesions to malignancy was noted. Animals were sacrificed
when moribund or when tumors exceeded 1.0 cm^3 in size. Representative benign skin tumors and all carcinomas diagnosed grossly were
excised, fixed in 10% formalin and blocked in paraffin. Slides
were prepared and stained with hematoxylin and eosin for histo-
pathological diagnosis.

For each observation interval, the number of new tumors was
divided by the average number of mice alive to obtain the rate of
tumor occurrence. The rates were added cumulatively to obtain the
yield of tumors in tumors per mouse (cumulative hazard) as a
function of time.

Figure 2 shows the yield of papillomas and carcinomas in
mice receiving only TPA thrice weekly. These data are based on
63 mice. Median survival was 550 days and there were 7 mice left
at 650 days. Papilloma formation began at 150 days after the
start of promotion and increased continuously thereafter. All
carcinomas appeared from preexisting papillomas. The conversion
of papillomas to carcinomas was initially evident at 350 days
and continued thereafter with a ratio of papillomas to carcinomas
at about 7:1. No tumors were observed in 40 acetone treated
mice during the same period of time.

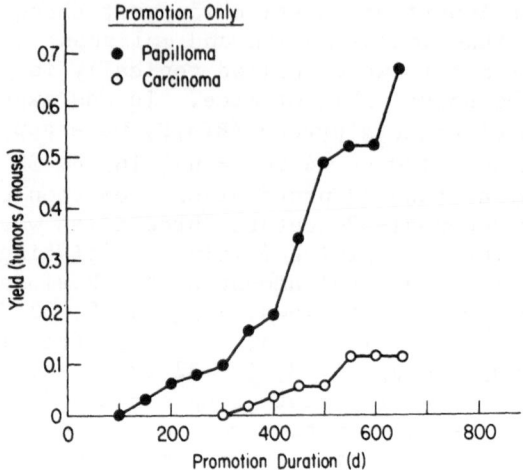

Figure 2. The yield of papillomas and carcinomas in mouse (Ha/1CR) skin treated only with 5 µg TPA in 0.2 ml acetone 3 times weekly.

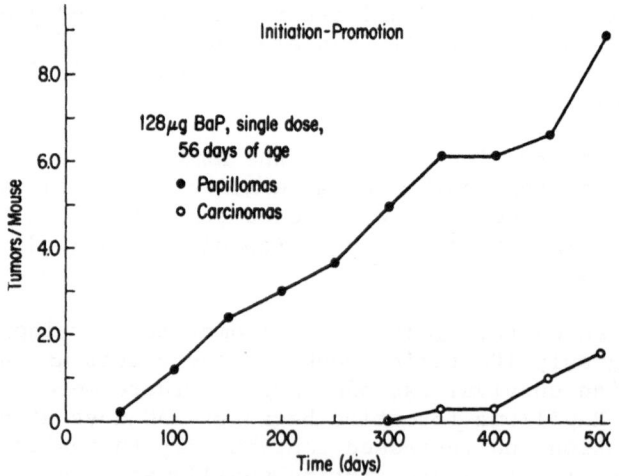

Figure 3. Cumulative yield of skin papillomas and of skin carcinomas after topical treatments. A single dose of 128 µg B(a)P administered at 56 days of age was followed by treatment three times weekly with 5 µg TPA in 0.2 ml acetone.

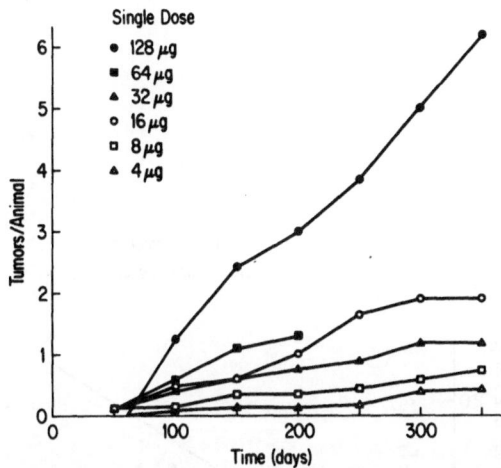

Figure 4. The yield of skin papillomas per mouse as a function of time after treatment involving initiation with various doses of benzo(a)pyrene (B(a)P), followed by promotion with 5.0 µg TPA thrice weekly.

Figure 4 shows the temporal pattern of papilloma formation after single doses of B(a)P ranging from 4 µg to 128 µg. Tumor formation began at about 50 days with the slope of the curves generally increasing in proportion to dose.

Figure 3 shows the papilloma and carcinoma yield after a single initiating dose of 128 µg B(a)P followed by TPA thrice weekly. The temporal pattern is typical of that for other initiating doses of B(a)P. Papilloma formation began at about 50 days and continued fairly steadily thereafter. A few carcinomas developed from preexisting papillomas beginning at about 350 days.

Figure 5 shows the dose-response relationships for papilloma yield at 200 days based on the data in Figure 4. The pattern is consistent with a linear dose-response function.

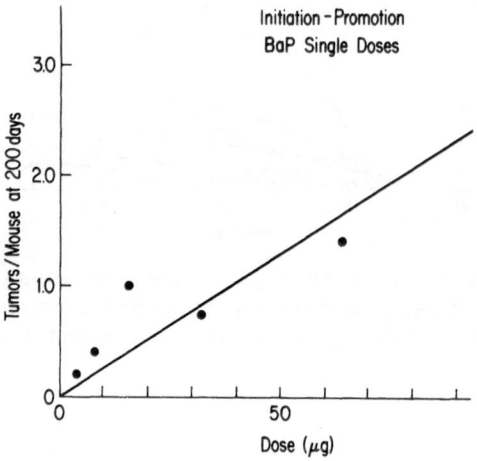

Figure 5. The yield of skin papillomas per mouse as a function of the initiating dose of B(a)P at 200 d after the start of promotion with 5.0 µg TPA three times weekly. All chemicals were applied in 0.2 ml acetone.

The temporal pattern of tumor formation after single and multiple applications of B(a)P as an initiating agent are similar. These data are shown in Figure 6.

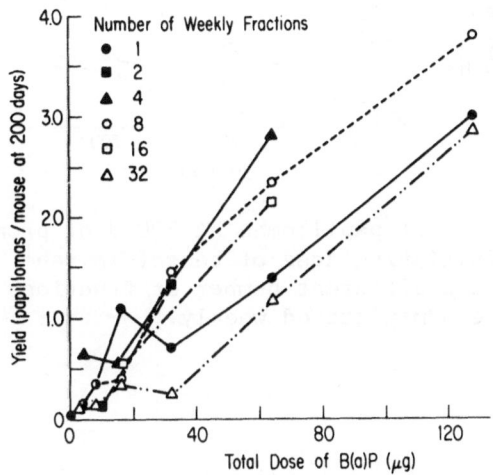

Figure 6. Cumulative yield of skin papillomas and skin carcinomas observed after topical carcinogen treatments. A total dose of 128 µg of B(a)P was administered in 32 weekly fractions of 4 µg per week. This treatment was followed one week after the last B(a)P dose by treatment with 5.0 µg TPA three times weekly. Time zero was the start of the TPA treatments.

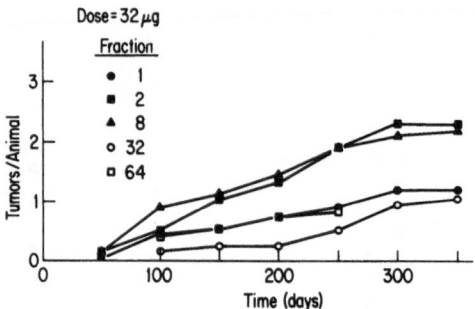

<u>Figure 7.</u> The yield of papillomas at 200 d of promotion as a
function of the initiating dose of benzo(a)pyrene. Each set
of data represents a different number of fractions as indicated.
The fractions were administered weekly.

The dose-response relationships for single and fractionated
B(a)P initiation at 200 days of TPA promotion are shown in
Figure 7. Within a factor of about two there is no effect of
fractionating the initiating dose of B(a)P on subsequent tumor
induction.

The lack of fractionation effect permits the display shown
in Figure 8 of the tumor response per fractional dose. For
example, if 128 μg were given in 8 fractions with a tumor incidence

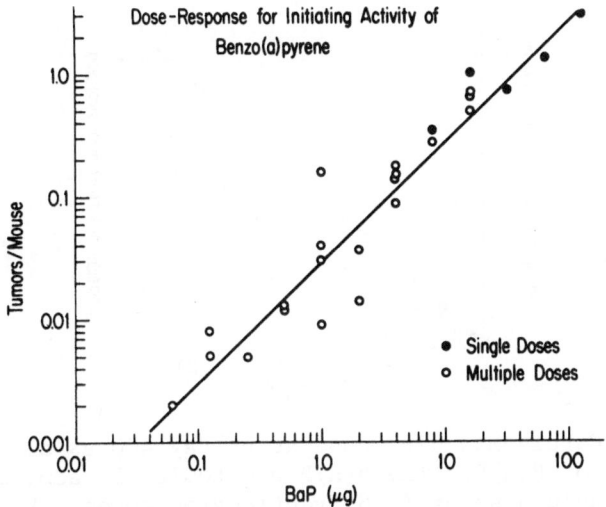

Figure 8. A log - log plot of the yield of papillomas per fraction as a function of the dose per fraction. The solid line was fitted by regression analysis and indicates a very good linear fit (exponent 0.9).

of 5.3 tumors/mouse at 200 days, the net tumor yield per fraction ($\frac{5.3-0.06}{8}$ = 0.66) would be plotted against the dose per fraction ($\frac{128}{8}$ = 16). Figure 8 shows this data for all single and fraction-ated exposures. The regression line drawn through the data points has a slope of 1.08. The data support the linear dose-response relationship of papilloma formation for B(a)P iniation throughout a dose range extending 3 orders of magnitude. The slope is such that one initiated tumor site is produced by each 30 µg dose of B(a)P.

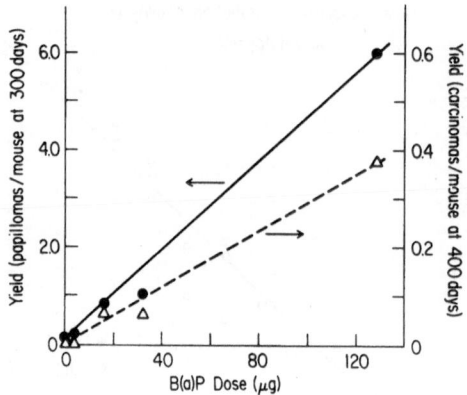

Figure 9. Carcinomas per mouse as of day 400 as a function of total doses of B(a)P. The B(a)P was topically administered as either a single dose or in 8 fractionated doses. Promotion with 5 µg TPA three times weekly began one week after the last B(a)P treatment. Time zero was the start of the TPA treatments.

The linearity of carcinoma induction as well as papilloma formation is shown in Figure 9 for the experiment involving the indicated total B(a)P doses given in 8 fractions twice a week.

The data presented in Figures 2-9 strongly support the linear non-threshold character of the dose-response relationships for the initiation of carcinogenesis by B(a)P in the mouse skin. A linear non-threshold dose-response was also obtained from B(a)P in the skin of Sencar mice using 2 µg TPA twice a week[14]. The lack of a fractionation effect is consistent with the linear response to single carcinogen exposures and implies a mechanism based on a single irreversible event.

If each papilloma is considered to be a clonal expansion of an initiated cell, and an initiated cell is the first stage in carcinogenesis, the above data permit an evaluation of $K_1 = a_1 + b_1 D$. For example, from the data in Figure 2, $a_1 = \frac{0.5}{575}$ transitions/mouse/D and from the data in Figure 5, $b_1 = \frac{2}{1600}$ transitions/mouse µg day. The pattern of papilloma induction and conversion of papillomas to carcinomas in the uninitiated mice treated thrice weekly with TPA suggests that the skin has a background of initiation equivalent to about (4000/575) µg of B(a)P, i.e., a_1/b_1. Since the area of mouse skin treated contains about 3×10^6 epidermal cells, the corresponding transition constants in units of transitions per cell per day are $a_1 = \frac{0.5}{575(3)} \times 10^{-6}$ and $b_1 = \frac{2}{(16,000)3} \times 10^{-6}$ transitions/cell µg day.

DNA Binding

The dose dependency of the binding of benzo(a)pyrene (B(a)P) with DNA of mouse epidermis was investigated. B(a)P-conjugated epidermal DNA was isolated and enzymatically degraded to deoxyribnucleosides. The B(a)P-DNA adducts were separated by Sephadex LH-20 column or high-performance liquid chromatography. Two major B(a)P-DNA adducts were found. One was in the region of the elution profile that contained polycyclic aromatic hydrocarbons adducted to deoxyribonucleosides. The other adduct was eluted from Sephadex LH-20 and high-performance liquid chromatography columns before the deoxyribonucleosides and after deoxyribonucleotides. Both adducts of B(a)P in epidermal DNA reached a maximum 7 hours after a single skin application, and subsequently little, if any, loss of adducts was observed for 49 hours. Both adducts varied as a linear function for topical doses in the range from 0.01 to 300 µg/mouse. The formation of DNA adducts by B(a)P occurred in proportion to dose at doses several orders of magnitude below those that are feasible to test for carcinogenicity.

When B(a)P is applied to mouse skin[15], added to cell culture[16], or indubated in the presence of microsomes and DNA[17], electrophilic metabolites are formed that covalently bind to DNA. The initiation of carcinogenesis by polycyclic aromatic hydrocarbons is believed

to involve covalent binding to cellular macromolecules, and there
appears to be an especially good correlation between their
carcinogenic potency and DNA binding[15]. Thus, the binding to
DNA might serve as a sensitive indicator of carcinogenicity since
analytical techniques are available to detect such binding at
extremely low doses. Actually, the formation of a number of
different DNA adducts as well as tritium exchange onto the bases
is possible. Thus, specific B(a)P:DNA adducts could serve as a
better marker for biological potency than the total amount of
binding in B(a)P-conjugated DNA. The major hydrophobic B(a)P
adduct to deoxyribonucleosides formed in vivo has been identified
and studied extensively[18,19]. Hydrophilic B(a)P:DNA adducts
present in the elution profiles obtained from the chromatography
systems used in the isolation of B(a)P:deoxyribonucleoside adducts
remain to be characterized[20].

Promotion in Combination with a Carcinogen

Promoters have important consequences in determining the
temporal pattern of cancer induction by accelerating the development
of neoplasia. Promoters may act by stimulating clonal expansion
of potentially cancerous cells or they may stimulate the expression
of a neoplastic event or they may actually produce neoplastic
events. In order to determine the temporal effect of promoters on
carcinogenesis, mouse skin was exposed to weekly doses of benzo-
(a)pyrene either alone or in combination with various twice weekly
doses of TPA. The cancer yield as a function of time when B(a)P
was given alone is shown in Figure 10. As the B(a)P dose increased
from 16 μg weekly to 128 μg weekly, the tumor curves were displaced
progressively to earlier times in such a manner that n/m in the
expression, $dt_{50}^{n/m}$ = constant, was about 2.1; where d was
weekly dose and t_{50} was time to 50% prevalence.

The results when various weekly doses of TPA were added
to a given weekly dose of B(a)P are shown in Figure 11. As the
TPA dose was increased, the cancer yields were progressively
displaced to earlier times, although there seemed to be a plateau-
effect in the sense that the increase from 0.5 to 5.0 μg per
week produced much less displacement than the increase from 0.05
to 0.5 μg per week. There is little doubt from these data that
TPA, a promoter of papillomas, accelerated the development of
carcinomas. The maximum degree of temporal displacement (the
highest TPA dose) was equivalent to a 4-fold increase in B(a)P
dose. These data suggest that part of the temporal displacement
associated with different doses of B(a)P could be derived from the
promoting action of B(a)P.

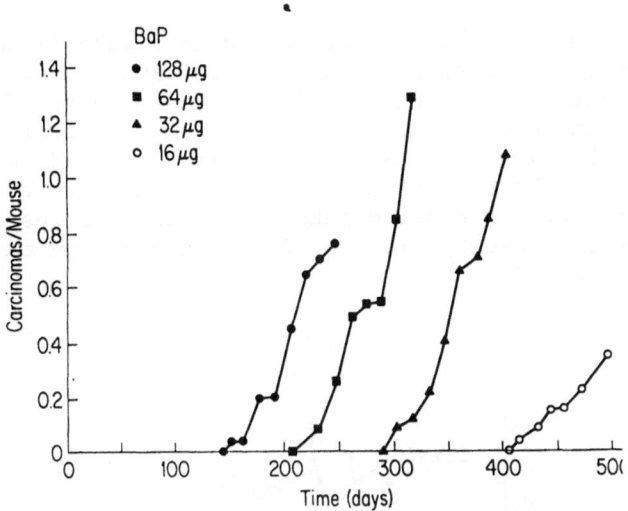

Figure 10. Cumulative yield of skin carcinomas per mouse. Numbers
identifying each curve indicate the topically applied weekly dose
of B(a)P treatment at 56 days of age.

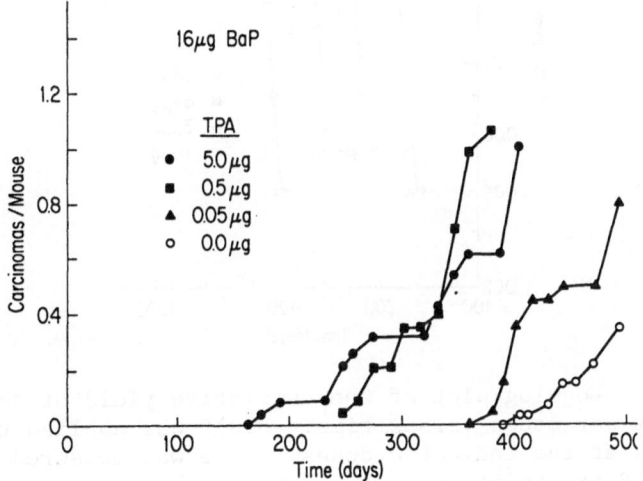

Figure 11. Cumulative yield of skin carcinomas per mouse. Each
animal received weekly treatments of 16 µg B(a)P (Monday) plus
twice weekly treatments of either 0, 0.05, 0.5 or 5.0 µg TPA
(Wednesday and Friday). Chemicals were topically applied in
0.2 ml acetone.

The carcinoma data has been replotted in Figure 12 on log-log coordinates in order to show the temporal onset pattern more clearly. Straight lines on such a plot represent power functions of the form ct^m where c is a constant and m the exponent can be estimated from the slope[10]. As indicated in Figure 12, m ranges from 7.8 to 10.0. These patterns are quite typical of those observed for exposure of other organs to carcinogens, especially, rat liver exposed to diethylnitrosamine and human lung exposed to cigarette smoke[11,12].

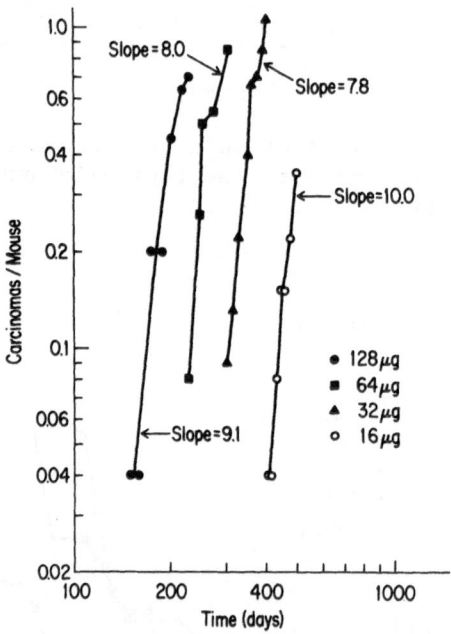

Figure 12. Log-log plot of the cumulative yield of skin carcinomas per mouse versus time. B(a)P was applied topically every week at the indicated doses. Time was measured from the first B(a)P treatment as in Figure 11.

A dose-effect relationship for carcinoma induction under conditions of repeated weekly B(a)P exposure can be generated by considering the tumor yield at a specific point in time, specifically 300 d after the B(a)P was started. These data are shown in Figure 13. In the absence of TPA the cancer yield increased sharply with dose consistent with a squared or cubed function. However, when TPA was added weekly along with B(a)P, the dose effect function shifted markedly to the left, i.e., to lower B(a)P doses, and more importantly lost the squared or cubed dose dependence and became nearly linear.

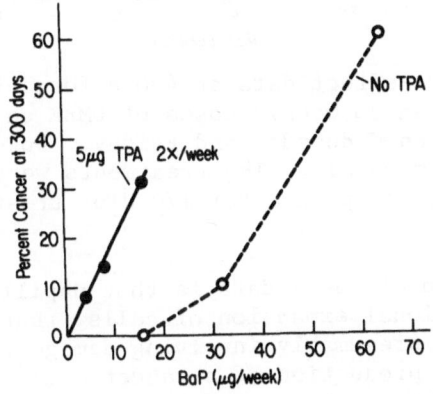

Figure 13. The dose-effect data at 350 d for carcinoma induction in mouse skin exposed to a weekly dose of B(a)P on Monday with or without 5.0 µg TPA on Wednesday and Friday. Doses refer to the amount of B(a)P given per week. The treatments were started at 56 d of age.

   A similar result was obtained when 7,12 dimethylbenz(a)anthra-
cene (DMBA) was used instead of benzo(a)pyrene. These data are
shown in Figure 14 for 5 µg of TPA twice weekly added to various
weekly doses of DMBA as indicated. All treatments were stopped
at 175 d and the data shown are cancer yields at 400 d. Again,
here the addition of TPA shifted the curves to much lower doses
of DMBA and changed a sharply increasing function into one that
was nearly linear.

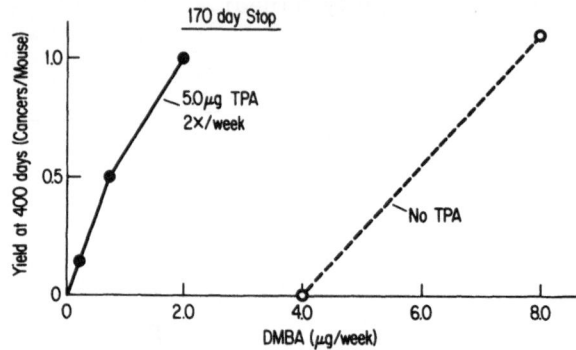

Figure 14. The dose-effect data at 400 d for carcinoma induction
in mouse skin exposed to weekly doses of DMBA on Monday with or
without 5.0 µg TPA on Wednesday and Friday. Doses refer to the
amount of DMBA given weekly. The treatments were started at
56 d of age and were stopped after 170 d of treatment.

   One explanation of these data is that papillomas contain
cells, probably a clonal expansion of cells, that have undergone
one or more events, presumably involving damage to DNA, that are
early events in the production of a cancer cell. It is not
suggested here that every event presumed to be involved in
carcinogenesis necessarily produces cells that are expandable
into clones by the action of phorbol ester. Neither can we
eliminate the possibility at the present time that the promoter
may have effects in addition to stimulation of clonal expansion,
although such events must differ from initiator-induced events.

One hypothesis consistent with the ideas outlined here
could be called the cell generation theory. In this theory one
or two events, e.g., chromosome breaks, produced either directly
or indirectly by the action of a carcinogen causes an instability
leading to the accumulation of additional changes, possibly as
many as 4-6[21]. Presumably any or all of these events may occur
spontaneously which is necessary to explain the occurrence of
'spontaneous' cancer in untreated animals and the conversion of
persisting papillomas to cancers without further treatment. The
clonal expansion implicit in the growth of a papilloma greatly
increases the chance that cancer will occur because each papilloma
cell has a spontaneous risk of occurrence of later events, including
some that could be produced by action of a carcinogen. The
promoter may also fix the initiation since short exposure to a
promoter followed by a mitotic stimulation will produce tumors,
whereas mitotic stimulation alone will not.

The shapes of the dose-effect functions for carcinoma induction
with and without promotion can be explained in terms of the above
ideas as follows. In the absence of promotion the carcinogen
must act directly and repeatedly on target cells to produce what-
ever number of events are necessary for a malignant cell to occur
(possibly 2 or 3); hence the yield of cancers is proportional to
(dose rate)$^{2-3}$ and a relatively high total dose is needed to
produce a given yield. If the tissue is promoted, clonal expansion
of some intermediate state leads to a greatly increased overall
risk of malignancy because each initiated cell in a papillomatous
clone is assumed to have acquired some risk, albeit small, of the
occurrence of additional events that would complete the transition
to malignancy. Cancers derived from such papillomas would be expected to follow the dose-response characteristic of the papillomas,
since second and subsequent events would occur spontaneously without the necessity for action by the carcinogen. The cancer yield
for a given dose of carcinogen would be much higher with promotion
than without because of the risk multiplication inherent in clonal
expansion.

The data in Figure 2 shows that the rate of conversion of
spontaneous papillomas to carcinomas was about 1/300 per day,

while the data in Figure 3 shows the comparable rate for induced
papillomas was about the same (1/350 per day). If all papilloma
cells are at risk, these values reduce to transition rates of
about (1/300-350) x 10^{-6} per cell per day since there are about
10^6 cells per papilloma. In our model the latter quantity is an
estimate of a_2; the spontaneous rate of transition of papillomas
to a cell type that has a high risk of further events in the
progression to cancer.

From the dose-response function in the absence of TPA in
Figure 13, one can derive an estimate of b_2 by assuming the dose
of carcinogen to be high enough that a_1 and a_2 can be neglected.
Then the yield of cancers should conform to the expression
$Y = Kb_1(b_2t)d^2$. From the curve in Figure 13, $Kb_2 = \dfrac{1}{128}$ cancers/
transition µg.

Interactions between Initiators

Given that the neoplastically-related cellular damage is
not precisely known and that carcinogenic chemicals are chemically
diverse, it is important to establish whether cells initiated
neoplastically by one carcinogen exhibit differences in their
interaction with a second carcinogen (21). Since single initiated
cells cannot yet be isolated and studied, it is necessary to study
interactions by applying carcinogens to whole tissues. The
initiation-promotion system in mouse skin is one of the most
useful for studies of this type (7). The objective of the study
described here was to determine how the several chemically-diverse
initiators interacted when applied at different times to the same
region of dorsal mouse skin.

The purpose of these experiments was to determine whether
different classes of chemical carcinogens produce additive yields
of papillomas when applied sequentially to mouse skin. The
carcinogens were benzo(a)pyrene (B(a)P), nitroquinoline oxide (NQO)
and beta-propriolactone (BPL) applied topically to the shaved
dorsal skin of mice (Ha/ICR) in 0.2 ml acetone. The papilloma
yield as a function of promotion time is shown by the open
triangles in Figure 15 for mice that received 12 mg BPL and 16 µg
B(a)P. The summation of the yields for separate groups of mice
that received 12 mg BPL or 16 µg B(a)P as single doses is indicated
by the closed triangles. The combined exposure produced about
twice as many papillomas as expected from the summation of the
individual single doses. No carcinomas were observed.

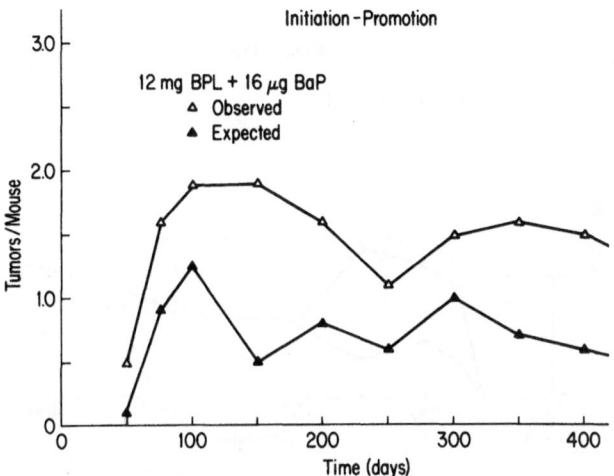

Figure 15. The curve identified as 'observed' shows the yield of skin papillomas per mouse following initiation with 12 mg BPL plus 16 µg B(a)P. The curve identified as 'expected' shows the numerical summation of the yields in groups of mice given single doses of 12 mg BPL or 16 µg B(a)P. All animals were promoted with 5 µg TPA three times per week.

The results for 6 mg BPL and 16 μg B(a)P are shown in
Figure 16. The papilloma yield for mice receiving both chemicals
is indicated by the open triangles, while the summation of yields
of separate groups of mice given single doses of either BPL or

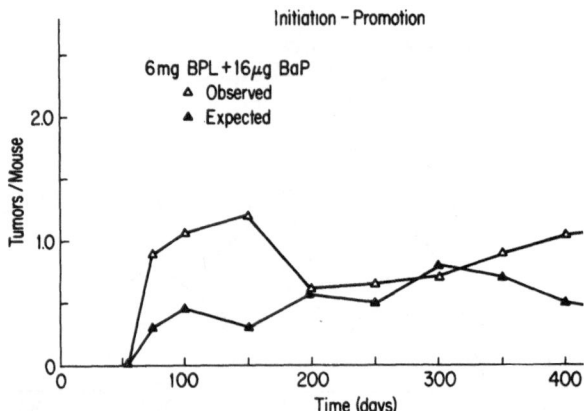

Figure 16. The curve identified as 'observed' shows the incidence
of skin papillomas per mouse following initiation with 6 mg BPL
plus 16 μg B(a)P. The curve identified as 'expected' shows the
numerical summation of the yields in groups of mice given single
doses of 12 mg BPL or 16 μg B(a)P. All animals were promoted
with 5 μg TPA three times per week.

B(a)P is indicated by the closed triangles. The combined exposure
to both chemicals produced a higher yield of papillomas than the
summation of yields from groups exposed to only one of the two
individual chemicals. No carcinomas were observed.

The papilloma and carcinoma yields for 400 µg NQO and 16 µg B(a)P are shown in Figure 17. Here the sequence of administration markedly affected the yield of tumors. NQO prior to B(a)P produced about the same yield of papillomas as the summation of the yields for the individual exposures. However, the yield of carcinomas was much greater than expected from the summation of yields from the individual exposures. When the sequence was reversed (B(a)P first), the yield of papillomas was about the same as that produced by either a single dose of NQO or B(a)P alone. Only about 50% of the yield expected from the summation of the single-dose yields was realized by administering B(a)P before NQO. In marked contrast to the NQO-first sequence, no carcinomas were observed.

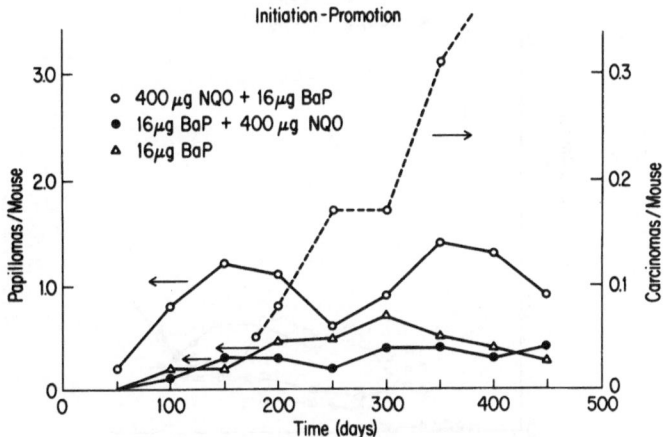

Figure 17. Incidence of skin papillomas (on left) and carcimonas (on right) per mouse observed following skin painting. Topical carcinogen treatments involved either a single dose of B(a)P or a single dose of either NQO or B(a)P followed two weeks later by another single dose of either NQO or B(a)P (whichever had not been applied the first time). Thrice weekly topical treatments with 5 µg TPA began one week after initiation.

The yield of papillomas as a function of promotion time is shown in Figure 18 for single and split doses of NQO. A single dose of 400 µg produced about the same yield of papillomas as a single dose of 800 µg. When a given dose was split into two doses, the yield of tumors declined to about 50% of the yield of the corresponding single dose.

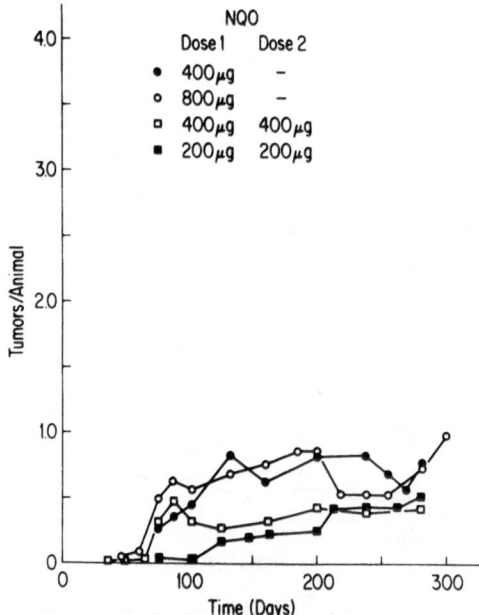

Figure 18. The yield of papillomas (average number of tumors per animal) as a function of promotion time for single and split doses of NQO. The split doses were separated by one week. Amounts indicated were delivered topically in 0.2 ml acetone.

The papilloma yield as a function of promotion time is shown in Figure 19 for single doses of BPL as indicated. The yield reached a peak at about 100 d and declined slowly thereafter until a fairly stable level was reached beyond 250 d. The 48 mg yield was about twice as great as the 24 mg yield throughout the experiment. Carcinomas began to appear after 350 d.

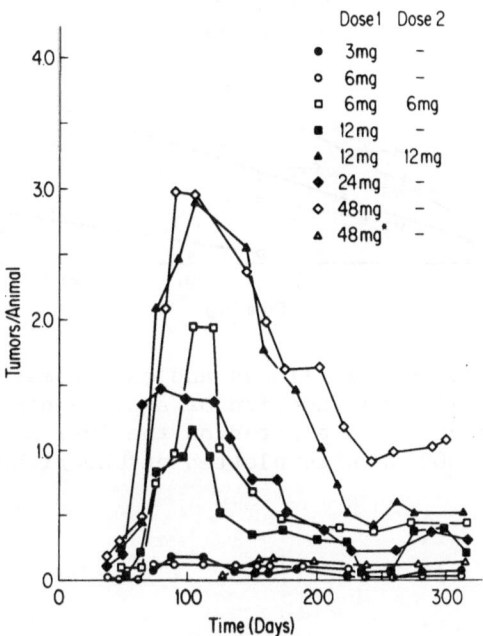

Figure 19. The yield of papillomas (average number of tumors per animal) as a function of promotion time. Single doses of beta-propiolacetone (BPL) were given at 56 d of age followed by promotion with 5 µg TPA three times weekly.

The dose response at 200 d of promotion for single and split doses of BPL is shown in Figure 20. The yield of papilloomas versus dose is reasonable well fitted by a linear function, and the split doses produced up to 70% more papillomas than the corresponding single dose. Split doses produced as many as 10 fold more carcinomas than corresponding single doses.

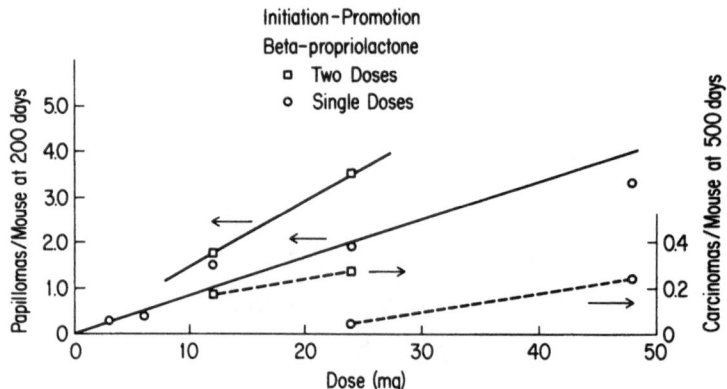

Figure 20. The yield of papillomas and carcinomas (average number of tumors per animal) as a function of applied dose of BPL. The papilloma yield at 200 d is plotted on the left scale and the carcinoma yield at 500 days is plotted on the right scale.

The results reported here suggest that different carcinogens given far enough apart in time that chemical interaction is unlikely may interact in complex ways depending on the carcinogens. Even the same carcinogen may interact with earlier doses of itself to either enhance, as for BPL, or inhibit, as for NQO, the induction of papillomas by a promoter. Extensive evidence reported elsewhere indicates that polycyclic aromatic hydrocarbon, benzo(a) pyrene, (B(a)P), produces papillomas in proportion to dose even when the dose is split into as many as 32 different fractions. From these results, B(a)P appears not to interact with earlier doses of itself.

When NQO preceded B(a)P, the papilloma results were additive, but a marked enhancement of carcinomas was noted. When B(a)P was given before NQO, the papilloma yield was approximately the same as that produced by either a single dose of NQO or B(a)P alone. No carcimonas developed after treatment with B(a)P prior to NQO. BPL, a compound that produced a slightly enhanced response with itself also exhibited enhancement when combined with B(a)P, whereas another alkylating compound, NQO, that produced an inhibitory response with itself, exhibited a similar inhibitory effect when given subsequent to the B(a)P. When NQO was applied before B(a)P, the tumor response showed mere additivity, although a marked enhancement of carcinomas was seen.

It is difficult to explain results as seemingly diverse as these without considering the component processes of the carcinogenic mechanism (7). If initiation were the only effect being produced, the order of administration of two carcinogens ought not to matter. However, if one compound, e.g., NAQ, were to have promoting activity relevant to B(a)P, then NQO prior to B(a)P ought to be more effective than vice versa. This effect was observed, especially with regard to carcinoma incidence. On the other hand, B(a)P or BPL could have approximately equal promoting activity relative to one another, since they were more effective in producing papillomas when given together in comparison to the summation of their individual effects. Since the enhancement observed here is inducible by a single exposure to the second initiator, the events involved could be analogous to what has been called the second stage of promotion (22).

It is not likely that B(a)P, NQO or BPL applied to skin persist in significant quantities after a few days, so that very little is expected to be present after one or two weeks. However, since inducible enzyme systems may persist after the inducing chemical is gone, the subsequent application of another chemical requiring activation after a dose could be influenced by a residual inducible enzymes still present at the time of the second application. Direct acting carcinogens, e.g., BPL and NQO, do not

depend for their carcinogenic activity on enzyme activation, so
the enhanced yield seen with the combination of these chemicals
and B(a)P is probably not related to enzyme induction.

The Progression of Papillomas to Carcinomas

Papillomas are focal, benign lesions consisting of folded
layers of rapidly dividing cells that differentiate into squamous
keratinizing cells almost as rapidly as they are produced (23).
Such lesions may persist for many months growing slowly, others
may regress, and still others may develop into invasive carcinoma (24). The latter papillomas are especially interesting in
carcinogenesis. Generally about 5 to 7% of the papillomas underwent malignant conversion within the observation period.

Papillomas induced by initiation-promotion of mouse skin
exhibit a spectrum of neoplastic properties in their ability to
grow independently of the promoting chemical and their tendency
to undergo conversion to carcinomas. Not unexpectedly the
greatest tendency for conversion to carcinomas was found among
the papillomas with the greatest degree of autonomy, i.e., those
having the least tendency to undergo regression when the promoting
chemical is stopped.

Papillomas may be conceived of as clonal expansions of
initiated cells, and the results here indicate that such cells,
especially in autonomous papillomas, have a fairly high probability of undergoing malignant transition. It is not unreasonable
to postulate that the precursor cells of the papillomas, i.e.,
the original initiated cells, retain the same probability of
malignant transition as the cells in the papillomas. Since
papillomas contain at least 10^5 cells, their overall probability
of malignant transition would be at least that much greater than
that of single initiated cells, and corresponding cancers would
be expected earlier and with greater frequency in the papillomatous tissue. Obviously, more work is necessary to test such
ideas, but the skin papilloma clearly provides an excellent model
for studying the benign-to-malignant transition.

Conclusions

The model outlined here is tentative in the sense that
additional confirmatory studies are necessary to define more
precisely the distinction between carcinogen-induced and spontaneous events and the role of clonal growth in whole carcinogenesis, and its applicability to organs other than skin is
uncertain. Nevertheless, there are several important and testable
implications of the model at low carcinogen doses where considerable
regulatory concern currently exists. One inevitable implication

of the model is that as long as a_1 and a_2 are not zero, there must exist a region of dose where the dose-response function is linear. In the absence of promotion, the linear dose region is defined by the magnitude of the various transition constants, since the yield function has the form $y = $ constant $(a_1 + b_1 d)(a_2 + b_2 d) \sim (a_1 a_2 + a_2 b_1 + a_1 b_2)d)$. However, the clonal growth of cells containing the first transition effectively amplifies the value of a_1 and b_1 so that in the extreme as observed in our experiments the dose-response function becomes linear even at high doses. Clearly there must exist an intermediate situation where linear and dose-squared (or higher) terms coexist. The region of coexistence will be defined largely by the amount or intensity of the promotion. The model implies that the general dose-response function has the form $Y = $ (constant) $(A + B + Cd^2)$ where the magnitude of the constants A, B and C depend on promotion and/or clonal growth of one-event cells. Furthermore, the model implies that the constant may also be promoter dependent, because all additional non-independent events necessary to complete the transition to a cancer cell occur at a certain rate or probability in each cell generation, i.e., at each mitosis. Hence, an increased mitotic rate is expected to increase the rate of occurrence of such transitions.

In addition, clonal growth of 2-event cells could affect the time function so that extreme care must be exercised when interpreting the exponent on the time function in terms of the number of events in carcinogenesis. At best, the exponent represents the upper limit of the number of events that might be involved but to the extent that clonal growth of intermediate stages is involved the exponent could reflect such growth. Since clonal growth is presumably stimulated by the action of promoters, these ideas emphasize the overriding importance of promotion and promoters in the temporal functions of cancer incidence.

References

1. L. Foulds, Neoplastic Development-2. Academic Press, N.Y., (1975).
2. P. Armitage and R. Doll, The Age Distribution of Cancer and a Multistage Theory of Carcinogenesis. Brit. J. Cancer 8:1-12, (1954).
3. R. Peto and P.N. Lee, Weibull Distribution for Continuous Carcinogenesis Experiments. Biometrics 29:457-470, (1973).
4. J. German, Chromosomes and Cancer. John Wiley, New York, (1974).
5. J. Furth, Conditioned and Autonomous Neoplasms: Review, Cancer Res. 13:477-492, (1953).

6.   F.J. Burns, M. Vanderlaan, E. Snyder and R. Albert, Induction
     and Progression Kinetics of Mouse Skin Papillomas.   In:
     Carcinogenesis, Vol. 2 Mechanisms of Tumor Promotion and
     Co-Carcinogenesis. (T.J. Slaga, R.K. Boutwell and A. Sivak,
     Eds.), Raven Press, New York, N.Y., pp.91-96, (1978).
7.   I. Berenblum, Carcinogenesis as a Biological Problem,
     Frontiers of Biology, Vol. 34.   North Holland Publishing
     Co., Amsterdam, Oxford, (1974).
8.   A. Whittemore and J. Keller, Quantitative Theories of
     Carcinogenesis. S.I.A.M. Rev. 20:1-30, (1978).
9.   P.M. Iannaccone, R.L. Gardner and H. Harris, The Cellular
     Origin of Chemically-induced Tumors. J. Cell Sci. 29:
     249-269, (1978).
10. F.J. Burns and R.E. Albert, The Additivity of Multiple Doses
     of a Liver Carcinogen in Rats. Environ. International
     1:391-393, (1978).
11. H. Druckrey, Quantitative Aspects of Chemical Carcinogenesis.
     In: Potential Carcinogenic Hazards from Drugs, Evaluation
     of Risks, VICC Monograph Series Vol. 7, (R. Truhart, Ed.),
     Springer-Vergal, N.Y., pp. 60-78, (1967).
12. R.E. Albert and B. Altshuler, Considerations Relating to the
     Formulation of Limits for Unavoidable Population Exposures
     to Environmental Carcinogens. In: Radionuclide Carcino-
     genesis, (C.L. Sanders, R.H. Busch, J.E. Ballou and D.D.
     Mahlum, Eds.), AEC Symposium Series, CONF-720505, NTIS,
     Springfield, Virginia, June, 1973.
13. R. Peto, F.J.C. Roe, R.N. Lee, L. Levy and J. Clack,
     Cancer and Ageing in Mice and Men. Brit. J. Cancer 32:
     411-416, (1975).
14. T.J. Slaga, G.T. Bowden, J.D. Scribner and R.K. Boutwell,
     Dose-Response Studies on the Ability of 7,12-Dimethylbenz(a)
     anthracene and Benz(a)anthracene to Initiate Skin Tumors.
     JNCI 53(5):1337-1340, (1974).
15. P. Brookes and P.D. Lawley, Evidence for the Binding of
     Polynuclear Aromatic Hydrocarbons to the Nucleic Acids of
     Mouse Skin: Relation between Carcinogenic Power of Hydro-
     carbons and Their Binding to DNA. Nature (Lond.) 202:
     781-784, (1964).
16. M. Duncan, P. Brookes and A. Dipple, A Metabolism and
     Binding to Cellular Macromolecules of a Series of Hydro-
     carbons by Mouse Embryo Cells in Culture. Int. J. Cancer
     4:818-819, (1969).
17. H.V. Gelboin, A Microsomal-dependent Binding of Benzo(a)-
     pyrene to DNA. Cancer Res. 29:1272-1276, (1969).
18. P.L. Grover, A. Hewer, K. Pal and P. Sims. The Involvement
     of a Diol Epoxide in the Metabolic Activation of Benzo(a)-
     pyrene in Human Bronchial Mucosa and in Mouse Skin. Int. J.
     Cancer 18:1-6, (1976).

19. I.B. Weinstein, A.M. Jeffrey, K.W. Jennette, S.H. Blobstein, R.G. Harvey, C. Harris, H. Autrup, H. Kasai and K. Nakanishi, Benzo(a)pyrene Diol Epoxides as Intermediates in Nucleic Acid Binding in vitro and in vivo. Science 193:592-595, (1976).

20. T. Meehan, K. Strabu and M. Calvin, Benzo(a)pyrene Diol Epoxide Covalently Binds to Deoxyguanosine and Deoxyadenosine in DNA. Nature (Lond.) 269:725-727, (1977).

21. K.S. Crump, D.G. Hoel, C.H. Langley and R. Peto. Fundamental Carcinogenic Processes and Their Implications for Low Dose Risk Assessment. Cancer Res. 36:2973, (1976).

22. T.J. Slaga, S.M. Fischer, K. Nelson and G.L. Gleason, Studies on the Mechanism of Skin Tumor Promotion: Evidence for Several Stages in Promotion. PNAS 77:3659-3663, (1980).

23. F. Burns, M. Vanderlaan, A. Sivak and R. Albert, The Regression Kinetics of Mouse Skin Papillomas. Cancer Res. 36:1422-1427, (1976).

24. E.J. Andrews, The Morphological, Biological and Antigenic Characteristics of Transplantable Papillomas and Keratinous Cysts Induced by Methylcholanthrene. Cancer Res. 34: 2842-2851, (1974).

This work was supported by United States Department of Energy (Contract AT(11-1)2737) and by Center Grants from National Institute of Environmental Health Sciences, ES 00260 and National Cancer Institute, CA 13343.

PROGRESS IN THE STUDY OF IN VITRO NEOPLASTIC TRANSFORMATION

Paul O.P. Ts'o

Division of Biophysics
School of Hygiene and Public Health
The Johns Hopkins University
Baltimore, Maryland USA

INTRODUCTION

Since the pioneering work of Berwald and Sachs[1,2] in 1963-1965, much effort has been made to develop adequate and useful mammalian cell systems for the study of the basic mechanisms of neoplastic transformation in chemical carcinogenesis. This constitutes a major aspect of this chapter. More recently, advances have been made to characterize neoplastic transformation at the molecular level; i.e. the study on neoplastic transformation has advanced from the animal model to the cell system, and then to the molecular description. While this approach is still in its infancy, some promising results have begun to appear. The description of this future trend will be included at the end of this chapter.

In addition to the above "reductionalistic" approach, there is a new development for the study of different cell types from various tissues (i.e. fibroblast versus epithelial cells versus hematopoietic cells), as well as the study of cell types obtained from various differentiation stages and age of animals. This is a promising "constructionalistic" approach which links carcinogenesis to the differentiation process, such as embryonic development and aging. Finally, there is an urgent practical and scientific need for the study of neoplastic transformation of human cells. A few comments about this problem and the promise of this research will also be presented in this chapter.

In Vitro Neoplastic Transformation as a Model for the Study of
Carcinogenesis

The first and most fundamental issue is whether or not the in
vitro study of neoplastic transformation can provide the basic
understanding of carcinogenesis in animals or men. Clearly,
certain aspects of carcinogenesis, such as immunological defense
and hormonal control, would not be easily investigated through a
study of cells in culture. Nevertheless, the transformation of
cells observed in tissue culture can have the same
characteristics or can be governed by the same principles as the
transformation of cells in the intact host. However, we need to
choose the experimental system very carefully. In our
laboratories[3,4,5], we have chosen the early culture of Syrian
hamster embryo fibroblasts as pioneered by Sachs[1,2], DiPaolo[6,7,8]
and others. These cells are normal diploid cells and can
maintain their karyotype in culture. In passaging, these
fibroblasts will senesce with a very low rate of spontaneous
transformation. Since the laboratory Syrian hamster is highly
inbred, tumorigenicity can be studied quantitatively without
immunological interference. In many respects, normal diploid
human cells can also be used for similar study, except in testing
tumorigenicity, a subject to be discussed later.

Two major observations from our laboratory and other
laboratories indicate that in vitro neoplastic transformation,
using Syrian hamster embryo fibroblasts, can serve as a reliable
model for carcinogenesis:

1.   First, several abnormal growth properties of transformed
cells are closely associated with tumorigenicity. In this
experiment, a variety of clonally-devised cell lines with
varying degrees of tumorigenicity were established.[9] The
heritable and abnormal growth properties were then
quantitatively measured. A statistically significant
correlation between some of these abnormal growth properties and
tumorigenicity of these cells was established, notable
anchorage-independent growth (cloning efficiency in soft agar)
(Table I) A much more extensive investigation using this
approach is now near completion with cells transformed
spontaneously, as well as by physical and chemical means. The
data clearly indicate that certain heritable, abnormal cellular
properties observed in culture can be correlated to
tumorigenicity of these neoplastically transformed cells in
animals.

2.   Secondly, progression in neoplastic transformation in
vitro mimics the progression in carcinogenesis in vivo. One

major characteristic of carcinogenesis observed by pathologists[10,11] is the phenomenon of progression. Subpopulations of carcinogenic cells undergo a series of qualitative and quantitive changes, leading finally to neoplasia and malignancy. This process takes considerable time and many cell generations. Our work[4,5] and other studies clearly demonstrate that such a process also occurs in in vitro neoplastic transformation. Therefore, the phenomenon of progression in carcinogenesis can be studied in in vitro neoplastic transformation.

Table I. Correlation Among In Vitro Growth Properties and Tumorigenicity of Syrian Hamster Cell Lines[9]

Growth Parameters	Coefficient of Rank Correlation, τ[a]
Cloning efficiency, semisolid agar	0.986[b]
Fibrinolytic activity	0.754[c]
Generation time, 1% serum	0.754[c]
Cloning efficiency, liquid medium	0.638[c]
Organization of intracellular actin	0.570[c]
Saturation density, 10% serum	0.246
Generation time 10% serum	0.062

[a]Computation of the Kendall coefficient of rank correlation, τ, between the TD_{50} of the cell lines and their respective growth properties was performed.

[b]Significantly correlated at the 99% confidence level (p ≤ 0.01).

[c]Significantly correlated at the 95% confidence level (p ≤ 0.05).

The Relationship Between Somatic Mutation and Neoplastic Transformation

One area of rapid growth in cell biology is the study of somatic mutation of cells in culture, and one important hypothesis for carcinogenesis is the theory of somatic mutation. Thus, the relationship between these two phenomena of cells in cultures was investigated first. The initial step was to establish an experimental system in which somatic mutation and neoplastic transformation of the same cell culture could be investigated simultaneously after perturbation[3,12]. In the simultaneous studies of somatic mutation (point mutation), and neoplastic transformation, it is evident that while neoplastic transformation may be initiated by somatic mutation, somatic mutation is an inadequate biological model for the study of neoplastic transformation. One example of this problem is shown in Table II. In this table, somatic mutation and neoplastic transformation of diploid SHE cells were examined concomitantly. Mutations, induced by B(a)P and MNNG, were quantitated at the HGPRT and the Na^+/K^+ ATPase loci and compared to phenotypic transformations measured by changes in cellular morphology and colony formation in agar. Both cellular transformations had characteristics distinct from the somatic mutations observed at

Table II. Comparison of Phenotypic Changes of SHE Cells[12]

	Somatic Mutation	Morphological Transformation	Anchorage Independent Growth[a]
Observed frequency (spontaneous)	$<10^{-6}$	$\sim 10^{-4}$ [b]	$<1.4 \times 10^{-8}$
Observed frequency (carcinogen-treated)	$10^{-5} - 10^{-4}$	$10^{-3} - 10^{-2}$	$10^{-5} - 10^{-6}$
Expression/detection time[c]	6-8	≤ 8	32 - 75

[a]As measured by colony formation in soft agar.
[b]Six spontaneous, morphologically transformed colonies were observed per ~62,000 control colonies examined.
[c]Population doublings.

the two loci. Morphological transformation was observed after a time comparable to somatic mutation but a a frequency 25-540-fold higher. Transformants capable of colony formation in agar were detected at $10^{-5}-10^{-6}$ frequency, but not until 32-75 population doublings after carcinogen treatment. While this frequency of transformation is comparable to that of somatic mutations, the detection time required is much longer than the optimal expression time of conventionally studied somatic mutations. The main reason is that the type of somatic mutation chosen as a model system is the one in which the mutation of a single gene can be studied in a truncated manner, namely involving a one-step change from wild type to mutant, without inducing a cascading effect in a cell which leads to further consequences. In this context, it is difficult to study a gene mutation which will lead subsequently to other mutations, which in turn will affect the original mutation. To the contrary, one characteristic of neoplastic transformation is a phenomenon of a cascading effect of many interrrelated, highly coupled processes in the cell. Therefore, in using a highly simplified somatic mutation model (point mutation) to approximate the complex neoplastic transformation process, the information obtained is often inadequate and inappropriate[12]. However, the major issue remains, can neoplastic transformation be initiated by a single gene mutation? If it can, what would be the nature of such a mutation? This issue is complicated by the phenomenon of neoplastic progression. This question, therefore, can only be answered separately for each of the various steps between substages during progression. Nevertheless, somatic genetic analysis of neoplastic transformation, particularly of the progression process, is a worthwhile enterprise.

Somatic Genetic Studies of Neoplastic Transformation

1. The rate of spontaneous neoplastic transformation was analyzed by fluctuation analysis[13]. Several spontaneous transformation lines of Syrian hamster fibroblasts were developed in our laboratory from fibrinolytically active clones[4,5]. Upon prolonged culture, these clonal lines spontaneously generated soft-agar positive (Aga[+]) colonies, which were subsequently shown to be tumorigenic. It was further shown that acquisition of tumorigenicity of a culture can be strictly correlated to the appearance of the Aga[+] subpopulation. Through fluctuation analysis, (Luria-Delbruck analysis), the rate of spontaneous neoplastic transformation leading to Aga[+] colonies was found to be about the same as that of spontaneous somatic point mutations. It was first thought that perhaps at least two steps were required in neoplastic transformation. The first step could be an initiation of an autosomal recessive mutation, while the second step would be another mutation to

convert the original recessive mutation from a hemizygous state to a homozygous state. This hypothesis, while attractive at the time, was subsequently not supported by the following major observations[13,14]:

i.   It was found that these spontaneously transformed cells are aneuploid or nearly tetraploid; thus, these cells are very difficult to be induced to exhibit recessive mutation, including sex-linked, recessive mutation (HPRT locus). However, these cells can be induced to yield dominant mutations (Na^+/K^+ ATPase locus). Therefore, expression of recessive mutations in these cells is highly unfavorable.

ii.   As expected from the first observation, the frequency of Aga^+ colonies in these cultures cannot be increased through treatment by a variety of mutagens and carcinogens. Therefore, while the apparent rate of the appearance of Aga^+ in this spontaneously transformed line mimics that of a spontaneous point gene mutation rate, the data do not support the hypothesis that this is the underlying mechanism in progression. Neither observation supports the hypothesis that neoplastic transformation is a manifestation of a dominant mutation.

2.   At the same time, the chromosomal variabiity of this spontaneous line in culture was investigated. It was found that the spontaneous variation of karyotypes is very high, even after recloning. These results indicated that karyotypic heterogeneity with a high rate of nondisjunction is an intrinsic property of these cells. Quantitative calculations indicate that a high rate of nondisjunction, or a high tendency in karyotypic variability, could be an underlying mechanism of the spontaneous changes leading to the emergence of Aga^+ subpopulations.

3.   The investigation for the nature of the mutation was expanded by two different approaches, with the underlying assumption that somatic mutation can be a major cause for neoplastic transformation.

i.   The first approach was through intraspecies cell hybrids[14]. In these experiments, highly tumorigenic cells (BP6T) and the normal Syrian hamster fibroblasts were hybridized in culture. The results indicated that the Aga^+ property was immediately suppressed in the hybrid within several cell doublings after hybridization. But, the Aga^+ properties in the hybrid did reexpress upon further growth in culture after 10 to 25 cell doublings. The progenies from the hybrids exhibited a high degree of variability in the expression of Aga^+. The data revealed that the hybrid

formation initially suppressed the Aga[+]
property and that the Aga[+] property was then reexpressed upon
segregation. This investigation again points to the importance
of variability of chromosomes as an important aspect of
neoplastic transformation.

ii.   The second approach was the investigation based on
the effect of gene-dose, or ploidy[15]. In these experiments,
clones of diploid (2N) cells and clones of tetraploid (4N) cells,
were selected, and were then separately treated by mutagens and
carcinogens. The results clearly indicate that while diploid
clones can be induced to neoplastic transformation, the
tetraploid cells under an identical situation cannot be induced
to exhibit any neoplastic properties. The experiments clearly
indicate that if the response to perturbation is related to
somatic mutation, then the response has to be due to a recessive
mutation.

The conclusion in this investigation is that if chemically
induced neoplastic transformation is initiated by somatic
mutation under certain circumstances, the mutation has to be
recessive in nature. At present the underlying mechanisms for
the long period of progression is not yet clear, but this
progression is most likely due to the occurrence of chromosomal
variabilities, which may lead to two alternative consequences.

One possible consequence is the expression of the recessive
autosomal mutation through a process of converting the hemizygous
state into the homozygous state through karyotypic changes.
However, there is another possible consequence. After the
initial insult, which may or may not cause a mutation, chromosome
variability is needed to express phenotypically the neoplastic
characteristics by alteration of gene balances or the structure
of the genetic apparatus. The only way to resolve this problem
is to perturb experimentally the chromosome patterns of the cells
in order to generate clones and populations having various
chromosomal patterns in culture for further investigation.   An
experiment of this nature is currently in progress.

DNA as a Critical Target for Neoplastic Transformation

Although it may not be possible to directly investigate the
exact involvement of somatic mutation in neoplastic
transformation, experiments can be done to delineate whether DNA
is a critical target in the cells, the perturbation of which
alone will lead to neoplastic transformation.   In this
experiment, the most critical issue is to find means to perturb
DNA only, and not any other macromolecules in the cell.   This is

usually not the case in the chemical transformation experiment, since the metabolically activated carcinogens may attack many types of molecules within the cell.   Therefore, special experiments have to be designed.   Over the past five years in our laboratory, three sets of DNA-specific perturbation experiments have been done.

    1.   Incorporation of 5-bromodeoxyuridine into DNA, followed by near-UV irradiation[16,17].   This experiment leads to specific strand breaks in DNA where the 5-bromodeoxyuridine has been incorporated. This experiment was done with both unsynchronized and synchronized cell culture, demonstrating the cell cycle dependence of such a perturbation.   In fact, the somatic mutation and neoplastic transformation can only be induced by such a treatment at S phase and is particularly more effective in the mid-S phase.

    2.   Perturbation by incorporation of tritiated thymidine, using tritiated uridine as a control[18].   This experiment clearly showed that with similar dosages of radiation, tritiated uridine did not induce somatic mutation and morphological transformation, while tritiated thymidine did induce both somatic mutation and neoplastic transformation of cells in culture.

    3.   Perturbation by DNase I encapsulated in liposomes[19]. The cells were treated by pancreatic DNase I encapsulated in phosphotidylserine liposomes.   The treated cells exhibited DNA breaks, chromosome abnormalities, cell death, a certain type of somatic mutation, as well as neoplastic tranformation after a prolonged period of progression.   This data, based on perturbation by specific DNase, clearly indicates that damage to DNA alone by single strand breaks can initiate neoplastic transformation.

    The results of the above three sets of experiments reinforce each other in pointing to the conclusion that specific perturbation to DNA alone, possibly through strand breaks, is sufficient to initiate neoplastic transformation.   However, through such a perturbation to DNA, cell killing can be observed within a few cell divisions, and somatic mutation can also be observed within 5-10 population doublings, the required time for expression.   But neoplastic transformation as indicated by anchorage independent growth or tumorigenicity cannot be observed in this culture until 50-150 population doublings after the initial insult.   What kind of cellular process requires an expression time of some many cell divisions?   Apparently, this is one of the most challenging puzzles, and it becomes one of the crucial differences between neoplastic transformation and somatic mutation, even though both processes can be initiated by specific perturbation to DNA alone.

Relationship Between Differentiation and Neoplastic Transformation

The relationship between differentiation and neoplastic transformation can be investigated in part by studying the propensity toward neoplastic transformation of cells prepared from tissues at various stages of differentiation[20]. The skin fibroblasts of 5-8 month old Syrian hamsters (young adults) and 20 month old Syrian hamsters (aging), were established in culture. These cells, together with the 12-day-old embryonic fibroblasts, exhibited an inverse relationship between average maximum population doubling (PDL) and age of the donor: embryo cells, 20.3 PDL; 6 month old adults, 17 PDL; and 20 month old adults, 10.8 PDL. These cells were treated with MNNG or B(a)P, passaged in vitro, and analyzed for neoplasia-related phenotypic changes. All treated adult cell cultures after 20-30 PDL contained morphologically distinct cells, which continued to proliferate while the control cultures senesced. However, the treated adult cell cultures only infrequently exhibited Aga[+] properties, and appeared to enter a second crisis period, in contrast to the treated embryonic cells which became neopastically transformed and exhibited the Aga[+] property. Thus, carcinogenic treatment of adult hamster skin fibroblasts clearly can disrupt the senescence pattern, but only in rare cases does this lead to neoplastic transformation. These preliminary investigations further suggest that an inverse relationship exists between in vivo cellular age (age of donor animal) and frequency of neoplastic transformation in vitro.

In the study on early embryonic fibroblasts, it was found that there exist cellular subpopulations having two of the growth properties of neoplastically transformed cells---lack of post confluence inhibition of cell division (CI[-]) and anchorage independence of growth (the Aga[+] property)[21]. These subpopulations decrease with increasing gestation period of the embryo as well as with continuing passage in vitro. Careful investigation on the isolated clones suggests that these subpopulations did not lose proliferative capacity, but acquired the contact-inhibited phenotype or anchorage independent phenotype by cellular differentiation. The susceptibility of these subpopulations to become neoplastically transformed by MNNG

was investigated by employing the clonally isolated embryonic
fibroblasts lacking post-confluence inhibition of cell division
(CI⁻). The frequency of morphological transformation foci
formation, and neoplastic progression decrease in proportion to
the decrease of the original subpopulation of CI⁻ cells in the
treated culture. The data clearly indicates the CI⁻ cells are
many-fold more susceptible to neoplastic transformation than the
CI⁺ cells, suggesting that the susceptibility decreases with
cellular differentiation.

We may asked the question, would the neoplastic
transformation of cells from a young embryo be both qualitatively
and quantitatively different from that of cells of aged animals?
To provide a cellular model to study the basic mechanism relating
carcinogenesis to development, and finally, to aging, we have
considered this developmental process of the cells in three
stages:

1.   Cells that have full potential to replicate and have
little constraint of replication, such as cells from embryos that
replicate rapidly and seem to be not contact-inhibited[21].

2.   Cells that have replicating potential but are constrained
by other biological factors such as cell-cell contact, as is
expected of a differentiating tissue.

3.   Cells that now have lost their reproductive capability
and cease to divide, as in a terminally differentiated tissue.

It is now apparent that we can develop from the fibroblast
system these three cell types in different stages of development
in culture. We can ask whether the neoplastic transformation of
these three different cell types will involve similar or
different processes or mechanisms. Apparently, we have to block
the differentiation pathway for the embryonic cells to maintain
the cells in a state of continuing replication without
constraint, to achieve a state of neoplasia. Obviously we have
to reactivate the dormant reproductive capabilities in senescent
cells to allow a continuation of cell division and an escape of
senescence. Experiments are now in progress to answer to above
questions.

Future Directions

1.   Characterization of Neoplastic Transformation at the

Molecular Level.

Results described above have revealed the advantages in studying the basic mechanism in carcinogenesis through investigation of in vitro neoplastic transformation at the cellular level. When the problem is defined at the cellular level, we can begin to focus downward to the molecular level, asking the question, what are the molecular differences between normal and tumorigenic cells? Currently, there are two new directions in our laboratory:

i. Analysis of plasma membrane proteins from normal and highly tumorigenic cells by two-dimensional gel electrophoresis (pH 5-7 gradient followed by an SDS acrylamide gradient gel)[22]. In four independent preparations, there were about 500 resolvable polypeptides shown in the 2-D gels. In a comparison between the preparations from normal cells versus those from tumorigenic cells, about 10% of these polypeptides exhibited qualitative differences (presence or absence) and about 10% exhibited quantitative differences (increase or decrease). More definitive investigation in correlating the molecular differences and the cellular properties is currently being conducted.

ii. Previously, experiments indicated an extensive homology of nuclear RNA and polysomal-polyA-mRNA between normal and highly tumorigenic cells[23]. These results demonstrate that the phenotypic changes associated with neoplastic transformation induced by chemical carcinogens are accompanied by relatively few changes in the qualitative pattern of gene expression in cells cultured in vitro. Therefore, a more powerful technique with a higher power of resolution is needed to detect the differences in gene expression between normal and tumorigenic cells. By the use of recombinant DNA techniques, a genomic DNA library and a mRNA-cDNA library are being constructed. These libraries can be used to monitor the qualitative and quantitative changes of mRNA in tumorigenic cells versus the normal cells. When completed, this experiment will provide a description of the molecular properties of cells at the level of gene expression.

2. Specific Perturbations

One major contribution from our laboratory is the establishment of a strategy to perturb specifically one target macromolecule at a time inside the living cell. So far, the

target has been DNA, with the perturbation leading specifically
to DNA chain breaks. It will be of interest to perturb the
methylation of DNA or to perturb other non-DNA targets, such as
RNA, proteins, or other gene products. This approach is
especially important in order to understand the basic mechanism
in the establishment of heritable changes in the process of
differentiation.

3. Studies of Other Cell Types

So far in this chapter, only fibroblasts have been
discussed. The main reason for this is that fibroblasts are the
cell type that is most easy to grow and therefore can be more
readily analyzed in neoplastic transformation experiments. It is
clear that most of the naturally occurring cancer cells belong to
the epithelial cell type which is much more difficult to grow in
culture. More advances have been made in this area, particularly
in the study of epidermal cells.

In our laboratory, we have focused on the study of
hematopoietic tissue from bone marrow and spleen[24], in addition
to the fibroblasts. In this research, hematopoietic cells from
bone marrow and spleen of Syrian hamsters can now be cultured in
liquid medium for a considerble length of time and can still
contain stem cells for replication and differentiation. The
manipulation of this culture system in the study of replication
and differentiation, as well as the use of this system in
neoplastic transformation seems to have a very promising future
both from the standpoint of practical interest and the standpoint
of fundamental biology.

4. The Study of Neoplastic Transformation of Human Cells in Culture.

In our limited experience, and from the literature, it
has been indicated that the frequency of somatic mutation of
human cells and rodent cells is more or less the same (within a
factor of 2) when given the same set of mutagenic or carcinogenic
perturbations. However, it was generally recognized that
neoplastic transformation of human cells in culture is much more
difficult to obtain as compared to the neoplastic transformation
of rodent cells under a similar environment. In the case of the
animal system, however, the terms "tumorigenic cells" and "tumor
cells" can often be interchangeable, since we can conduct
tumorigenicity experiments with animals. Obviously, such is not
the case in the human system. Therefore, it is very difficult to
have a scientifically sound criterium of the neoplastic
transformation of human cells in culture.

In general, there are only two logical approaches. The
first approach is to characterize the growth characteristics and
requirements of a variety of human tumor cells obtained from
biopsies and autopsies. These growth properties could be used as
a general guide for the neoplastic cells. However, one problem
with this approach is that the tumor cells are obtained from
various tissues and various patients, which may or may not be
comparable for the cell type used in the neoplastic
transformation experiments in vitro. The second approach will be
to use the growth characteristics of the animal tumorigenic cells
as a guide. In this case, the most popular criterium is that of
xenotumorigenicity in nude mice, an animal in which immunological
defense has been compromised. It is known that in animals,
tumorigenicity and xenotumorigenicity can be cross-correlated and
therefore it is hoped that xenotumorigenicity of human cells in
nude mice could be considered as evidence for the presumptive
tumorigenicity in man. However, as described in preceding
paragraphs, the transformation of hman cells with undefined
criteria appear to be much more difficult than those of rodent
cells. For instance, the tumorigenic rodent cells are usually
immortal, while several xenotumorigenic human cells in the
laboratory turn out to senesce upon further growth in culture.
Thus, at the cell biology level there does not appear to be any
sound scientific criteria to define neoplastic transformation of
human cells in terms of tumorigenicity.

There is a possibility that this difficulty can be
overcome at the molecular biology level, particularly through the
study of gene expression at the mRNA level. It would be
important to describe the neoplastic transformation system in
animals through mRNA content. In this case, the
neoplasia-associated mRNA changes can be used to characterize the
phenotypic changes of neoplastic transformation in rodent cells.
These mRNA changes can then be developed as probes for the survey
of neoplastic transformation in animal cells. It is a likely
possibility that the human cells and the presumptive human
tumorigenic cells can also be described in the context of mRNA
content. In this case, mRNA probes for the human situation can be
developed, which however, may be much more difficult to obtain in
the human case. It will be an ideal situation, however, at least
for such a study, if the mRNA probes developed for rodent cells
are highly homologous in base sequence to the
neoplasia-associated mRNA of the human system. In this case, the
problem will be much easier to resolve.

In conclusion, the in vitro studies of neoplastic
transformation not only provide valuable information about

neoplastic transformation and differentiation, but also about
the fundamental mechanism in control and function of the
genetic apparatus.

Acknowledgement

The abstract is based on the results obtained from a
collaborative effort of many scientists in the Division of
Biophysics, School of Hygiene and Public Health, The Johns
Hopkins University. Specifically, the contributions of the
following colleagues are gratefully acknowledged: J. Carl
Barrett, Sarah A. Bruce, Wai Nang Choy, Brian D. Crawford,
Deborah L. Grady, Stanley Lin, David Morry, Robert K. Mozyis,
Shuji Nakano, Masahide Takii, Takeki Tsutsui, and Maria Zajac.

References

1. Y. Berwald and L. Sachs, In vitro cell transformation with
        chemical carcinogens, Nature 200:1182-1184 (1963).
2. Y. Berwald and L. Sachs, In vitro transformation of normal
        cells to tumor cells by carcinogenic hydrocarbons, J. Natl.
        Cancer Inst. 35:641-661 (1965).
3. J.C. Barrett, N.E. Bias and P.O.P. Ts'o, A mammalian cellular
        system for the concomitant study of neoplastic transform-
        ation and somatic mutation, Mutation Res. 50:121-136 (1978).
4. J.C. Barrett, B.D. Crawford, D.L. Grady, L.D. Hester, P.A.
        Jones, W.F. Benedict, and P.O.P. Ts'o, The temporal ac-
        quisition of enhanced fibrinolytic activity by Syrian
        hamster embryo cells following treatment with benzo(a)-
        pyrene. Cancer Res. 37:3815-3823 (1977).
5. J.C. Barrett and P.O.P. Ts'o, Evidence for the progressive
        nature of neoplastic transformation in vitro, Proc. Nat.
        Acad. Sci. USA 75:3297-3301 (1978).
6. J.A. DiPaolo and P.J. Donovan, Properties of Syrian hamster
        cells transformed in the presence of carcinogenic hydro-
        carbons, Exptl. Cell Res. 48:361-377 (1967).
7. J.A. DiPaolo, P.J. Donovan and R. Nelson, Quantitative studies
        of in vitro transformation by chemical carcinogens, J. Nat.
        Cancer Inst. 42:867-874 (1969).
8. J.A. DiPaolo, R.L. Nelson, and P.J. Donovan, Morphological,
        oncogenic, and karyological characteristics of Syrian
        hamster embryo cells transformed in vitro by carcinogenic
        polycyclic hydrocarbons, Cancer Res. 31:3573-3583 (1971).
9. J.C. Barrett, B.D. Crawford, L.O. Mixter, L. M. Schectman,
        P.O.P. Ts'o and R. Pollack, Correlation of in vitro growth
        properties and tumorigenicity of Syrian hamster cell lines,

Cancer Res. 39:1504-1510 (1979).

10. L. Foulds, The experimental study of tumor progression: A review, Cancer Res. 14:327-339 (1954).

11. L. Foulds, "Neoplastic Development, Vol. 1", Academic Press, London (1969) and "Neoplastic Development, Vol. 2", Academic Press, London (1975).

12. J.C. Barrett and P.O.P. Ts'o, The relationship between somatic mutation and neoplastic transformation, Proc. Nat. Acad. Sci. USA 75:3297-3301 (1978).

13. J.C. Barrett, B.D. Crawford, and P.O.P. Ts'o, The role of somatic mutation in a multistage model of carcinogenesis, in: "Advances in Modern Environmental Toxicology, Vol. 1, Mammalian Cell Transformation by Chemical Carcinogenesis", N. Mishra, V. Dunkel and M. Mehlman, eds., Senate Press, Inc., Princeton, N.J. (1981).

14. Brian D. Crawford, Ph.D. Thesis, School of Hygiene and Public Health, The Johns Hopkins University (1981).

15. David Morry, Ph.D. Thesis, School of Hygiene and Public Health, The Johns Hopkins University (1980).

16. J.C. Barrett, T. Tsutsui, and P.O.P. Ts'o, Neoplastic transformation induced by a direct perturbation of DNA, Nature 274:229-232 (1978).

17. T. Tsutsui, J.C. Barrett and P.O.P. Ts'o, Chromosomal aberrations, DNA damage and morphological transformation of synchronized Syrian hamster embryo cells: Effect of 5-bromodeoxyuridine and near ultraviolet radiation, Cancer Res. 39:2356-2365 (1979).

18. S.L. Lin, M. Takii and P.O.P. Ts'o, Somatic mutation and neoplastic transformation induced by [Methyl-^{3}H]thymidine, Radiat. Res., in press (1982).

19. M. Zajac and P.O.P. Ts'o, In vitro neoplastic transformation induced by DNase I encapsulated in liposomes, Eur. J. Cell Biol. 22:1585, p. 533, Abstract of Second International Congress on Cell Biology (1980).

20. S.A. Bruce and P.O.P. Ts'o, Senescence and neoplastic transformation of Syrian hamster embryo and adult fibroblasts in vitro, Eur. J. Cell Biol. 22:1642, p. 552, Abstract of Second International Congress on Cell Biology (1980).

21. S. Nakano and P.O.P. Ts'o, Cellular differentiation and neoplasia: Characterization of subpopulations of cells that have neoplasia-related growth properties in Syrian hamster embryo cell cultures, Proc. Nat. Acad. Sci. USA 78:4995-4999 (1981).

22. D.L. Grady, R.K. Moyzis and P.O.P. Ts'o, An analysis of plasma membrane proteins from normal and highly tumorigenic Syrian hamster embryo cells by two dimensional gel electrophoresis, J. Cell Biol. 91, No.2, Part 2, Abst.15061 (1981).

23. R.K. Moyzis, D.L. Grady, D.W. Li, S.E. Mirvis and P.O.P. Ts'o,
     Extensive homology of nuclear ribonucleic acid and poly-
     somal poly(adenylic acid) messenger ribonucleic acid
     between normal and neoplastically transformed cells,
     Biochemistry 19:821-832 (1980).
24. E.A. Arnold, W.S. Liaw and P.O.P. Ts'o, The use of cell
     cultures to assay the effects of chemicals on bone marrow,
     in:"Carcinogenesis: Fundamental Mechanisms and Environ-
     mental Effects," B. Pullman, P.O.P. Ts'o and H. Gelboin,
     eds., D. Reidel Publishing Company, Dordrecht, Holland
     (1980).

PULSE-CARCINOGENESIS BY ETHYLNITROSOUREA IN THE DEVELOPING

RAT NERVOUS SYSTEM: MOLECULAR AND CELLULAR MECHANISMS

Manfred F. Rajewsky

Institut für Zellbiologie (Tumorforschung)
Universität Essen (GH)
Hufelandstrasse 55, D-4300 Essen 1
Federal Republic of Germany

INTRODUCTION

The molecular and cellular mechanisms of malignant transformation and tumorigenesis can probably be best studied in so-called "pulse-carcinogenesis systems",[1,2,3] i.e., in systems where, after a single dose of a short-lived carcinogen sufficient to produce a high tumorigenic effect, the process proceeds autonomously without the complication of continued interaction of the target cell population(s) with the carcinogen. In such systems one can operationally separate the process of carcinogenesis into three phase (A,B,C): Phase A, period of carcinogen interaction with target cells; phase B, time interval between phase A and phase C; and phase C, period beginning with the onset of (clonal) proliferation of tumorigenic cells. More or less synonymous terms are "initiation" for phase A and "expression" (of malignant phenotypes) for phase B. In spite of its obvious importance, least is presently known about phase B which often constitutes the longest of the three phases. Phase B appears to encompass a sequence of phenotypic changes (including acquisition of the capacity for continuous proliferation) in the cells which ultimately become tumorigenic,[4,5,6] and represents the period during which, for instance, tumor promotors can exert their pleiotropic effects, i.e., modify gene expression and induce cell proliferation in the target cell population.[7,8,9,10]

Structural alterations of DNA in the chromatin of target cells are primary events in the multi-step process of malignant transformation and tumorigenesis by most chemical carcinogens.[11,12][13,14,15,16,17] In general, covalent binding occurs between nucleophilic centers (electron-rich N and O atoms) in cellular DNA

and highly reactive, electrophilic derivatives (ultimate
carcinogens) generated from the respective parent compounds
(pre-carcinogens) either by enzyme-catalyzed "metabolic activation"
or via non-enzymatic decomposition.[18,19] As a consequence of their
reaction with DNA most chemical carcinogens are also mutagenic.[20,21,22] However, the strong correlation of carcinogenicity and
mutagenicity does not constitute proof for an obligatory
requirement of mutation (nor even of modification of DNA structure
in general) for malignant transformation. Cellular macromolecules
other than DNA also contain multiple nucleophilic sites which can,
and indeed do, react with carcinogen-generated electrophiles.
Nonetheless, the central importance of DNA structure and
conformation for the expression of genetic information provides a
strong argument for a critical role of DNA alterations as a
prerequisite for the initiation of carcinogenesis by chemical
agents.

Carcinogen-modified DNA structures can, in principle, lead to
local alterations of nucleotide sequence[11,12,13,15,17,23] and
helical distortions,[13,24] possibly facilitate transition of the
B-form of the double helix to a left-handed conformation (Z-DNA),
[25,26,27,28] or, for example, interfere with the patterns of mRNA
processing (splicing)[29] and DNA methylation,[30,31,32,33] affect the
precision of DNA rearrangements (note that transpositional events
in the genome may be associated with development/differentiation
in mammalian cell systems),[34] cause inappropriate gene
amplification[35] and rearrangements at the chromosomal level,[34,36]
and perhaps induce error-prone DNA repair.[37] It is presently still
a matter of speculation, whether one or several of these mechanisms
are of a predominant importance in terms of malignant transformation.
However, there is little doubt that the common denominator is an
interference with the genetic programmes of target cells. More
information is, therefore, needed on the molecular control of
eucaryotic gene expression, on the mechanisms regulating phenotypic
differentiation and cell proliferation in developing and mature
cell systems, and on the particular combinations of genes involved
in these complex processes. Although it is theoretically not
excluded that malignant transformation is generally the consequence
of alterations in the same (few) specific gene(s), the wide spectrum
of differing phenotypes observed in cancer cells (and the specific
architectural and microenvironmental properties of each of the
respective normal tissues and cell systems of origin) seems to
argue against such a "unifying" possibility. The observed
variety of malignant phenotypes may indeed not only reflect the
different types of the corresponding normal cells of origin and
their developmental/differentiation stage and/or the particular
phenotypic "plasticity" of cancer cells in general; it could also
indicate that a variety of qualitatively different phenotypic
alterations may share the property of resulting in a malignant
behavior of cells in their respective tissue environment. The DNA

transfection approach recently introduced to define genes involved in the malignant transformation of mammalian cells may soon provide important information on this question.[38]

The late stages of the maturation of cells from the stem cell level to a terminally differentiated state are generally accompanied by a cessation of proliferative activity. In mature cells, the nonproliferative state can either be of an apparently irreversible nature (e.g., neurons), or be reversible ("G_O-cells") under special physiological conditions, such as the requirement for reparative or functional hyperplasia (e.g., parenchymal liver cells, astrocytes in the brain). Temporary nonproliferative states of part of the cell population are, however, also characteristic of stem cells, and probably of "precursor" cells at more advanced stages of maturation.[39,40]

Like UV-induced photoproducts in DNA,[41] certain carcinogen-DNA adducts can be specifically recognized, removed, and repaired by cellular enzymes.[2,41,42,43,44,45] The majority of non-repaired, persistent modifications introduced into DNA by carcinogens are likely to be localized in transcriptionally silent parts of the genome, and will become effective only in the course of gene activation, e.g., by the further progression of cells along the developmental/differentiation pathway, or by inducing cells to express specialized functions and to enter the cell cycle from a G_O-state (e.g., by the action of tumor promotors). No evidence is available which would indicate that cells can undergo malignant transformation after having reached a terminally differentiated, irreversibly nonproliferative state prior to carcinogen exposure.[3,38] Instead it appears that the expression of malignant phenotypes is much more readily induced in cells exposed to carcinogenic agents either during earlier proliferation-linked stages of their differentiation pathway or in a G_O-state.[39,46] Of particular interest is the question whether along the differentiation pathway of a given cell lineage specific stem cell and precursor cell stages exist where by interaction with a carcinogen the gene programme can be shifted to the expression of malignant phenotypes with higher than random probability.[2,37,48]

In terms of their reactive derivatives and reaction products with cellular DNA, the alkylating N-nitroso compounds are among the best characterized chemical carcinogens.[11,12,14,15,17,49] They include the alkylnitrosamines (which require enzymatic activation) and the alkylnitrosoureas and alkylnitrosoguanidines (which undergo rapid, non-enzymatic decomposition). The resulting electrophilic alkyl substituents are small compared with the bulky adducts derived from, e.g., carcinogenic hydrocarbons or aromatic amines. One of the alkylnitrosoureas, N-ethyl-N-nitrosourea (EtNU[50]) has become a model "pulse-carcinogen" in the rat, and the properties of this experimental system will be described in more detail in the following.

PULSE-CARCINOGENESIS BY ETHYLNITROSOUREA IN THE RAT

At the pH conditions prevailing in vivo, EtNU decomposes
non-enzymatically to a reactive ethyldiazonium ion with a half-life
< 8 min.[51] Therefore, after systemic application, nucleophilic
sites in cellular macromolecules (e.g., DNA) become ethylated to
a similar extent in all tissues (as shown by radiochromatographic
analyses of DNA exposed to radioactively labeled EtNU in vivo,[1,51,]
[52] or by radioimmunoassay,[53,54] and also by whole-body
autoradiography[55]). In spite of the initially very similar degree
of ethylation in all cells of the organism (phase A in the process
of carcinogenesis; see Introduction), a single pulse of EtNU
applied to fetal or newborn rats results in the death of a high
proportion of the animals with malignant neuroectodermal tumors,
while tumors in tissues other than the brain and peripheral nervous
system are rarely detected (neural tissue tropism of the
carcinogenic effect). Following a transplacental pulse of EtNU to
BDIX-rats, fetal brain cells subsequently transferred to a long-
term culture system undergo malignant transformation in vitro
after a time period similar to the time required for tumor
formation in vivo.[2,4,56] Tumor yield and latency period are
dose-[2,57] and strain-dependent.[58] The tumorigenic effect is,
however, also a function of the developmental stage of the nervous
system at the time of the carcinogen pulse (developmental/
differentiation stage dependence of the carcinogenic effect).
Tumorigenicity is highest after an EtNU-pulse during late prenatal
or early postnatal development, but decreases strongly in animals
exposed to the same dose of EtNU at later postnatal age. The
carcinogenic effect is thus inversely correlated with the
developmental/differentiation stage of the neural cell system, and
appears to require the presence of proliferative neural (precursor)
cells at the time of exposure to the carcinogen.[2,3] However, the
carcinogenic effect apparently also decreases sharply when a
transplacental EtNU-pulse is applied at developmental stages prior
to the 15th day of gestation. Thus no neuroectodermal tumors were
observed (in limited numbers of experimental animals) after
exposure to EtNU before the 11th day of gestation.[50,59] On day 11
of prenatal development the total number of brain cells has reached
a value of about 10^5 in the BDIX-rat.[54] Thus, in an experiment
with about 20 BDIX-rat embryos at this developmental stage, the
total (highly proliferative) neural target cell population amounts
to $\sim 2 \times 10^6$ cells.

The developmental period of maximum sensitivity in terms of
the neuro-oncogenic effect of EtNU appears to vary in different
species. For example only a low incidence of neural tumors has
been observed in a number of mouse strains after late prenatal and
neonatal administration of EtNU,[60,61] and postnatal application of

EtNU to Mongolian gerbils has resulted in malignant transformation
of cutaneous melanocytes (neural crest-derived) but not in tumors
of the brain or peripheral nervous system.[62]   However, mainly brain
tumors (besides kidney and ovary tumors) were observed when
immunologically competent (nu/+) or incompetent nu/nu mice (CBA/H
or BALB/c) were treated with EtNU on day 12-14 of prenatal
development, while in animals treated on day 16-18 most tumors were
found in the lung, liver (males), and kidney.[63]   Similarly, EtNU
caused predominantly neural tumors in rabbits when applied during
early phases of prenatal development, whereas exposure to EtNU
during later fetal stages lead mainly to kidney tumors.[64,65,66]
It appears, therefore, that the "localization" of phases of
increased carcinogenic risk during development/differentiation of
a given cell system in different species requires careful
monitoring by narrowly-spaced carcinogen exposure.

A comparison of different alkylating carcinogens indicates a
positive correlation between their carcinogenicity and the relative
extent of alkylation on O-atoms (e.g., O^6-alkyldeoxyguanosine)
versus N-atoms (e.g., 7-alkyldeoxyguanosine) in DNA.   Thus for the
potent carcinogen EtNU the initial O^6-ethyldeoxyguanosine
(O^6-EtdGuo)/7-ethyldeoxyguanosine (7-EtdGuo) ratio is ∿ 0.7,[1,67]
while the corresponding value for the weakly carcinogenic
diethylsulfate is ∿ 0.003.[68]   The relative extent of alkylation on
O-atoms in DNA is a function of the reaction mechanism of the
respective agent.   A bimolecular nucleophilic substitution (SN2)
reaction will result in a lower O/N alkylation ratio than an SN2
mechanism with a tendency towards a unimolecular (SN1) reaction.[11,69]

Highly sensitive analytical methods are required for the
detection of alkylation products in the DNA of target tissues and
cells.   The sensitivity of radiochromatographic techniques commonly
used to quantitate alkylation products in DNA[70] is limited mainly
by the specific radioactivity of the respective [^{3}H]- or [^{14}C]-
labeled carcinogens.   Under favorable conditions these procedures
will detect one alkylated base in ∿ 10^6 molecules of the
corresponding normal base, and relatively large amounts of DNA
(i.e., large numbers of cells) are necessary for analysis.   Since
radiochromatography requires the use of radioactively labeled,
laboratory-synthesized carcinogens, analysis of DNA from (e.g.,
human) tissues and cells exposed to low doses of non-radioactive
(e.g., environmental) agents is not possible.   In this regard,
recently developed immunoanalytical procedures using high-affinity
"conventional" and monoclonal antibodies (antibody affinity
constants, 10^9 to > 10^{10} 1/mol) specifically directed against
defined alkylation products in DNA, have opened new possibilities.
[71,72]   Thus Müller and Rajewsky[53,73] have developed a sensitive
competitive radioimmunoassay (RIA) for the quantification of
O^6-EtdGuo in DNA exposed to EtNU in vivo or in vitro.   At present

$\sim$ 0.04 pmol of O^6-EtdGuo can be detected by RIA at 50 % tracer-antibody binding, thus permitting quantification of O^6-EtdGuo at an O^6-EtdGuo/deoxyguanosine molar ratio of $\sim$ 3 x 10^{-7} in a hydrolysate of 100 μg of ethylated DNA (corresponding to $\sim$ 10^7 diploid cells). The detection limit can be lowered even further if the alkyl-deoxynucleosides to be quantitated are separated from the DNA hydrolysate by high performance liquid chromatography (HPLC) prior to the RIA. The spectrum of available high-affinity monoclonal antibodies specific for different DNA alkylation products[71],[72] is presently being expanded,[74],[75],[76] and their application is extended to the use of immunostaining techniques for detection and quantification of alkylation products in the DNA of individual cells (Adamkiewicz, Ahrens and Rajewsky, in preparation) and in isolated DNA molecules (Nehls, Adamkiewicz, Spiess and Rajewsky, in preparation).

The different ethylation products formed in DNA after exposure to EtNU have been carefully analyzed.[11],[17],[49],[67],[77],[78] They are produced with equal relative frequencies, regardless of whether the reaction with EtNU occurs in vivo, in cell culture, or with purified DNA in vitro.[1],[52],[67] The following ethylation products have been detected in DNA: (a) Ethylation on O-atoms ($\sim$ 80 % of all ethylation products in DNA): O^6-EtdGuo ($\sim$ 10 %), O^2-ethyldeoxythymidine ($\sim$ 7 %), O^2-ethyldeoxycytidine (O^2-EtdCyd; $\sim$ 4 %), O^4-ethyldeoxythymidine (O^4-EtdThd; $\sim$ 3 %), and ethylphosphotriesters ($\sim$ 56 %). (b) Ethylation on N-atoms: 7-EtdGuo ($\sim$ 14 %), 3-ethyldeoxyadenosine (3-EtdAdo; $\sim$ 5 %), 7-ethyldeoxyadenosine ($\sim$ 4 %), 1-ethyldeoxyadenosine (1-EtdAdo; $\sim$ 0.3 %), 3-ethyldeoxycytidine (3-EtdCyd; $\sim$ 0.2 %), 3-ethyldeoxyguanosine ($\sim$ 0.1 %), and 3-ethyldeoxythymidine (3-EtdThd; $\sim$ 0.1 %). The alkyl groups of O^6-EtdGuo, O^2-EtdCyd, O^4-EtdThd, 3-EtdThd, 3-EtdCyd, and of 1-EtdAdo, are localized on atoms normally involved in Watson-Crick base-pairing. The relative O^6-EtdGuo content in DNA has been determined by RIA in chromatin of different folding levels, isolated from fetal rat brain cells and briefly exposed to EtNU in vitro.[79],[80] Compared with naked DNA (relative value, 1.0), the degree of ethylation on the O^6 of deoxyguanosine decreases from the DNA of extended (histone H1-free) chromatin fibers ($\sim$ 0.6) to the DNA in nucleosomes (core particles; $\sim$ 0.5), and is lowest in the DNA of condensed chromatin fibers ("superbeads",[81] $\sim$ 0.4). Independent of the chromatin folding level, nucleophilic sites located in the major and minor groove, and in base-pairing regions of the DNA double helix, are equally accessible (or equally protected by the basic structural proteins) to the reactive ethyldiazonium ion generated from EtNU.[79],[80] Chromosomal DNA preferentially digested with DNase I (transcribable conformation[82],[83]) was found to have a higher O^6-EtdGuo content than chromosomal DNA less susceptible to this enzyme (non-transcribable genome regions).[79],[80]

The initial degree of ethylation by EtNU in the DNA of pre-
and postnatal rat brain (high carcinogenic risk) is not
significantly different from that found in the DNA of other
"low-risk"-tissues.[1,51,52,54] However, as shown by kinetic
analyses after a pulse of radiolabeled EtNU to 10-day-old BDIX-
rats, the content of O^6-EtdGuo decreases very rapidly in liver
DNA (and less rapidly in the DNA of other tissues) but much more
slowly in brain DNA. The difference in the elimination rates of
O^6-EtdGuo from brain versus, e.g., liver DNA is so dramatic that
a specific enzymatic recognition and elimination mechanism had
to be assumed for this particular alkylation product.[1,2,52] In
contrast, ethylation products such as 3-EtdAdo and 7-EtdGuo
disappear from the DNA of brain and other tissues at much faster
rates than does O^6-EtdGuo from brain DNA, and significant
differences in tissue-specific elimination rates are not apparent
for these ethylation products. Very similar elimination rates of
O^6-EtdGuo and 7-EtdGuo are observed when the EtNU-pulse is applied
to rats on the 20th day of prenatal development.[84] In a
semilogarithmic plot, the elimination kinetics of O^6-EtdGuo have a
bi (or multi)-componential appearance. Several mechanisms, alone
or in combination, could account for this phenomenon: (i) An
enzyme - or (one of) several enzymes - is initially present in
excess, consumed upon reaction, and is synthesized at relatively
low rate; (ii) Differential accessibility of O^6-EtdGuo in the DNA
of chromatin of different folding levels (see above); and (iii)
the tissue is composed of subpopulations of cells with different
capacities for the enzymatic elimination of O^6-EtdGuo.

O^6-EtdGuo not eliminated from DNA prior to a subsequent round
of DNA replication can, like O^4-EtdThd,[85] lead to anomalous base-
pairing,[77,86] i.e., cause an alteration of nucleotide sequence in
the daughter strand. EtNU is presently considered the most potent
point-mutagen in eukaryotic systems.[87,88,89] It is possible that
persistence of O^6-EtdGuo in brain DNA, and the high rate of DNA
replication of the neural precursor cells during the transformation-
sensitive period of brain development, are among the factors
responsible for the neural tissue tropism of the carcinogenic
effect of EtNU in the rat.[1,2,52]

Considerable efforts have been made by various research groups
to identify the enzyme(s) responsible for the removal of
O^6-alkylguanine from DNA. In E. coli an "adaptive response" has
been discovered which is inducible by low concentrations of simple
methylating agents.[90,91] This response involves the expression of
a system capable of transferring a methyl group (possibly also an
ethyl group) from the O^6 of deoxyguanosine in DNA to a cysteine
residue in an acceptor protein which is thereby apparently
inactivated.[92,93,94,95] It is not excluded that an intermediate
methyltransferase may be involved; however, it seems likely that

the alkyl group is bound directly to the acceptor protein (which
would then itself have the properties of a DNA methyltransferase).
Interestingly, similar enzymatic activities (with transfer of methyl
and ethyl groups from the O^6 of deoxyguanosine in DNA to cysteine
residues in acceptor proteins) have recently been described for
mouse and rat liver.[96,97] An active fraction specifically reducing
the O^6-alkyldeoxyguanosine content of DNA had previously been
isolated from rodent and human liver homogenates.[98,99,100]
Furthermore, evidence has been obtained indicating that the enzyme
reducing the O^6-methyldeoxyguanosine content of rat liver DNA has
an elevated activity during the S-phase (and possibly the $[G_2-M]$-
phase) of the cell cycle as compared to the G_1-phase and to the
G_0-state.[101,102] Finally, it is now well established that the
enzymatic elimination of O^6-alkylguanine from liver DNA is less
efficient after high carcinogen doses ("saturation" of the enzyme
system[103]), and that in different species this saturation effect
occurs at different carcinogen dose levels. Thus the liver of the
Syrian golden hamster has a much lower "saturation threshold" than
rat liver.[104,105,106] Correspondingly, hamster liver is sensitive
to the induction of hepatocellular cancer by a single dose of,
e.g., dimethylnitrosamine but rat liver is not.[107]

It has yet to be established whether, in addition to a
constitutive O^6-alkylguanine eliminating enzyme(s), there is also
an inducible enzyme activity in mammalian systems, analogous to
the inducible DNA methyltransferase in E. coli. Several groups
have reported an elevated elimination capacity in rat liver in
response and to pretreatment with low doses of dimethyl - or
diethylnitrosamine, 1,2-dimethylhydrazine, N-acetylaminofluorene,
or 3,3-dimethyl-1-phenyltriazene (reviewed in ref.[106]). However,
the relatively low increase in elimination activity appears
equally compatible with an increased fraction of proliferating
hepatocytes in S-phase,[101,102] i.e., a regenerative hyperplasia
in response to the carcinogen pretreatment.[38] The important
question of cell type- and developmental/differentiation
stage-dependent differences in the capacity for enzymatic
elimination of critical alkylation products from DNA has not
yet been investigated; except for the case of parenchymal versus
non-parenchymal rat liver cells after treatment with 1,2-
dimethylhydrazine, which induces hemangiosarcomas but not
hepatocellular carcinomas in rats. Here it was found that
O^6-methyldeoxyguanosine accumulated selectively in the non-
parenchymal cells.[108] This approach will in the future be
facilitated by the use of high-affinity monoclonal antibodies in
conjunction with sensitive immunostaining procedures. Moreover,
these techniques will permit the study of enzymatic repair
processes in small amounts of cells, e.g., during prenatal stages
of development. In the EtNU - rat brain system, it will thus be
of interest to investigate whether in early stages of prenatal
development (with an apparently lower carcinogenic risk; see

above) the capacity of neural precursor cells for the elimination of O^6-EtdGuo from their DNA is equally low, or higher than in later(high risk)developmental stages.[54]

ACKNOWLEDGEMENTS

This report is based on a presentation at an International Workshop on Modified Nucleosides and Cancer, held in Freiburg i.Br., Fed. Rep. of Germany, 28 September - 2 October, 1981. The author gratefully acknowledges support by the Deutsche Forschungs-gemeinschaft (SFB 102) and the Fritz Thyssen Stiftung (1980/2/41).

REFERENCES

1. R. Goth and M. F. Rajewsky, Molecular and cellular mechanisms associated with pulse-carcinogenesis in the rat nervous system by ethylnitrosourea: Ethylation of nucleic acids and elimination rates of ethylated bases from the DNA of different tissues, Z. Krebsforsch. 82:37 (1974).
2. M. F. Rajewsky, L. H. Augenlicht, H. Biessmann, R. Goth, D. F. Hülser, O. D. Laerum, and L. Ya. Lomakina, Nervous system-specific carcinogenesis by ethylnitrosourea in the rat: Molecular and cellular mechanisms, in: "Origins of Human Cancer," Book B: "Mechanisms of Carcinogenesis," H. H. Hiatt, J. D. Watson and J. A. Winsten, eds., Cold Spring Harbor Laboratory, Cold Spring Harbor, N.Y., p. 709 (1977).
3. M. F. Rajewsky, Possible determinants for the differential susceptibility of mammalian cells and tissues to chemical carcinogens, Arch. Toxicol., Suppl. 3:229 (1980).
4. O. D. Laerum and M. F. Rajewsky, Neoplastic transformation of fetal rat brain cells in culture following exposure to ethylnitrosourea in vivo, J. Natl. Cancer Inst. 55:1177 (1975).
5. J. C. Barrett and P. O. P. Ts'o, Evidence for the progressive nature of neoplastic transformation in vitro, Proc. Natl. Acad. Sci. USA 75:3761 (1978).
6. T. Kakunaga, K.-Y. Lo, J. Leavitt, and M. Ikenaga, Relationship between transformation and mutation in mammalian cells, in: "Carcinogenesis: Fundamental Mechanisms and Environmental Effects," B. Pullman, P. O. P. Ts'o, and H. Gelboin, eds., Reidel, Dordrecht, p. 527 (1980).
7. I. Berenblum, Sequential aspects of chemical carcinogenesis: Skin, in: "Cancer: A Comprehensive Treatise," Vol. 1, F. F. Becker, ed., Plenum Press, New York, p. 323 (1975).
8. T. J. Slaga, A. Sivak, and R. K. Boutwell, eds., "Carcinogenesis. A Comprehensive Survey," Vol. 2, "Mechanisms of Tumor Promotion and Cocarcinogenesis," Raven Press, New York (1978).

9.   I. B. Weinstein, R. A. Mufson, L.-S. Lee, P. B. Fisher,
     J. Laskin, A. D. Horowitz, and V. Ivanovic, Membrane and
     other biochemical effects of the phorbol esters and their
     relative to tumor promotion, in: "Carcinogenesis:
     Fundamental Mechanisms and Environmental Effects," B.
     Pullman, P. O. P. Ts'o, and H. Gelboin, eds., Reidel,
     Dordrecht, p. 543 (1980).

10. E. Hecker, ed., "Carcinogenesis: Biological Effects of Tumor
     Promotors," Raven Press, New York (1981).

11. P. D. Lawley, Carcinogenesis by alkylating agents, in:
     "Chemical Carcinogens," C. E. Searle, ed., ACS Monograph
     No. 173, American Chemical Society, Washington, D.C.,
     p. 83 (1976).

12. A. E. Pegg, Formation and metabolism of alkylated nucleosides:
     Possible role in carcinogenesis by nitroso compounds and
     alkylating agents, Adv. Cancer Res. 25:195 (1977).

13. D. Grunberger and I. B. Weinstein, Conformational changes in
     nucleic acids modified by chemical carcinogens, in:
     "Chemical Carcinogens and DNA," P. L. Grover, ed., CRC
     Press, Boca Raton, p. 59 (1979).

14. P. L. Grover, ed., "Chemical Carcinogens and DNA," CRC Press,
     Boca Raton (1979).

15. B. Singer, N-nitroso alkylating agents: Formation and
     persistence of alkyl derivatives in mammalian nucleic
     acids as contributing factors in carcinogenesis, J. Natl.
     Cancer Inst. 62:1329 (1979).

16. B. Pullman, P. O. P. Ts'o, and H. Gelboin, eds.,
     "Carcinogenesis: Fundamental Mechanisms and Environmental
     Effects," Reidel, Dordrecht (1980).

17. M. F. Rajewsky, Specificity of DNA damage in chemical
     carcinogenesis, in: "Molecular and Cellular Aspects of
     Carcinogen Screening Tests," R. Montesano, H. Bartsch,
     and L. Tomatis, eds., IARC Scientific Publications No. 27,
     International Agency for Research on Cancer, Lyon, p. 41
     (1980).

18. E. C. Miller and J. A. Miller, The metabolism of chemical
     carcinogens to reactive electrophiles and their possible
     mechanisms of action in carcinogenesis, in: "Chemical
     Carcinogens," C. E. Searle, ed., ACS Monograph No. 173,
     American Chemical Society, Washington, D.C., p. 737 (1976).

19. J. A. Miller and E. C. Miller, Perspectives on the metabolism
     of chemical carcinogens, in: P. Emmelot and E. Kriek, eds.,
     "Environmental Carcinogenesis," Elsevier/North-Holland
     Biomedical Press, Amsterdam, p. 25 (1979).

20. J. McCann, E. Choi, E. Yamasaki, and B. N. Ames, Detection of
     carcinogens as mutagens in the Salmonella/microsome test:
     Assay of 300 chemicals, Proc. Natl. Acad. Sci. USA
     72:5135 (1975).

21. M. Nagao, T. Sugimura, and T. Matsushima, Environmental mutagens and carcinogens, Ann. Rev. Genet. 12:117 (1978).

22. M. Hollstein, J. McCann, and F. A. Angelosanto, Short-term tests for carcinogens and mutagens, Mutat. Res. 65:133 (1979).

23. R. P. P. Fuchs, N. Schwartz, and M. P. Daune, Hot spots of frameshift mutations induced by the ultimate carcinogen N-acetoxy-N-2-acetylaminofluorene, Nature (Lond.) 294:657 (1981).

24. R. P. P. Fuchs, J. F. Lefévre, J. Pouyet, and M. P. Daune, Comparative orientation of the fluorene residue in native DNA modified by N-acetoxy-N-2-acetylaminofluorene and two 7-halogeno derivatives, Biochemistry 15:3347 (1976).

25. A. H. Wang, G. J. Quigley, F. J. Kolpak, J. L. Cranford, J. A. Van Boom, G. Van der Macel, and A. Rich, Molecular structure of a left-handed double helical DNA fragment at atomic resolution, Nature (Lond.) 282:680 (1979).

26. E. Sage and M. Leng, Conformation of poly (dG-dC)·poly (dG-dC) modified by the carcinogens N-acetoxy-N-acetyl-2-aminofluorene and N-hydroxy-N-2-aminofluorene, Proc. Natl. Acad. Sci. USA 77:4597 (1980).

27. R. M. Santella, D. Grunberger, I. B. Weinstein, and A. Rich, Induction of the Z conformation in poly (dG-dC)·poly (dG-dC) by binding of N-2-acetylaminofluorene to guanine residues, Proc. Natl. Acad. Sci. USA 78:1451 (1981).

28. A. Nordheim, M. L. Pardue, E. M. Lafer, A. Möller, B. D. Stollar, and A. Rich, Antibodies to left-handed Z-DNA bind to interband regions of Drosophila polytene chromosomes, Nature (Lond.) 294:417 (1981).

29. F. Crick, Split genes and RNA splicing, Science 204:264 (1979).

30. J. N. Lapeyre and F. F. Becker, 5-Methylcytosine content of nuclear DNA during chemical hepatocarcinogenesis and in carcinomas which result, Biochem. Biophys. Res. Commun. 87:698 (1979).

31. T. L. Boehm and D. Drahovsky, Hypomethylation of DNA in Raji cells after treatment with N-methyl-N-nitrosourea, Carcinogenesis 2:39 (1981).

32. M. Ehrlich and R. Y.-H. Wang, 5-Methylcytosine in eukaryotic DNA, Science 212:1350 (1981).

33. A. Pfohl-Leszkowicz, C. Salas, R. P. P. Fuchs, and G. Dirheimer, Mechanism of inhibition of enzymatic deoxyribonucleic acid methylation by 2-(acetylamino)fluorene bound to deoxyribonucleic acid, Biochemistry 20:3020 (1981).

34. J. Cairns, The origin of human cancers, Nature (Lond.) 289:353 (1981).

35. S. Lavi, Carcinogen-mediated amplification of viral DNA sequences in simian virus 40-transformed Chinese hamster embryo cells, Proc. Natl. Acad. Sci. USA 78:6144 (1981).

36. J. German, ed., "Chromosomes and Cancer," Wiley, New York
     (1974).
37. M. Radman, Is there SOS induction in mammalian cells?
     Photochem. Photobiol. 32:823 (1980).
38. R. A. Weinberg, Use of transfection to analyze genetic
     information and malignant transformation, Biochem. Biophys.
     Acta 651:25 (1981).
39. M. F. Rajewsky, Proliferative parameters of mammalian cell
     systems and their role in tumour growth and carcinogenesis,
     Z. Krebsforsch. 78:12 (1972).
40. L. G. Lajtha, Stem cell concepts, Differentiation 14:23 (1979).
41. P. C. Hanawalt, P. K. Cooper, A. K. Ganesan, and C. A. Smith,
     DNA repair in bacteria and mammalian cells, Annu. Rev.
     Biochem. 48:783 (1979).
42. T. Lindahl, DNA glycosylases, endonucleases for apurinic/
     apyrimidinic sites, and base excision repair, Progr. Nucleic
     Acid Res. Mol. Biol. 22:135 (1979).
43. G. P. Margison and P. J. O'Connor, Nucleic acid modification
     by N-nitroso compounds, in: "Chemical Carcinogens and DNA,"
     Vol. 1, P. L. Grover, ed., CRC Press, Boca Raton, p. 111
     (1979).
44. A. R. Lehmann and P. Karran, DNA repair, Int. Rev. Cytol.
     72:101 (1981).
45. E. Seeberg and K. Kleppe, eds., "Chromosome damage and repair,"
     Plenum Press, New York (1981).
46. G. F. Saunders, ed., "Cell Differentiation and Neoplasia,"
     Raven Press, New York (1978).
47. T. Graf and H. Beug, Avian leukemia viruses: interaction with
     their target cells in vivo and in vitro, Biochim. Biophys.
     Acta 516:269 (1978).
48. W. Jaenisch, Retroviruses and embryogenesis: Microinjection of
     Moloney leukemia virus into midgestation mouse embryos,
     Cell 19:181 (1980).
49. P. J. O'Connor, R. Saffhill, and G.P. Margison, N-nitroso
     compounds: Biochemical mechanisms of action, in:
     Environmental Carcinogenesis," P. Emmelot and E. Kriek,
     eds., Elsevier/North-Holland Biomedical Press, Amsterdam,
     p. 73 (1979).
50. S. Ivankovic and H. Druckrey, Transplacentare Erzeugung
     maligner Tumoren des Nervensystems. I. Äthylnitrosoharnstoff
     (ÄNH) an BDIX-Ratten, Z. Krebsforsch. 71:320 (1968).
51. R. Goth and M. F. Rajewsky, Ethylation of nucleic acids by
     ethylnitrosourea-1-^{14}C in the fetal and adult rat, Cancer
     Res. 32:1501 (1972).
52. R. Goth and M. F. Rajewsky, Persistence of O^6-ethylguanine in
     rat brain DNA: Correlation with nervous system specific
     carcinogenesis by ethylnitrosourea, Proc. Natl. Acad. Sci.
     USA 71:639 (1974).

53. R. Müller and M. F. Rajewsky, Immunological quantification by
    high affinity antibodies of O^6-ethyldeoxyguanosine in DNA
    exposed to N-ethyl-N-nitrosourea, Cancer Res. 40:887 (1980).
54. R. Müller and M. F. Rajewsky, submitted for publication (1982).
55. E. J. Johansson-Brittebo and H. Tjälve, Studies on the
    tissue-disposition and fate of N-(^{14}C)ethyl-N-nitrosourea
    in mice, Toxicology 13:275 (1979).
56. O. D. Laerum, Å. Haugen, and M. F. Rajewsky, Neoplastic
    transformation of foetal rat brain cells in culture after
    exposure to ethylnitrosourea in vivo, in: "Neoplastic
    Transformation in Differentiated Epithelial Cell Systems
    in Vitro," L. M. Franks and C. B. Wigley, eds., p. 190
    (1979).
57. H. Druckrey, B. Schagen, and S. Ivankovic, Erzeugung
    neurogener Malignome durch einmalige Gabe von Äthyl-
    nitrosoharnstoff (ÄNH) an neugeborene und junge BDIX-
    Ratten, Z. Krebsforsch. 74:141 (1970).
58. H. Druckrey, C. Landschütz, and S. Ivankovic, Transplacentare
    Erzeugung maligner Tumoren des Nervensystems.
    II. Äthylnitrosoharnstoff an 10 genetisch definierten
    Rattenstämmen, Z. Krebsforsch. 73:371 (1970).
59. M. F. Rajewsky, Structural modifications and repair of DNA in
    neuro-oncogenesis by N-ethyl-N-nitrosourea. J. Cancer Res.
    Clin. Oncol., Suppl., in press (1982).
60. R. H. Denlinger, A. Koestner, and W. Wechsler, Induction of
    neurogenic tumors in C3HeB/FeJ mice by nitrosourea
    derivatives: Observations by light microscopy, tissue
    culture, and electron microscopy, Int. J. Cancer 13:559
    (1974).
61. E.L. Jones, C. E. Searle, and T. W. Smith, Medulloblastomas
    and other neural tumours in mice treated neonatally with
    N-ethyl-N-nitrosourea, Acta Neuropathol. 36:57 (1976).
62. P. Kleihues, J. Bücheler, and U. N. Riede, Selective induction
    of melanomas in gerbils (meriones unguiculatus) following
    postnatal administration of N-ethyl-N-nitrosourea, J. Natl.
    Cancer Inst. 61:458 (1978).
63. O. Stutman, Transplacental carcinogenesis in athymic nude
    mice, Path. Res. Pract. 165:170 (1979).
64. D. Stavrou, T. Hanichen, and I. Wriedt-Lübbe, Onkogene Wirkung
    von Äthylnitrosoharnstoff beim Kaninchen während der
    pränatalen Periode, Z. Krebsforsch. 84:207 (1975).
65. D. Stavrou, E. Dahme, and B. Schröder, Transplacentare
    neuroonkogene Wirkung von Äthylnitrosoharnstoff beim
    Kaninchen während der frühen Graviditätsphase, Z.
    Krebsforsch. 89:331 (1977).
66. R. R. Fox, B. A. Diwan, and H. Meier, Transplacental induction
    of primary renal tumors in rabbits treated with 1-ethyl-1-
    nitrosourea, J. Natl.Cancer Inst. 54:1439 (1975).

67. B. Singer, W. J. Bodell, J. E. Cleaver, E. H. Thomas, M. F.
     Rajewsky, and W. Thon, Oxygens in DNA are main targets for
     ethylnitrosourea in normal and Xeroderma pigmentosum
     fibroblasts and fetal rat brain cells, Nature (Lond.)
     276:85 (1978).
68. L. Sun and B. Singer, The specificity of different classes of
     ethylating agents toward various sites of HeLa Cell DNA
     in vitro and in vivo, Biochemistry 14:1795 (1975).
69. C. K. Ingold, "Structure and Mechanism in Organic Chemistry,"
     Chapter 7, Cornell Univ. Press, Ithaca-New York (1953).
70. W. M. Baird, The use of radioactive carcinogens to detect DNA
     modifications, in: "Chemical Carcinogens and DNA," P. L.
     Groover, ed., CRC Press, Boca Raton, p. 59 (1979).
71. M. F. Rajewsky, R. Müller, J. Adamkiewicz, and W. Drosdziok,
     Immunological detection and quantification of DNA components
     structurally modified by alkylating carcinogens
     (ethylnitrosourea), in: "Carcinogenesis: Fundamental
     Mechanisms and Environmental Effects.", B. Pullman,
     P. O. P. Ts'o, and H. Gelboin, eds., Reidel, Dordrecht,
     p. 207 (1980).
72. R. Müller and M. F. Rajewsky, Antibodies specific for DNA
     components structurally modified by chemical carcinogens,
     J. Cancer Res. Clin. Oncol. 102:99 (1981).
73. R. Müller and M. F. Rajewsky, Sensitive radioimmunoassay for
     detection of O^6-ethyldeoxyguanosine in DNA exposed to the
     carcinogen ethylnitrosourea in vivo or in vitro, Z.
     Naturforsch. 33c:897 (1978).
74. J. Adamkiewicz, W. Eberhardt, U. Langenberg, R. Müller, and
     M. F. Rajewsky, Monoclonal antibodies for the specific
     detection and quantification of DNA components structurally
     modified by alkylating carcinogens, Proc. Sect. Exp. Cancer
     Res. German Cancer Soc., J. Cancer Res. Clin. Oncol.
     99:A21 (1981).
75. R. Saffhill and J. M. Boyle, Detection of carcinogen-DNA
     adducts by radio-immunoassay, Abstr. Proc. 22nd Ann. Gen.
     Meeting Brit. Assoc. Cancer Res., Br. J. Cancer 44:275
     (1981).
76. J. Adamkiewicz and M. F. Rajewsky, submitted for publication
     (1982).
77. A. Loveless, Possible relevance of O^6-alkylation of
     deoxyguanosine to the mutagenicity and carcinogenicity of
     nitrosamines and nitrosamides, Nature (Lond.) 223:206
     (1969).
78. B. Singer and M. Kröger, Participation of modified nucleosides
     in translation and transcription, Progr. Nucl. Acid Res.
     Mol. Biol. 23:151 (1979).
79. P. Nehls and M. F. Rajewsky, Ethylation of fetal rat brain
     chromosomal DNA by ethylnitrosourea, Proc. Sect. Exp.
     Cancer Res. German Cancer Soc., J. Cancer Res. Clin.

Oncol. 99:A38 (1981).

80. P. Nehls and M. F. Rajewsky, submitted for publication (1982).

81. M. Renz, P. Nehls, and J. Hozier, Involvement of histone H1 in the organization of the chromosome fiber, Proc. Natl. Acad. Sci. USA 74:1879 (1977).

82. H. Weintraub and M. Groudine, Chromosomal subunits in active genes have an altered conformation, Science 193:848 (1976).

83. A. Garel and R. Axel, Selective digestion of transcirptionally active ovalbumin genes from oviduct nuclei, Proc. Natl. Acad. Sci. USA 73:3966 (1976).

84. M. J. W. Chang, R. W. Hart, and A. Koestner, Retention of promutagenic O^6-ethylguanine in the DNA of various rat tissues following transplacental inoculation with ethylnitrosourea, Cancer Lett. 9:199 (1980).

85. P. J. Abbott and R. Saffhill, DNA synthesis with methylated poly (dA-dT) templates: Possible role of O^4-methylthymine as a pro-mutagenic base, Nucleic Acids Res. 4:761 (1977).

86. P. J. Abbott and R. Saffhill, DNA synthesis with methylated poly (dC-dG) templates. Evidence for a competitive nature of miscoding by O^6-methylguanine, Biochim. Biophys. Acta 562:51 (1979).

87. W. L. Russell, E. M. Kelly, P. R. Hunsicker, J. W. Bangham, S. C. Maddux, and E. L. Phipps, Specific-locus test shows ethylnitrosourea to be the most potent mutagen in the mouse, Proc. Natl. Acad. Sci. USA 76:5818 (1979).

88. E. Vogel and A. T. Natarajan, The relation between reaction kinetics and mutagenic action of mono-functional alkylating agents in higher eukaryotic systems. I. Recessive lethal mutations and translocations in Drosophila, Mutat. Res. 62:51 (1979).

89. E. Vogel and A. T. Natarajan, The relation between reaction kinetics and mutagenic action of mono-functional alkylating agents in higher eukaryotic systems. II. Total and partial sex-chromosome loss in Drosophila, Mutat. Res. 62:101 (1979).

90. L. Samson and J. Cairns, A new pathway for DNA repair in Escherichia coli, Nature (Lond.) 267:281 (1977).

91. P. Jeggo, M. Defais, L. Samson, and P. Schendel, An adaptive response of E. coli to low levels of alkylating agents: Comparison with previously characterized DNA repair pathways, Mol. Gen. Genet. 157:1 (1977).

92. P. Karran, T. Lindahl, and B. Griffin, Adaptive response to alkylating agents involves alteration in situ of O^6-methylguanine residues in DNA, Nature (Lond.) 280:76 (1979).

93. R. S. Foote, S. Mitra, and B. C. Pal, Demethylation of O^6-methylguanine in a synthetic DNA polymer by an inducible activity in Escherichia coli, Biochem. Biophys. Res. Comm. 97:654 (1980).

94. M. Olsson and T. Lindahl, Repair of alkylated DNA in E. coli:
     Methyl group transfer from O^6-methylguanine to a protein
     cysteine residue, J. Biol. Chem. 255:10569 (1980).
95. T. Lindahl, DNA methyl transferase acting on O^6-methylguanine
     residues in adapted E. coli, in: "Chromosome Damage and
     Repair," E. Seeberg and K. Kleppe, eds., Plenum, New York,
     in press (1981).
96. J. M. Bogden, A. Eastman, and E. Bresnick, A system in mouse
     liver for the repair of O^6-methylguanine lesions in
     methylated DNA, Nucleic Acids Res. 9:3089 (1981).
97. J. R. Mehta, D. B. Ludlum, A. Renard, and W. G. Verly, Repair
     of O^6-ethylguanine in DNA by a chromatin fraction from
     rat liver: Transfer of the ethyl group to an acceptor
     protein, Proc. Natl. Acad. Sci. USA 78:6766 (1981).
98. A. E. Pegg and G. Hui, Formation and subsequent removal of
     O^6-methylguanine from DNA in rat liver and kidney after
     small doses of dimethylnitrosamine, Biochem. J. 173:739
     (1978).
99. A. E. Pegg and B. Balog, Formation and subsequent excision
     of O^6-ethylguanine from DNA of rat liver following
     administration of diethylnitrosamine, Cancer Res. 39:5003
     (1979).
100. A. E. Pegg, M. Roberfroid, H. Bresil, A. Likhachev, and R.
     Montesano, submitted for publication (1982).
101. H. M. Rabes, R. Kerler, R. Wilhelm, G. Rode, and H. Riess,
     alkylation of DNA and RNA by [^{14}C] dimethylnitrosamine
     in hydroxyurea-synchronized regenerating rat liver, Cancer
     Res. 39:4228 (1979).
102. A. E. Pegg, W. Perry, and R. A. Bennett, Effect of partial
     hepatectomy on removal of O6-methylguanine from alkylated
     DNA by rat liver extracts, Biochem. J. 197:195 (1981).
103. P. Kleihues and G. P. Margison, Exhaustion and recovery of
     repair excision of O6-methylguanine from rat liver DNA,
     Nature (Lond.) 259:153 (1976).
104. G. P. Margison, J. M. Margison, and R. Montesano, Methylated
     purines in the deoxyribonucleic acid of various Syrian-
     golden-hamster tissues after administration of a
     hepatocarcinogenic dose of dimethylnitrosamine, Biochem.
     J. 157:627 (1976).
105. R. Stumpf, G. P. Margison, R. Montesano, and A. E. Pegg,
     Formation and loss of alkylated purines from DNA of hamster
     liver after administration of dimethylnitrosamine, Cancer
     Res. 39:50 (1979).
106. R. Montesano, Alkylation of DNA and tissue specificity in
     nitrosamine carcinogenesis, J. Supramolec. Struct. Cell
     Biochem., in press (1982).
107. L. Tomatis and F. Cefis, The effects of multiple and single
     administration of dimethylnitrosamine to hamsters,
     Tumori 53:447 (1967).

108. J. G. Lewis and J. A. Swenberg, Differential repair of
     O^6-methylguanine in DNA in rat hepatocytes and non-
     parenchymal cells, Nature (Lond.) 288:185 (1980).

CHROMATIN, NUCLEI AND WATER: ALTERATIONS AND MECHANISMS FOR CHEMICALLY- INDUCED CARCINOGENESIS

Nicolini, C., Brambilla, G., Beltrame, F., Capitani, S., Carlo, P., Cavazza, B., Chiabrera, A., Finollo, R., Grattarola, M., Manzoli, A., Maraldi, N., Martelli, A., Parodi, G., Patrone, E., Ridella, S., Trefiletti, V., Viviani, R.

Interdisciplinary Group of Biostructure, University of Genova, Italy and National Research Council, Italy
Temple University, Department of Biophysics and Physiology Philadelphia, USA

In recent years experimental evidences (1-5) have been accumulating on the orderly organization of the chromatin-DNA within mammalian cells from the Watson-Crick double helix (secondary structure) through successive higher order DNA foldings (nucleosome and super-nucleosome) up to a quinternary level (5), being postulated as drapery-like regular packing of 300 A° "solenoid-like" or "rope-like" fibers. While uncertainty still exists on the exact three-dimensional geometry 'in situ' of the latter two superstructures, there is general agreement on both the tertiary structure (wrapping of DNA around octamer histones to form the nucleosome) and on the modulation of the overall chromatin structure during cell transformation and cell proliferation. Namely the native higher order structure (5, 6, 7,) has been conclusively linked to DNA replication and mitotic condensation, through abrupt structural transitions induced by enzymatic modifications of H1 histones, ions and generally by the neutralization of DNA phosphate charge (as strikingly expected from polyelectrolyte theory (8)). An increase of chromatin condensation has been also consistently associated with cell transformation (either induced by virus, chemical or spontaneously), suggesting that an higher order chromatin superpacking and a reduced chromatin template (9, 4) are a prerequisite for the expression of the transformed phenotype. This apparent paradox is however complicated by the significant chromatin modulation occuring during cell cycle progression of both normal and transformed cells, which

obscure the increased condensation. It would seem indeed that only the
degree of coupling between changes in nuclear morphometry (chromatin
higher order structure) and changes in cell morphometry is uniquely low for
individual transformed cell, being quite high for every fibroblast or normal
cell (5, 10). In transformed cell, the absence of any coupling would let
chromatin to progress through its cycles of condensation and decondensation
regardless the shape assumed by the intact cell, including a round one as in
suspension or as induced by cell-cell interaction, nutritional deprivation or
cell-substrate interaction. The mechanism by which cell geometry and cell
growth are respectively coupled in normal and uncoupled in transformed
cells (10) was indeed suggested to be the physically
(microtubules-microfilaments) or chemically induced coupling and
uncoupling between nuclear morphometry and cell geometry, with the higher
degree of fiber superpacking being also related to the expressions of
transformed phenotypes. It would be then interesting to verify if these
findings can be generalized to cell transformation induced by chemical
carcinogens in VIVO, but prior to characterize its significance and specific
structural-functional modification induced by chemical carcinogens (as
originally reported time ago (11)), it is mandatory to know more about
chromatin itself. Unperturbed rat liver cells and rat liver chromatin were
mainly used as experimental models; for the purpose of comparison
complementary measurements on calf thymus chromatin have been carried
out.

The aim of this chapter is to summarize all evidences in favor of a
rope-like model for quaternary chromatin structure and of its quinternary
drapery-like organization (involving also nuclear pores), in native conditions
and after the administration of a chemical carcinogen IN VIVO. These
studies have been conducted by means of computer-enhanced image analysis
of electron micrographs (to a level not obtainable by human observers) and
correlated freeze-etching, visco-elastometry, microcalorimetry, scanning
and flow cytometry. Other parallel changes occuring as early events in the
carcinogenic process, at the level of cytoskeleton, nuclei and intact cell (12)
(and their coupling) are also given and reviewed in conjuction with changes
in the amount of physical state of water and ions, as monitored by a
recently implemented measurement of nuclei complex dielectric constants.
Possible molecular mechanisms, in terms of polyelectrolyte theory (8) and
mean field theory (13), determining chromatin structral transitions and
related to the control of chemical-induced neoplastic transformation are
futhermore presented.

PREPARATION OF RAT LIVER NUCLEI AND CHROMATIN

Unless otherwise stated animals used were Sprague Dawley male rats
(200-250g body weight, 8-10 weeks old). Liver perfusion through portal vein
was carried out by injecting 120 ml of cold 0.027 M sodium citrate in
calcium magnesium free phosphate buffered solution. The use of trypsin
was omitted to avoid possible chromatin-DNA alterations. Liver cell
suspensions were obtained with six strokes of the pestle of a loose fitting
homogenizer and cells were collected by centrifuging for 4 min. at 150 X g.

The pellet was resuspended in 9 volumes of 0.75% Triton X-100 in dissociation medium (0.075 M NaCl, 0.024 M Na_2EDTA; pH 7.5) and incubated for 4 min. The suspension was centrifuged for 2 min. at 150 X g. This step was repeated once without further incubation.

The average range of ratios by weight among DNA, RNA and protein for these nuclei preparations was about 1:0.2:3.0 was about 1:0.2:3.0. For electron microscopy rat liver chromatin was obtained by diluting the nuclear pellet with low-salt media (0-2 mM Li_2SO_4, Tris-HCl buffer, pH 7.5). The final DNA concentration was 41g/ml. The same swelling procedure was used for calf thymus chromatin; nuclei were isolated according to the method described by Panyim et Al. with minor modifications (18). For microcalorimetry calf thymus chromatin was pelleted by ultracentrifugation (40,000 rpm for 24 h in a Beckman 60 Ti model rotor) at different salt concentrations (from 0 to 600 mM NaCl), in 1 mM Tris-HCl buffer, pH 8. The surnatant was decanted weighted (50 g) amounts of the pellet transferred into large volume (75 l) calorimetry capsuls; a known amount of the starting solvent added, the capsules sealed, and equilibration achieved by keeping the system at $4^{o}C$ for 5 h. The DNA content of these preparations was determined by measuring the absorbance at 260 m under alkaline conditions (pH 13.5); proteins and RNA contributions to the spectra were subtracted. Intact rat liver nuclei were studied under physiological conditions and harvested at 25,000 rpm for 3 h in a Beckman SV 50 L model rotor.

Treatment of rats with DMNA or AAF

DMNA (dimethylnitrosamine) was dissolved in 0.9% NaCl, and AAF (2-acetylaminofluorene) was suspended in 0.9% NaCl-1% carboxymethylcellulose, just before use, in a concentration that could be administered on the basis of 0.01 ml/g of body weight. Controls received the same volume of the same vehicle. Animals were sacrified always 4 or 14 hrs after treatment. DMNA was used at the doses of 5.4 mg/kg and 48.6 mg/kg; AAF at the dose of 50 mg/kg. Both carcinogens were injected i.p. in a single dose.

Occasionally rats were killed 18 hrs. after removal of 2/3 of the liver (partial hepatectomy), to monitor the effect of induced cell proliferation.

PROBES FOR HIGHER ORDER DNA STRUCTURE

Electron Microscopy

High resolution photographs of unfixed-unstained chromatin isolated in native conditions from intact swollen nuclei of rat liver and calf thymus were obtained by means of a recently introduced electron microscopic technique, involving a phospholipid monolayer (14). As previously pointed out the chromatin images acquired are absent of distortion or artifacts, due to fixation and/or staining, and present a limited acceptable level of background noise.

Computer-enhanced image analysis

Nuclear images were acquired and analyzed by means of the ACTA system built and installed at the Biophysical and Eletronic Engineering Section, Institute of Electrotecnic, University of Genova (Italy).

The E.M. pictures were imaged through a macroepidioscope (optical magnification=3.5-6x) on a European standard TV scanner target, equipped with a Plumbicon tube.

The Plumbicon tube ensures a highly linear transfer function between light intensity and electrical signal, therefore allowing a uniform discretization of the analog video signal in gray levels and to perform a standard calibration procedure which makes measurements repeatable. The analog video signal is fed through a fast A/D conversion group (8 bit, 30 MHz, a monolithic integrated circuit) and each video frame can be stored in real time on a memory according to the format 512x512 pixels, 8 bit resolution per pixel. Several routes were then possible and alternatively followed.

Images were transferred on a mass-memory device, such as magnetic tape or disk, interfaced to HP 21MX minicomputer (which controls the ACTA system); the very same images could also be sent back form the mag-tape to the fast memory for further processing. The digital video signal originating from the memory is sent through a look-up table system and D/A conversion to Black/White and color TV monitor.

Specifically, look-up tables, being under program control, allow us to use pseudocolor techniques to further enhance the images. Geometric and densitometric analysis are also carried out on the acquired images, by means of an interactive procedure involving a variable frame, program controlled for position and X-Y dimensions.

Final images are obtained after subtraction and equalization of the background due to optical and electronic noise determined in equivalent region outside the fiber.

Microviscometry

The apparatus has been previously described in its details (15). Basically, the viscometer consists of an oscillating crucible suspended by a wire and containing the liquid under study in a half-filled U-shaped circular channel. The parameter measured is the armonic damped oscillation of the crucible. This damping depends upon the frictional torque exerted by the liquid on the internal walls of the circular channel. The oscillations are started by a rotating device which gives a starting torsion to the nickel-chromium wire by which the crucible is suspended. The damped oscillation of the crucible is registered by a spot-follower whose mobile equipment receives the light beam reflected by a little mirror attached to the axis of the doughnut. A copper container, completely immersed in a water bath, isolates a region of constant temperature ($\pm$ 0.1°C) where the crucible oscillates. Two resistance thermometers, placed in the proximity of the doughnut, monitor temperature variations during the experiment.

The basic theory of the instrument, which has already been described by Gallina et al. (16), shows that for a toroidal channel we can relate the observed damping coefficient δ(logarithmic decrement of oscillations) to the coefficient of viscosity of the liquid by this relationship:

$$\frac{I}{4\pi^3 a^2 R^3 \rho} \frac{\{\delta - \delta_0\}}{} \sqrt{2} \{ 1 + \frac{T^2}{T_o^2} \} = G_1(q) - \delta \, G_2(q) + \frac{a^2}{R^2} G_3(q) \qquad (1)$$

where I is the moment of inertia of the oscillating system; T and T_o are the periods with and without the liquid, respectively; ρ is the density of the liquid; η the viscosity of the liquid; a the inner radius of the channel (3.5 mm in our instrument); q the dimentionless paramenter given by a $(2\pi\rho/\eta\, T)^{1/2}$; G_1 the universal function of q, the tabulation of which was given by Gallina et al. (16). As previously shown (15), in our experimental conditions the value of q falls in the left par of the G_1 (q) curve, where the variation of ($\delta - \delta_0$) for different η is maximum and results in a higher sensitivity of the instrument. Equation (1) gives absolute values of η only for a completely filled toroidal channel and for measurement made under vacuum. For our half-filled U-shaped circular channel we can obtain absolute values of η from ($\delta - \delta_0$) by standardizing our viscometer against glycerol solutions for different concentration.

In our viscosimetric assays the U-shaped circular channel of the crucible was indeed partially filled with a constant liquid volume of 10 ml and all the experiments were carried out at 22°C (15, 17); DNA viscosity was studied either in alkaline or in neutral condition at both high and low ionic strength, by adding successively in the circular channel of the crucible 4 ml of lysing solution (0.02 M Na_2EDTA, 0.138 M sarcosyl) + 1 ml of nuclear suspension in dissociation medium (0.075 M NaCl, 0.024 M Na_2EDTA).

Microcalorimetry

Differential scanning calorimetry (DSC) is a straight-forward technique allowing the determination of both temperature and enthalpy change associated with any given transition; moreover, pressure resistant sample capsules may be used, a further distinct improvement in the field of thermal analysis of aqueous solutions, allowing the investigation of conformational changes well above 90°C. To date, the low sensitivity of commercial instruments prevented their applicaton to biological systems. A more sensitive DSC apparatus has now become available (Perkin-Elmer DSC II) and we started a systematic study of the melting behaviour of both calf thymus chromatin and intact rat liver nuclei. In this report we describe some new, interesting findings, throwing light on the interpretation of the structural changes of native chromatin induced by salts or by DNA-damaging agents.

Because the enthalpy differences involved in the conformational transitions of biopolymers are of the order of few Kcal. per residue mole, and the higher effective sensitivity of our instrument is 0.5 mcal./sec, it is clear that in order to obtain a significant response the concentration of chromatin must be rised near or above its physiological value (2% by weight).

A critical, although apparently trivial point of our procedure is the way of filling the capsules. Contamination of their external wall results in large, spurious thermal effects. The simple instrument shown in ref. 18 was designed to manipulate pellets having different physical properties; in fact at low salt concentration the material is a swollen, viscous gel, but above 50 mM it becomes thick and rubber-like. The instrument consists of a stainless steel hollow punch, bearing a central plunger; the external body has a sharp tip, its external diameter (0.5 cm) being slightly smaller than the opening of the capsules. By rising the plunger, the soft gels may be easily withdrawn into the internal channel; hard gels are layered on a clean glass surface and sampled by gently pressing the hollow punch on them. For sensitivities equal to 0.5 mcal./sec or higher, the use of the autozero device of the calorimeter leads to quite large errors; by cutting out the device a curved baseline results. We have adopted the following scanning procedure. The sample capsule, equilibrated for heat capacity with the references, is heated from ~20°C up to ~ 120°C, and the thermal profile recorded. The temperature is then lowered down to its initial value, and a second scan is carried out on the denatured sample. As may be seen in Fig. 9 the baseline, although curved, can be defined with a reasonable accuracy, owing to the very small difference of specific heat (once excluded the sharp conformational transitions) between native and denatured chromatin. The error of the determinations depends chiefly on the concentration of the sample, which is a function of the ionic strength. We may roughly estimate that an uncertainty of $\pm$ 15% affects the determinations carried out in 1-5 mM salt, while better results ($\pm$ 5%) are obtained above 50 mM. The transition enthalpies are obtained form the areas of the thermograms, according to the standard formula

$$\Delta H = \frac{K \; A \; R}{W \; S}$$

where ΔH is the enthalpy change expressed in cal/g of DNA, W is the weight of DNA in mg, R is the sensitivity range in mcal./sec mm, S is the chart speed in mm/sec, and A is the area of the thermal peak in mm^2. The instrument calibration constant K was found to be equal to 1 under our experimental conditions.

Probe for RNA, DNA, and membrane

Previous studies (19) which concerned the staining of intact cells with acridine orange (AO) in solution, demonstrated that nuclear DNA and cytoplasmic RNA emit respectively on the green and in the red, when the ratio (M AO/ MDNA) is about 4 and final AO concentration is equal to 2.5×10^{-5} M (as in this study). Unfixed or alcohol-fixed liver cells were suspended in 5mM Tris pH 7 prior to staining and analysis. Fluorescasmine a dye covalently linked to primary amine, has been used to monitor nuclear and cell membranes (20).

Cell fluorescence (green, red) and low angle forward light scatter were simultaneously measured on a Becton Dickinson FACS II (at Temple University, USA), with a 4 watts ion laser, on line with a PDP 11/40 computer (19, 20), and displayed directly on a bidimensional array (Expt. I). Alternatively (Exp. II) flourescence distribution was acquired by a Phybe cytometer (Ortho Instruments, USA) at 488 nm excitation wavelength and stored on tape form for subsequent reduction and display by a HP digital computer. In the two different experiments two different human lymphocytes populations were used, fixed either with 2% glutaraldehyde (Expt. I) or with 90% alcohol (Expt. II).

PROBE FOR NUCLEAR AND CELL MORPHOMETRY

The isolated cells were fixed (3:1 mixture of ethanol and acetic acid) and either Feulgen or triple stained on slides as previously shown (21, 22). Each slide was analyzed with the automated image analyzer ACTA (24) or with the quantimet 720D (22, 23).

Descripton of the Quantimet-PDP11 configuration has been given at length in numerous publications and few reviews (23, 5); here we will summarize only the ACTA system.

Each slide was put under a 100 x objective (oil immersion) of a Leitz microscope. The images of the Feulgen stained nuclei were detected by an high sensitivity plumbicon tube and digitized in real time via a fast A/D converter with the format of 512X512 picture points/frame and 8 bits gray resolution for each picture point. Under the adopted magnification, each picture point corresponded to about .08 x .08 .

The digitized image was stored in real time in a 256 Kbyte memory (512x512 bytes, VDC 501 Tesak System). Each image, "frozen" in the memory was recorded on tapes and then analyzed off line by means of a minicomputer HP 21 MX.

The analysis was performed on image previously corrected for non homogenity and aberrations due to the optics. A fixed gray level window was then chosen for all the filtered images as a border discrimination between the nuclear images and the background.

The area (A), the integrated optical density (IOD) and the average optical density (AOD=IOD/A) of the nuclear image, was measured by proper thresholding discriminating the background. Finally the collected data were statistically analyzed and the resulting histograms displayed.

PROBE FOR WATER AND IONS

Dielectric constants were measured for the nuclear pellets placed in a proper sample holder (26, 25) in the 100-2000 MHz (step 50 MHz) frequency band, using an HP 8542A automatic network analyzer, controlled by an HP2116 computer.

The relative dielectric constant is the quantity that mainly characterize the response of a material to an EM field, in the frequency domain. It can be put into the form $\varepsilon = \varepsilon' - j\varepsilon''$ where ε' and ε'' are both real positive numbers, frequency-dependent; mainly ε'', which is shown in Fig. 14 for three samples, is particularly significant, since it relates directly to the conductivity of the material through the well known equation

$$\sigma = \pi f \varepsilon_0 \varepsilon'' \, 2 \qquad\qquad (\Omega\, m)^{-1}$$

where f is the EM frequency in MHz, ε_0 is the vacuum permittivity equal to 8.86×10^{-12} F.m.$^{-1}$. In all these measurements a reference solution of 4 mM NaCl is used routinely (N=4), to test the accuracy and the drift of the calibration (25).

For our electrical modelling purpose the nuclei are solutions of DNA, RNA, proteins, lipids and ions (salts) in water, with the additional property that fractions of water are bound to macromolecules in a quasicristalline state and have a dielectric behaviour ice-like or halfway between ice and water. Since the model has 39 complex values, the first problem is to summarize this large amount of information in as few physically meaningful parameters as possible, to help the understanding of the phenomena and alterations which can be monitored. By analogy with previos theoretical treatment of protein electric date (26), a model of nuclei permittivity is built on the following assumptions (27): 1) most part of the nuclear suspension is made of an electrolytic solution of free water (WF) and free ions (N) whose permittivity values are well charcterized by Stogryn formula (26). 2) two additional water layers around each macromolecules can be identified (26), namely an inner tightly bound (T) and an outer loosely bound vicinal (WB) water, the latter having a dielectric behaviour similar to free water but with a smaller relation frequency F; 3) being the nucleic acid and proteins in suspension, the Frickle equation for a mixture is used to compute the dielectric constant of the whole suspension

$$(\epsilon - \epsilon_m)/(\epsilon + x \epsilon_m) = v (\epsilon_p - \epsilon_m)/(\epsilon_p + x \epsilon_m)$$

where ϵ_m and ϵ_p are respectively the complex dielectric constant of suspending medium and of the suspended particles, x and v are the shape factor (x=2 for sphere) and volumetric fraction of overall suspended particles.

A detailed analysis (26) has shown that in this case the complex dielectric constant of the suspension is the ratio between two polynomials of third degree of the complex frequency, whose coefficients are function of a quantity P, which is a linear combination of tightly bound water (T) and suspended macromolecules $v_D + v_R + v_p$), of the quantity of vicinal bound water WB, its relaxation frequency (F) and of the ionic concentration in the suspension nuclear medium (N, expressed in equivalent NaCl normality). The volumetric fractions of DNA (V_D), RNA (V_R) and proteins (V_p) are given in Table IV. The four unknown P, WB, F and N of the model are calculated by an optimization algorithm (26) which minimizes the sum over all frequencies of the squared magnitude of the differences between the measured and calculated.

PROBE FOR NUCLEAR PORES

Freeze-etching electron microscopy was used to probe for number and distribution of pores in the nuclear membrane envelope. Isolated rat liver nuclei were fixed in 2.5% glutaraldheide in 0.1 M phosphate buffer, pH 7.2 for 1 hour and then rinsed in 0.15 M phosphate buffer. The nuclear pellet has been resuspended in 30% glycerol in distilled water for 30 minutes, freezed in Freon and processed for cleaving and replication in a Blazers 360 M Freeze-Etch device (28).

NATIVE CHROMATIN

Although it is generally agreed that the basic chromatin-DNA fiber (tertiary structure) is about 110 A in diameter and is composed of closely apposed nucleosomes (1) different expeimental findings have led to several models for the formation of higher order structure in native chromatin at the quaternary (2, 3) and quinternary (5) level.

The concept of regular and irregular folding of the nucleofilament into a solenoidal (2) or a two-order super-helical (3) fiber 250-300 A^o wide has been challenged by recent electron microscopic observations obtained on a phospholipid monolayer (14), suggesting that the same fiber is rather formed of up to four nucleofilaments properly interlinked. In the following lines we will produce new detailed evidences on the quaternary and quinternary structure (and nuclear pores) obtained by means of the newly developed or upgraded biophysical undestructive probes.

Quaternary Structure

In the nucleus of unperturbed rat liver as well as calf thymus cells two kinds of fibers are typically present at the earliest times after swelling, having a width of either about 250 A° or about 360A° (Fig. 1). An unfolding of these native fibers then takes place at successive time intervals after initial nuclear swelling; for the latest time (2.5 hours) the original fiber progressively branches in fibers of progressively smaller size, as shown in Fig. 1B-C down to a nucleofilament (100 A° wide). Figure 1D shows the computer-enhanced images of typical chromatin fibers from calf thymus nuclei shadowed with platinum. After background subtraction representative frequency distribution of gray level for these fibers is displayed in Figure 2. The multimodal distribution reveals about 3 levels of light absorbance, two of which ("black" and "white") are expected from the angle of fiber shadowing with platinum, but the third intermediate ("gray") level reflects subtle, discrete and discontinous distribution of biological material not ready apparent by visual inspection of the electron micrographs. Actually from the computer-enhanced image, discrete distribution of chromatin bodies ("black" regions of constant height) appear evident (Fig. 2) in either the native fiber or in any of the fibers resulting from spontaneous unfolding (Fig. 1A) breaking (Fig. 1B) or DNA-se induced nicking (Fig. 1D).

The discrete distribution of dark regions equally spaced by "light" regions, is readily quantifiable in terms of gray level intensity as function of distance along individual line crossing the fiber longitudinally (Fig. 3). Four parellel lines yield an highly reproducible pattern with peaks of gaussian distribution (70-110 A° wide) and hollows (18-80 A°) regularly alternating at an average interval of 140 A° (Fig. 3). Curiously (see Table 1) "dark bodies" are either 70 or 110 A° wide and frequently they appear as closely spaced pairs (equal or less than 18 A° apart) such that a superficial inspection of the computer-enhanced image suggests the existence of 175A° "dark bodies" with an apparent interdistance of about 82 A°.

This apparent interdistance progressively decreases from 82 A° ("tetrafilament", or 350 A° fiber) to 63 A° ("trifilament", or 245 A° fiber), 45 A° ("bifilament", or 175 A° fiber) and 23 A° ("mononucleofilament"); at the same time the size of the dark bodies (nucleosome-like) remain constant (29). Similar shrinkage (decreased pitch) is occuring whenever the apparent diameter of the fiber decreases, with the size of the "dark bodies" being invariant within any given fiber before and after its branching (see figures 1 A-D). It would then appear that the quaternary chromatin-DNA structure consists of a regular folding of four nucleofilaments (with the dark "bodies" being the nucleosomes) helically twisted (rope-like) to yield the frequently reported fiber: this conclusion is strongly supported by freeze-etching of the same fiber (Fig. 4). Circular nucleosome-like structure 65 A° diameter appears zig-zag arranged and equally spaced within the fiber (Fig. 4) apparently resulting from two

TABLE I

F.W.H.H. dimensions (A°) of high ('dark") and low ("gray") absorbance regions in the computer-enhanced image from rat liver. Measurements are taken directly from the frequency distribution of Fig. 3, progressing from left to right.

Region number	"Dark" region	"Gray" region
1	108	27
2	72	72
3	108	36
4	72	45
5	108	36
6	117	27
7	72	80
8	108	36
9	72	18
10	108	72
11	90	18
12	108	54
13	117	80
14	72	36
15	108	72
16	108	9
17	63	54
18	108	18
19	72	80
20	72	18
21	117	27
22	99	36
23	63	18
24	108	-

Under our operating condition the dimension of a pixel is 9 A°, which then reflects the resolution and accuracy of our measurements.

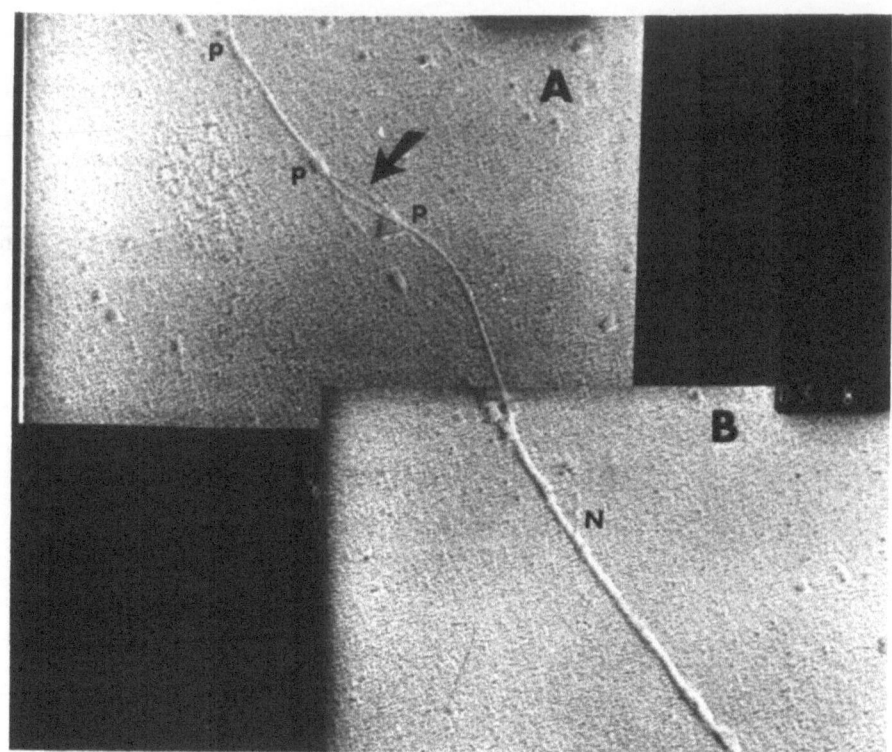

Figure 1 A) Rat liver chromatin fiber with typical example of the
spontaneous unfolding of the native fiber into two subfibers (arrow) and
their successive refolding occuring between pieces of biological material
periodically attached to the chromatin fiber (P). Branching of a 120 A°
wide 'nucleofilament' from the native 330 A° wide fiber can also be
visualized (N) as likely due to a spontaneous DNA strand breaking induced by
isolation procedure. B) An other portion of the 2 microns long liver
chromatin fiber, platinum shadowed few minutes after swelling of the
nucleus. C) Calf Thymus Chromatin fiber 1 hour after nuclear swelling,
displaying a spontaneous unfolding of native fiber into successively narrower
subfibers down to the "nucleofilament". D) (Right panel) Calf Thymus
Chromatin fiber resulting from mild micrococcal nuclease digestion (5
Units/ml for 20 seconds); A computer-enhanced image of the same fiber
shows the typical "discrete" distribution of the darkest pixels for both the
dark and white regions resulting from the platinum shadowing.

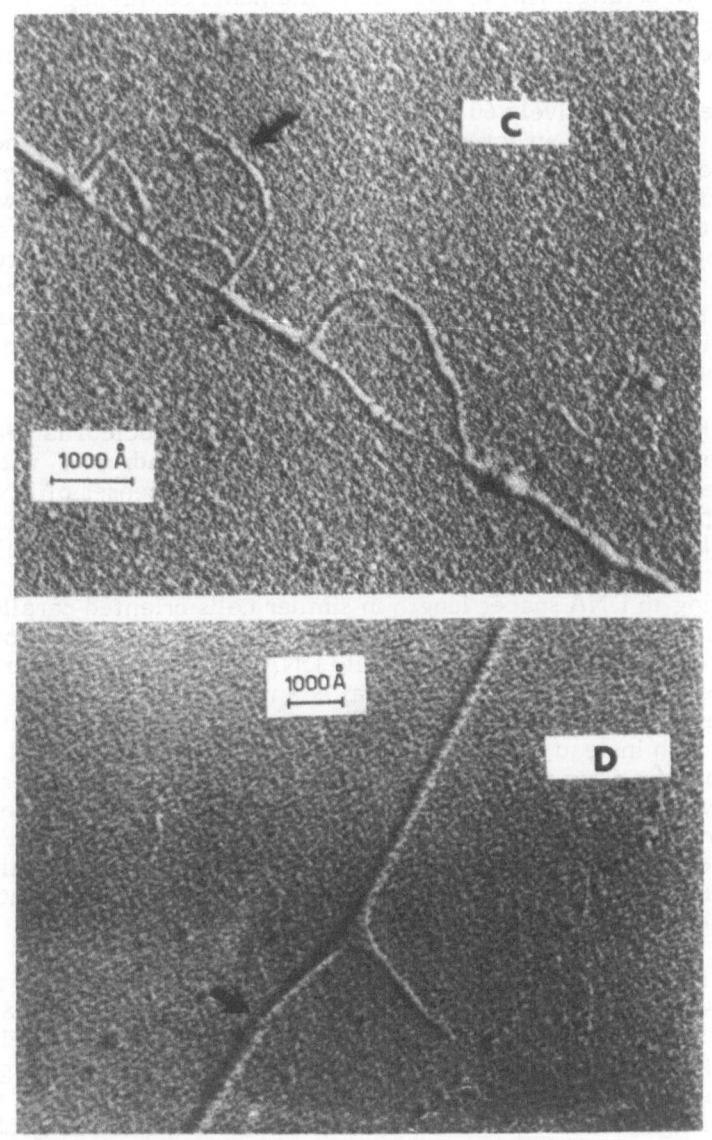

identical unfolded fibers of regularly alternating wide (230 a^o) and narrow (158 A^o) regions. At careful examination each subfiber (of size equivalent to the bifilament described in Fig. 1) seems formed by double-helical arrangement of two nucleofilaments containing nucleosome-like structures regularly intertwisted. Relaxation of the multinucleofilament fiber toward a larger diameter appears moreover associated with an increased spacer distance among "putative nucleosomes," respectively 60 and 120 A^o apart in the narrow and wide groove. The rope-like structure (Fig. 5) for the native fiber can then be inferred from the spontaneous unfolding of up to four nucleofilaments (Figs. 1 and 4) and from the gray level distribution (Fig. 2) in the 'white' shadow of the computer enhanced fiber image, where 'gray' regions (likely shadow projection of the 'dark bodies') are alternating with white regions and out of phase of a constant 45° angle, independently of fiber position respect to the illuminating source. This inclination could then result from the twisted rope-like path taken by the nucleofilaments and forced upon the incoming light.

With the formation of binucleofilament and tetranucleofilament, the internucleosomes distance respectively doubles and quadruples, with nucleosome size remaining unchanged, likely at the expenses of DNA strand wrapped around the octamer (Fig. 5). In the 110 A^o fiber the size of the "dark bodies" is indeed about 65 A^o, corresponding to the height of the nucleosome disc and the distance among them is about 23 A^o, corresponding to DNA spacer length in similar cells oriented parallel to the nucleofilament axis. Whenever two nucleofilaments merge they form a fiber apparently highly stable, since mild DNAse digestion (29) and H1 histone selective removal do cause local istanteneous unfolding of the tetrafilament into two bifilaments rather than into four nucleofilaments (110 A^o), which instead occurs subsequently for longer exposure of the native chromatin fiber to low (1mM Tris) ionic strength. This later phenomenon is compatible with the known fact that only addition of divalent cations or of higher amount of monovalent cations (as in the nucleus where the ionic strenght is likely 0.15 M NaCl) can maintain the native fiber, or any higher order superfolding of the nucleofilament, as also predicted by polyelectrolyte theory (8).

Fig. 6 shows the heat capacity (dq/dT) versus temperature, in the range 300-400° K, for isolated chromatin in 1 mM Tris-HCl, pH 8, at 0, 10, 30, 50, and 600 mM NaCl. Three transitions (I, II, III) are clearly and reproducibly identifiables, whose temperature values slightly change with salt concentration. As shown in Fig. 7 and summarized in Table II the enthalpy changes for isolated chromatin are instead dramatically changing with salt concentration: namely the enthalpy changes are decreasing between 0 and 10 mM to then remain constant for the transition I, are steadily increasing for the transition III, while sharply increasing up to 50 mM to then sharply decrease at 600 mM for the transition II.

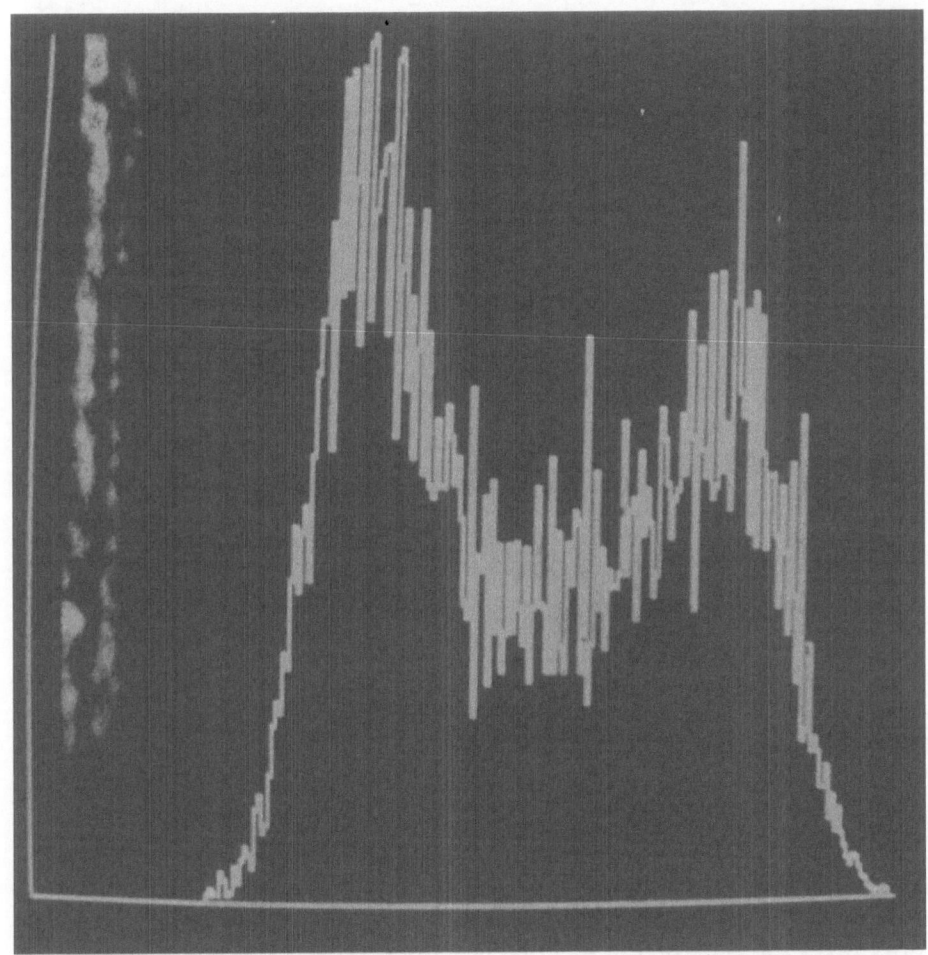

Figure 2 (Left) A computer-enhanced image of typical 330 A° native fiber shadowed with platinum. The dark and white regions are the result of the two platinum shadowing 90° apart. (Right) Frequency distribution of pixel gray levels from the same fiber.

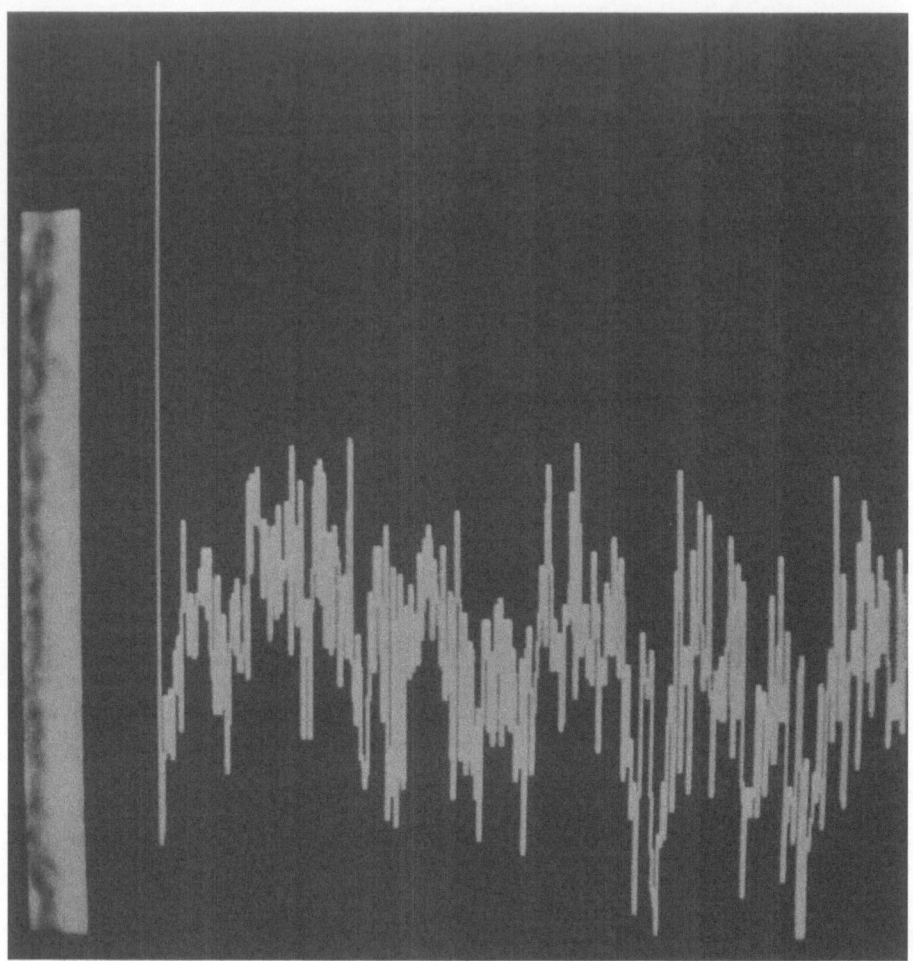

<u>Figure 3</u> The same 330 A° native fiber as Figure 2 (left panel), with the gray level for each of the 423 pixels sequentially taken along a line crossing the same fiber longitudinally from bottom to top (right pannel).

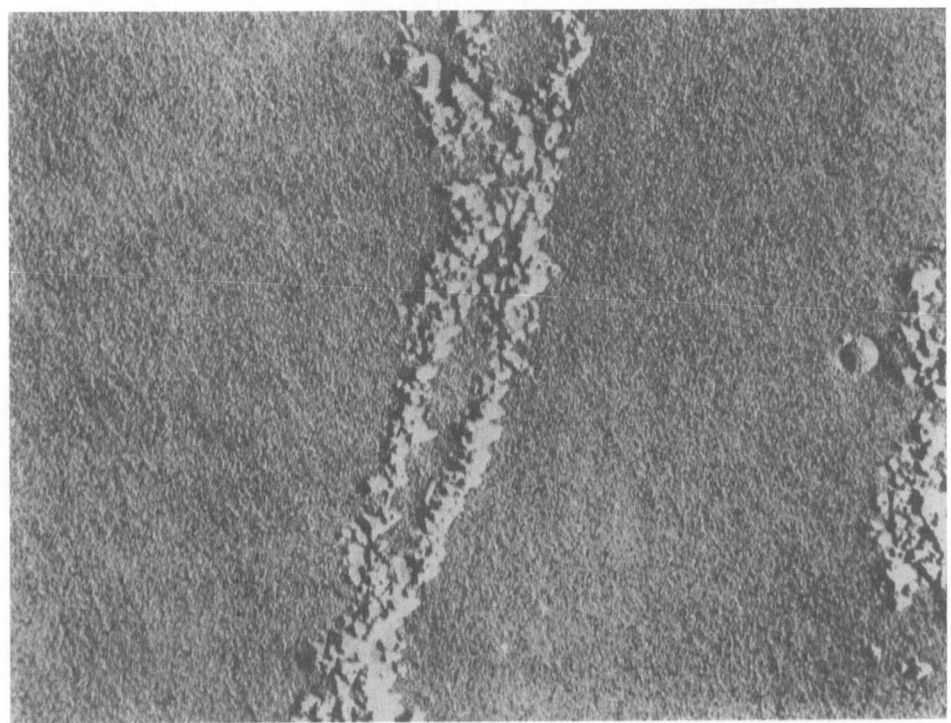

Figure 4 Freeze-etching electron microscopy of chromatin fiber from
'exploding' liver nuclei. The unfolding of the two subfibers closely parallels
the unfolding apparent in Figure 1 by the phospholipid monolayer
technique; furthermore the two subfibers appear to converge toward two
regions similarly apart of about 5000 A° (arrows).

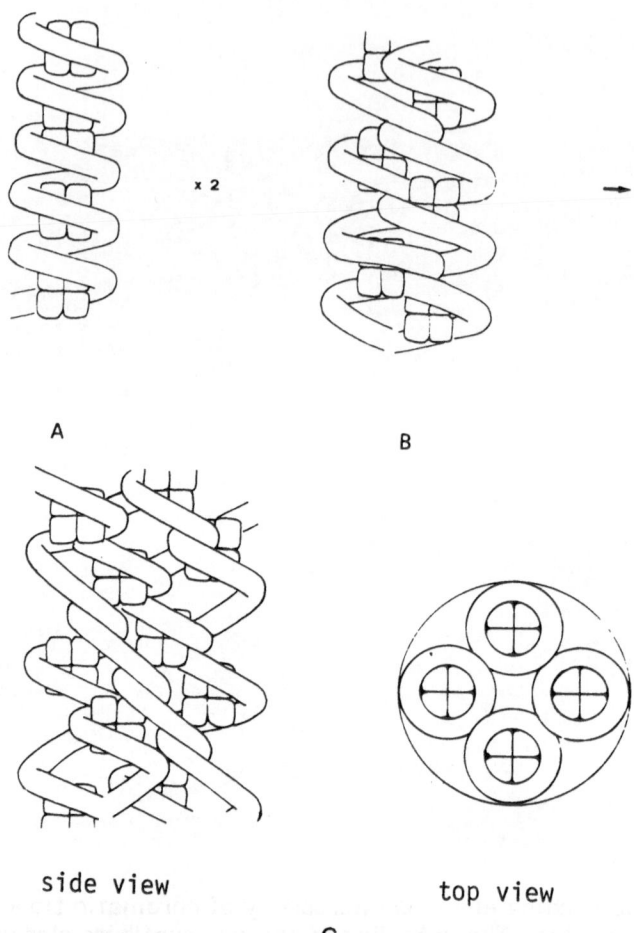

x 2

A   B

side view   top view

C

Figure 5 Rope-like model for quaternary chromatin-DNA structure formed by four nucleofilaments properly intertwisted. The successive formation of wider fibers from the nucleofilament (A) through the bifilament (B) up to the tetrafilament or typical "300 Aº' fiber (C) is also shown. As suggested by the experimental data, the internucleosome distance appears to increase with increasing fiber width.

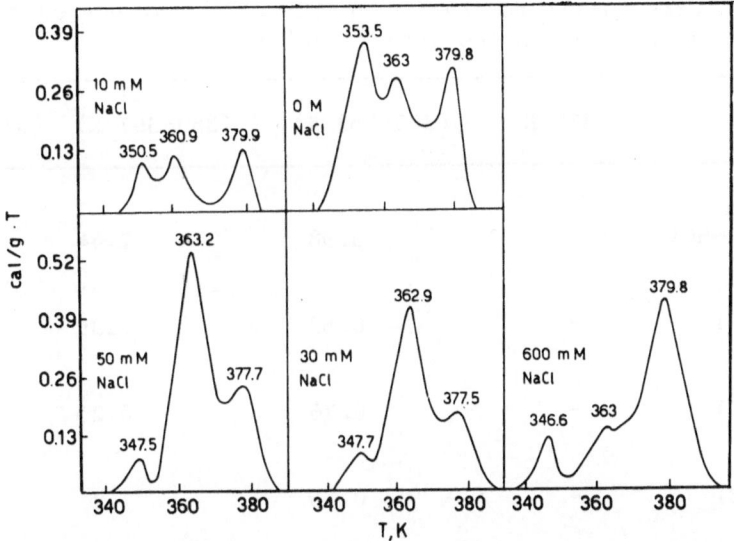

Figure 6 Heat capacity versus temperature of liver chromatin at different salt concentrations. All the sample were buffered in 1 mM Tris–HCl, pH 8. These data were obtained after subtracting from the measured heat capacity at each temperature the background value obtained for the very same sample after denaturation up to 400 °K.

TABLE II

Enthalpy (ΔH_m) changes in cal/g at the various transition
temperatures (0-III for native chromatin at various salt
concentrations and in the intact nuclei.

	0 (332 K)	I (346-353 K)	II (360-367 K)	III (376-384 K)
Chromatin 0 mM Trix-HCl	–	3.98	2.44	2.63
Chromatin 10 mM NaCl	–	0.57	1.39	1.14
Chromatin 30 mM NaCl	–	0.76	6.25	1.85
Chromatin 50 mM NaCl	–	0.75	7.2	2.86
Chromatin 600 mM NaCl	–	0.97	1.47	7.48
Nuclei (Rat liver)	1.89	3.61	7.56	11.26

Previous studies on rat liver chromatin, using circular dichroism and thermal denaturation, have shown that several conformational transitions could be identified from the derivative plot of chromatin molar ellipticity versus temperature (30):

a)   one above 92ºC, characterized by decrease in molar ellipticity, is related to helix-coil conformational transition;

b)   two or more, characterized by increased molar ellipticity, and occurring between 50ºC and 90ºC, are apparently related to the so-called "superhelix to helix" transition.

The calorimetric data here presented do confirm these assignments, further clarifying and quantifying thermodynamically the various levels of DNA structure.

Namely, the effect of 600 mM NaCl wash, known to remove the H_1 histone from chromatin and to disrupt the quaternary structure, combined with the critical dependence on ionic strength as expected also from polyelectrolyte theory (8), points to a possible assignment for the transition II to the quaternary rope-like structure (Fig. 5). For the third (III) transition its melting temperature, combined with the salt dependence of the enthalpy (Fig. 7), and with the effect of carcinogen (see later Fig. 16 and Table II) which alters chromatin structure toward a more disperse uncoiled state (18) apparently causing a rearrangement of part of the genome from the rope-like structure (II transition) to a lower order structure (III transition), points to a possible assignment of the third (III) transition to the nucleosomal DNA, i.e. helix-coil stabilized in the nucleofilament. This assignment is compatible with the C.D. and O.D. thermal profiles (30, 31) which show that above 365º K helix-coil dominates the denaturation process.

The first (I) transition in isolated chromatin cannot be related to the linker DNA as previously suggested, not only because of its independence from salt concentration (which instead should stabilize this type of structure), but namely because its pronounced increase (18) of the enthalpy of transition in isolated nuclei (Fig. 19), where the DNA present in the linker conformation, if any, should decrease. Tentatively this transition and the other (0) consistently observed at lower temperature (332º K) only in native nuclei, could then be related to the quinternary, drapery-like chromatin structure (0) and to the melting of macromolecules (i.e. membrane lipids-proteins and chromosomal proteins) strongly bound to native chromatin (I).

It is therefore comforting to notice that the highly flexible and elastic chromatin fiber is apparently connected at fixed points, apparently located at periodic intervals, on the nuclear pores membrane, where the four nucleofilaments form strong bonds among each other and with the

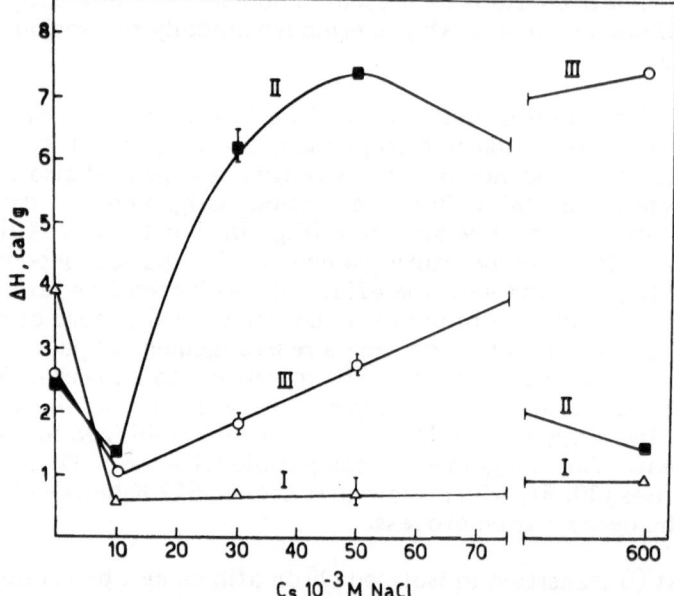

Figure 7 The dependence of the melting enthalpy ΔH_m on NaCl concentration for the liver chromatin thermal transitions corresponding to the first (I), second (II) and third (III) peaks in the thermal profiles of Figure 6.

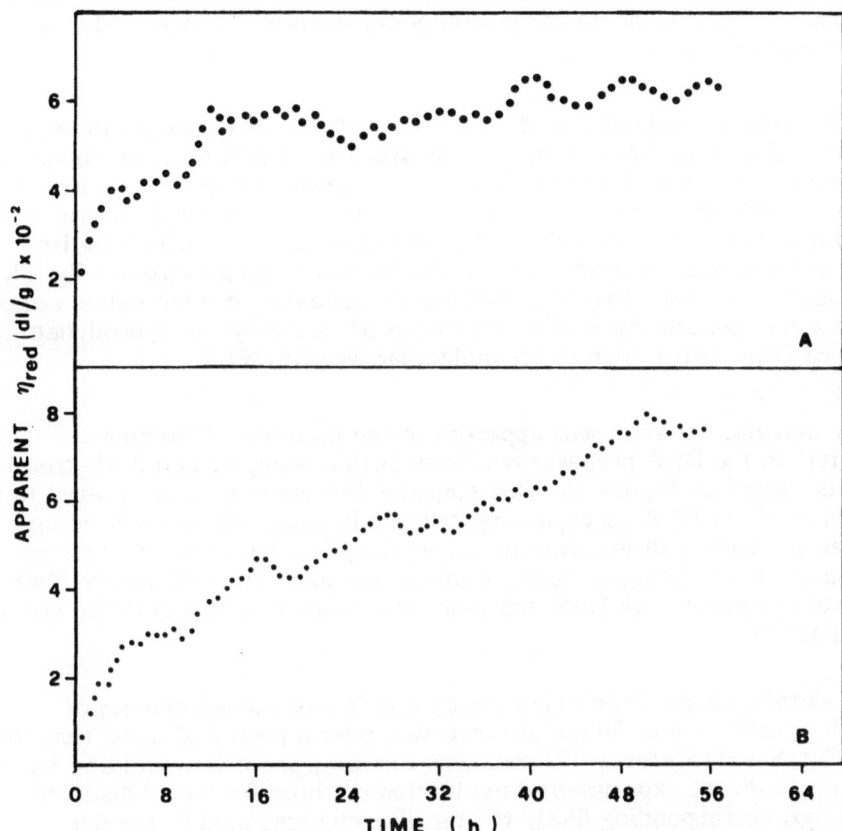

Figure 8 Apparent value of reduced viscosity n $_{red}$, as function of incubation time in lysing neutral solution (pH 8) of high ionic strength for liver nuclei obtained from a rat treated i.p. with 50 mg/kg of AAF (A), and from a control rat (B).

lipoproteic envelope, being capable to maintain the highly twisted superstructure predicted by a rope-like model (Fig. 5). This configuration, similar to what earlier suggested by a drapery-like model for quinternary chromatin-DNA structure (5), would require that the total DNA length between the fixed points (apparently corresponding to membrane attachements (Fig. 9)) be constant and any increase on internucleosomes distance may take place only at the expenses of DNA strand wrapped around the octamer, as could be caused by the mutual interpenetration of nucleosomes from adjacent nucleofilaments whenever a larger fiber is being formed (Fig. 5).

The data recently obtained on the time-dependent changes in intrinsic viscosity of nuclear DNA under non-denaturating conditions are compatible with the existence of the three levels of structures which chromatin has to undergo whenever slowly unfolds from the highly supercoiled structure (of low η) in native nuclei to a relaxed DNA (with high η , considering its larger surface volume ratio), after many hours in lysing solution (Fig. 8). It has indeed been found that the viscoelastic behavior of mammalian cellular DNA for non-denaturing lysis conditions is affected by the hydrodynamic radius of DNA rather than by its molecular weight (17).

A stepwise behavior was apparent in the increase of "intrinsic viscosity" in the DNA preparations from both resting G0 and AAF-treated rat liver cells (see Figure 8). This stepwise increase could be related to the various levels of DNA superpacking present in native chromatin, being apparently at least three, namely the tertiary (nucleosome), quaternary (rope-like superhelical polynucleosomes), and quinternary (drapery-like), as suggested by early work (1-5) and more conclusively in the detailed study here reported.

A detailed analysis, carried out by continuous measurements of viscosity performed at 30 minute intervals over a period of more than 48 hour (Fig. 8 and reference 17) confirms this interpretation, yielding for the first time a direct experimental evaluation of three (or more) discrete unfoldings, corresponding likely to step-like changes in higher order superstructures.

A derivative plot of the fifth order polynomial function best fitting the viscosity time-dependent increase confirms these transitions (not shown), averaging for the noise present in the measurement due to experimental artifacts or fluctuations. In addition to the lack of homogeneity in the suspended nuclear lysate, the inherent elasticity of the DNA fiber contributing to the "apparent" dynamic viscosity is likely the source of the observed fluctuations; the measuring frequency of our oscillating crucible is indeed abot 0.04 reciprocal seconds and yields a period of oscillation possibly close to the retardation time for our chromatin-DNA molecule.

Quinternary Structure

Interestingly the folding and unfolding occuring in the giant chromatin-DNA molecule (we have measured up to several micron long fibers) never propagate along the entire length, but remain confined to narrow regions limited by fixed points (Fig. 1A) identifiable as irregular pieces of "nuclear membrane" periodically attached along the chromatin fiber. As previously shown (14, 29) these highly irregular pieces may be recomposed by successive attempts to yield a continum suggesting that they were likely coming from the same cell component (i.e. nuclear envelope) to which chromatin fibers are linked and which is broken during the swelling of the nucleus.

The freeze-etching data here reported on the liver nuclei (Fig. 9) corroborate the drapery-like model for the regular folding of the 260 A° fiber within the nucleus, clearly showing the attachment sites for these fibers in correspondence of nuclear pores.

Strikingly the computer enhanced image (Fig. 9) clearly shows 260 A° fibers attached drapery-like to the nuclear envelope in correspondence to the pores. Curiously and comforting the overall total length of each fiber from pore to pore is about 4000 A° which is also the average distance along the same fiber between pieces of nuclear membrane apparent by phospholipid monolayer technique (Fig. 1).

A detailed analysis of the pore distribution on the nuclear membrane, as shown by the freeze-etching microphotographs (Fig. 10), displays an interesting feature which corroborates the critical role of pores in maintaning the quinternary drapery-like structure; the frequency distribution of the closet distances among successive pores reveals that over the total 250 pores in the nuclear hemisphere 236 have a mean distance among them of about 450 A°, with only 14 having a distance of 2000 A° or greater (Fig. 11A). A mathematical algorithm searching for the clustering in the pore distribution confirms indeed that about 12-14 clusters are apparent in the same nuclear hemisphere, yielding a total number for the overral nuclear envelope close to the total number of interphase chromosomes (23) present in the same liver cells. Interestingly, 22-26 islands are present in similar cells feulgen-stained and three-dimensionally reconstructed (32).

The distribution of distances among all pores following a "minimum spanning tree" algorithm shows furthermore (Fig. 11B) that most pores are regularly and periodically distributed on the nuclear envelope, displaying an otherwise unsuspected architecture. It would then appear that clusters of nuclear pores corresponding to clustering of chromatin fibers chromosone-sized (up to few microns long, or about 2×10^9 Daltons) can be identified on the nuclear envelope in a number very close to the actual number of chromosomes in rat liver cells, giving a possible linkage between the highly ordered structure of interphase chromatin-DNA and the

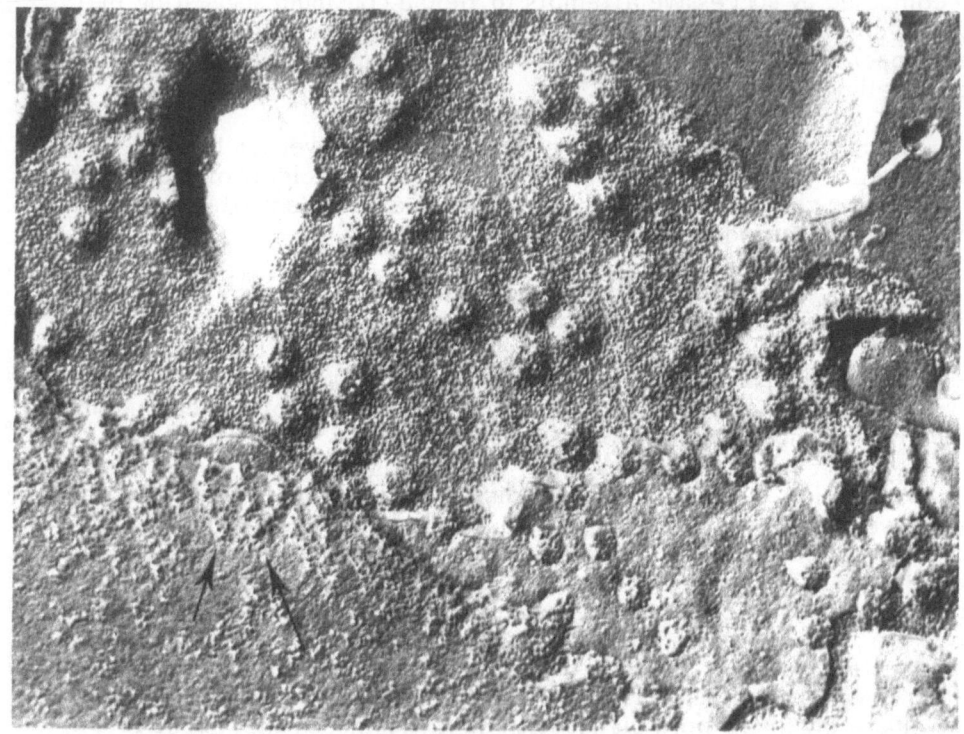

Figure 9 Freeze-etching electron microscopy of liver nuclei. The fracture makes apparent drapery-like chromatin fibers attached to the nuclear membrane at the pores.

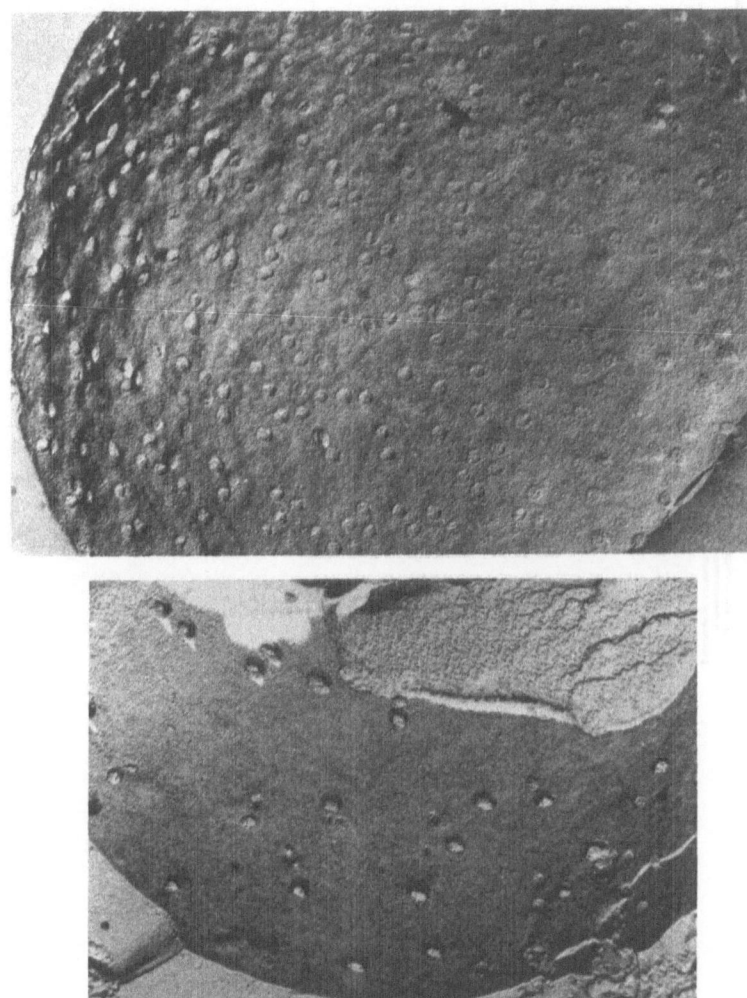

Figure 10 Freeze-etching of nuclear membrane from rat liver prior to (GO, above) and after liposome stimulation (G1, below). A dramatic decrease in the number of nuclear pores is apparent after stimulation in this preliminary experiment, which causes at the same time an increase in RNA synthesis and a dramatic relaxation of chromatin-DNA (see Figure 12).

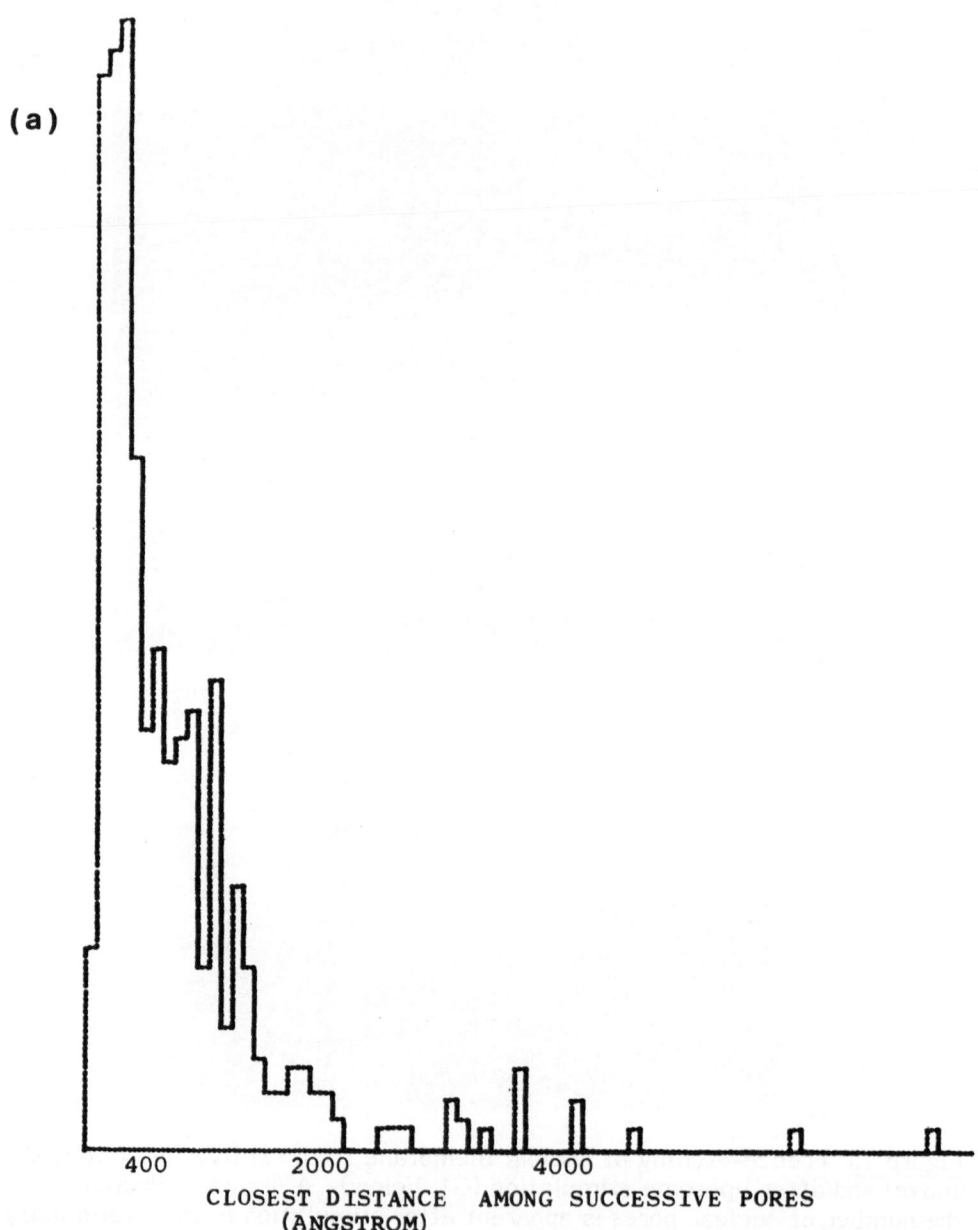

(a)

CLOSEST DISTANCE   AMONG SUCCESSIVE PORES
(ANGSTROM)

<u>Figure 11</u> (a) Frequency distribution of closet distance among
successive nuclear pores, as obtained by analyzing the image shown
in Figure 10, after computer enhancement and with proper algorithm.
(b) Frequency distribution of interpores distance along a spanning
tree from the same control nuclear membrane, as obtained with
proper computer algorithm.

(b)

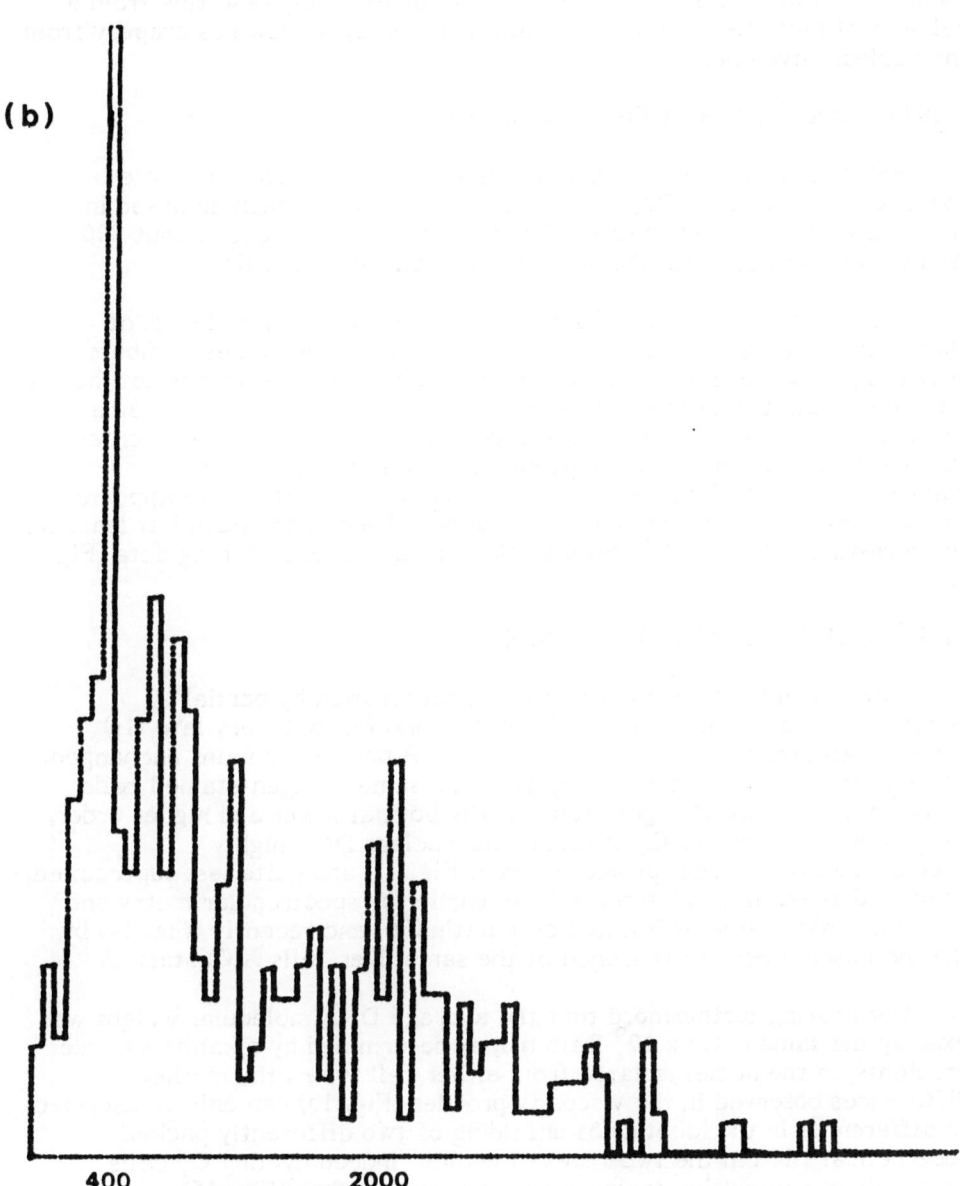

INTERPORES DISTANCES ALONG A SPANNING TREE
(ANGSTROM)

formation of individual metaphase chromosomes, likely resulting from a collapse of localized ropelike chromatin fibers laying down as drapery from the nuclear envelope.

THREE DIMENSIONAL RECONSTRUCTION

500 A sections (Fig. 12) of liver nuclei from untreated rat were specifically stained for DNA with uranyl actetate and then analysed in terms of gray level distribution of nuclear pixels, being each about 200 A^o in diameter (less than the size of individual rope-like fiber).

The resulting frequency distribution yields two distinct levels of chromatin condensation, as shown in Fig. 12A: the two types of fibers previously reported for the same rat liver nuclei do then reflect not merely different width for an identical superpacking, but two distinct chromatin superpackings. Namely an increased condensation relates to an increase number of nucleosomes per superhelical turn, as apparent in the computer-enhanced image of Figures 1 and 4. Chromatin DNA appears furthermore confined mostly toward the periphery of the nuclei at least for these resting GO cells (32), compatible with the freeze-etching data (Fig. 9).

EFFECT OF CELL PROLIFERATION

When rat liver cells are induced to proliferation by partial hepatectomy (at 4 hours (early G1) and) 18 hrs. (early S-very late G_1) after hepatectomy, while the amount of DNA per cell remains unchanged, as verified by densitometric analysis of the same Feulgen-stained cells, chromatin structure changes dramatically both at lower and higher order, to yield with respect to G_O control cells nuclear DNA highly decondensed (i.e., larger projected area, Fig. 13) and quite less supercoiled, as probed at tertiary-quaternary level earlier by spectropolarimetry and thermal denaturation of isolated chromatin (30) and recently (Fig. 14) by the increased green fluorescence of the same liver cells A.O. stained.

Considering furthermore that the average DNA molecular weight was exactly the same (1.5×10^9 Daltons), as determined by alkaline sucrose gradients, in the nuclei isolated from either cell types, the marked differences observed in the viscosity profiles (Fig. 15) can only be ascribed to differences in the kinetics of unfolding of two differently packed superhelical DNA in the two types of nuclei. Indeed cycling G_1 cells have only one transition taking place at very fast rate (Fig. 15). Interestingly, and contrary to resting G_O cells, chromatin from the same cycling G_1 liver cells appears to be only in one highly decondensed state as shown by the pixel gray level distribution of feulgen-stained nuclear DNA G1 image at the light microscope level (32).

Similarly at the electron mircoscope level (where in 500 A^o liver

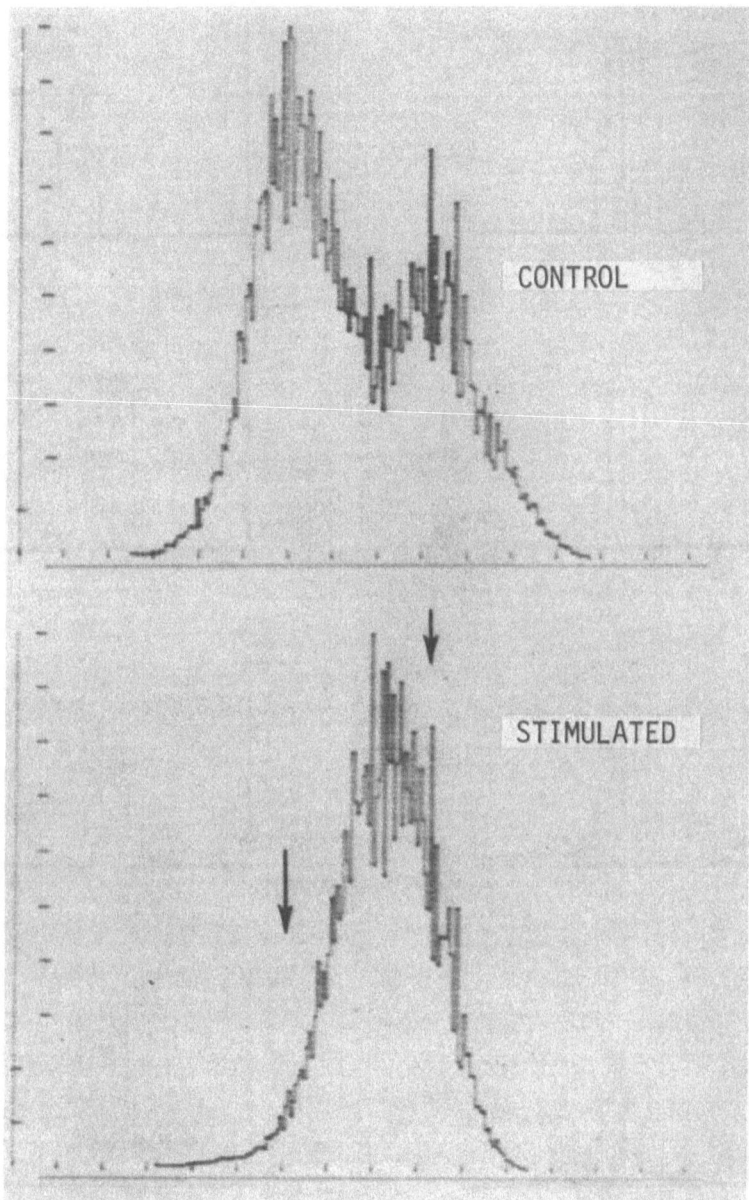

Figure 12 Number of pixels with given transmittance us function of transmittance for 500 A° thick nuclear sections, stained with uranyl acetate, from rat liver nuclei before (GO, above) and after (G1, below) liposomes stimulation.

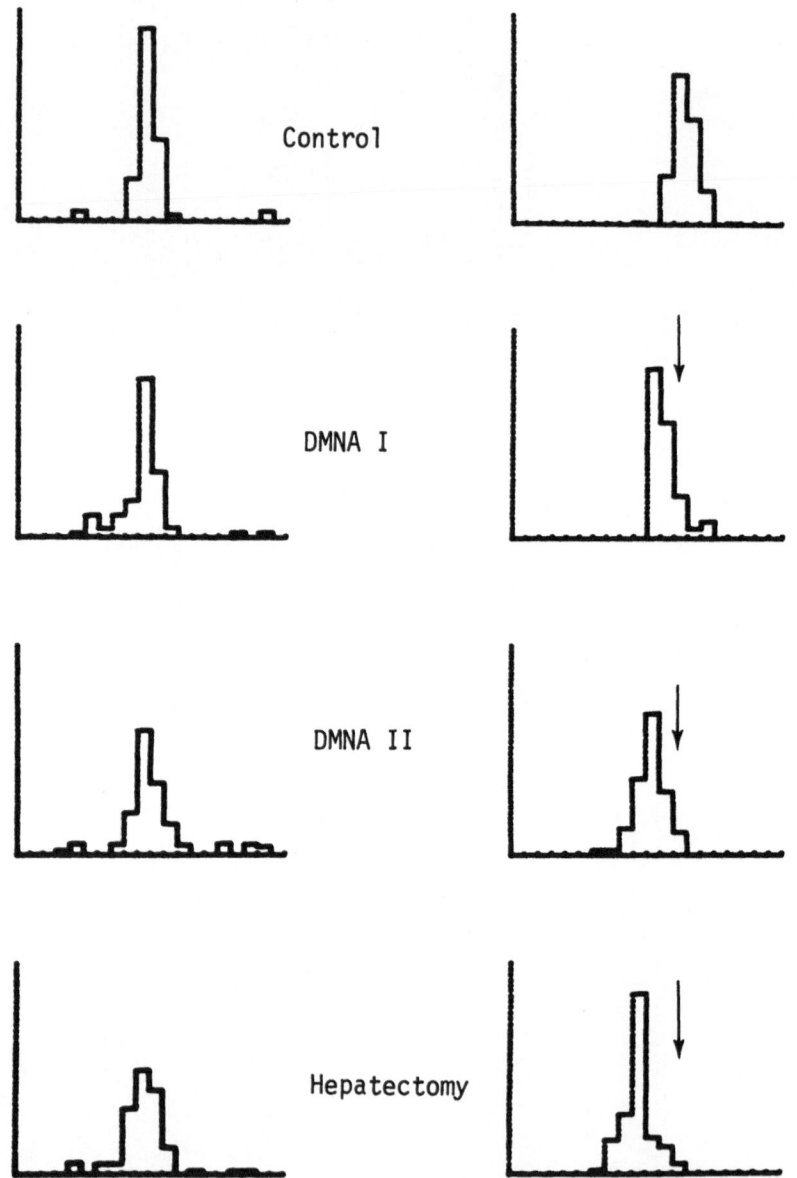

Figure 13 Frequency distribution of integrated optical density (IOD, related to DNA content) and average optical density (AVOD=IOD/Area, right pannels) of Feulgen stained liver nuclei from untreated control rat, from rats after a single injection of dimethylnitrosamine, 0.6 (DMNA I), or 5.4 mg/kg (DMNA II), and from rat after partial hepatectomy.

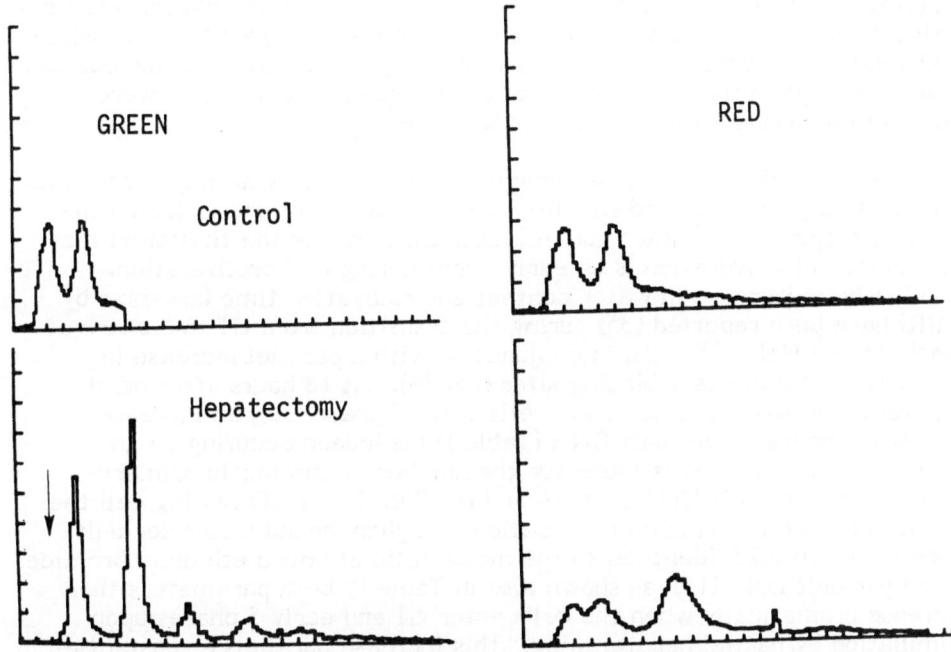

Figure 14 Monodimensional frequency distribution of green (left pannels and red (right pannels) fluorescence intensity per cell of liver cells suspension stained with Acribine Orange from untreated rat (A) and rat 18 hours after partial hepatectomy. Abscissa:fluorescence intensity per cell (channel number); ordinate:number of cells with given fluorescence intensity. Normalization and calibration of the hystrograms was carried out with alcohol fixed human lymphocytes.

sections the degree of chromatin supercoil can be monitored for individual fiber), 30 seconds stimulation by liposomes of the liver nuclei toward a more active state (Fig. 12 lower pannel) causes an abrupt shift of the more condensed chromatin toward the disperse state in a "quantum" transition (33) yielding an uniform distribution of DNA within the overall nuclear volume (Fig. 12, lower pannel) with chromatin "rope-like" fibers of larger width.

Specific enzymatic modifications in H1 histone and nonhistone proteins have been correlated (few even causally as for the phosphorilation) with chromatin alteration and gene expression (34), but search for possible modifications in water and ions, which make up to 90% of each nucleus and could also explain the involvement of overral genome and pores, were hampered by unavailability of adequate probes.

The intracellular water has long been known to play an important role in cellular organization and function, and the data here presented on the electric properties of intact nuclei (Table III) show for the first time that macromolecular hydration is an early event during cell proliferation. Previously, a decrease in water content and relaxation time (assessed by NMR) have been reported (35) during the transition from G1 to S phase of synchronized HeLa S3 cells, in conjunction with a parallel increase in chromatin-DNA primary binding sites (35, 36). At 18 hours after partial hepatectomy, when also our liver cells enter S phase (30), an increase in tightly bound water per unit DNA (Table IV) is indeed occuring on an amount similar to what is found for the number of chromatin primary binding sites per unit DNA (Fig. 14 and ref 30). For a GO resting cell the electrically derived volumetric fraction of tightly bound water per unit DNA is indeed 0.22, identical to the molar ratio of bound ethidium bromide (E.B.) per unit DNA (19); as shown also in Table IV both parameters then increase dramatically when the cells enter G1 and early S phases upon stimulation by partial hepatectomy. This increase parallels a substantial decrease in free (NF) and total (WT) water content and relaxation frequency (F), as also shown by NMR in a similar G1-S transition of synchronized He La (35) including a decrease in the relaxation times (increased bound water).

EARLY EFFECTS OF SINGLE ADMINSTRATION OF CHEMICAL CARCINOGENS

Structural alterations are known to occur in chromatin, either isolated (11) or "in situ" (37), after exposure to a relatively larger dose of a carcinogenic agent as DMNA.

Figures 16 and 17 show a comparison of viscosity profiles obtained at high ionic strength, in alkaline and neutral conditions respectively, with liver nuclei DNA from control rats and from rats treated i.p. with DMNA, a methylating carcinogen known to induce single-strand breaks. As recently shown (17) the changes in the initial viscosity value $(\eta)_0$ and in

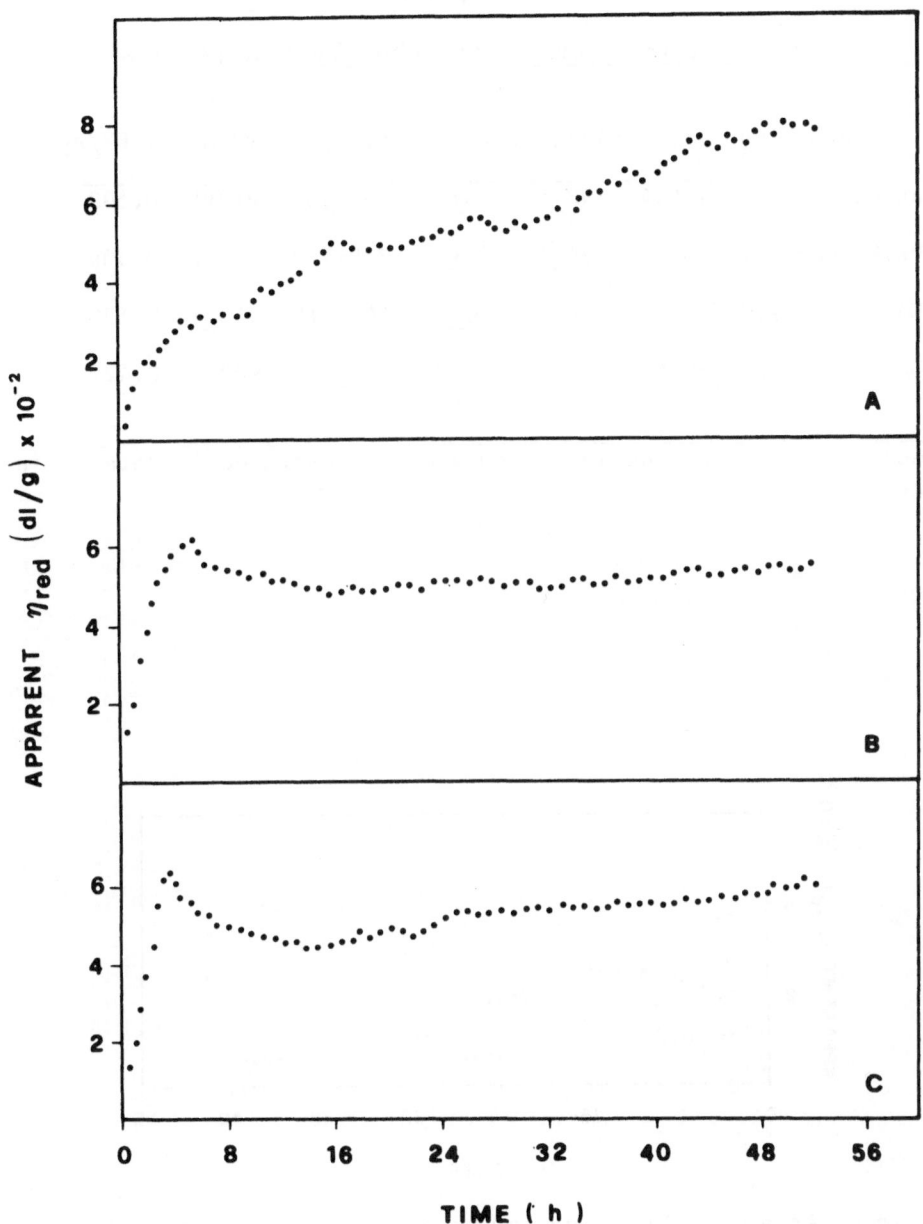

Figure 15 Apparent values of reduced viscosity, η_{red}, as function of incubation time in lysing neutral solution (pH 8) of high ionic strength for liver nuclei obtained from a control rat (A) and from rats 4 hours (B) and 18 hours (C) after partial hepatectomy. A typical experiment is shown for each condition.

TABLE III

A) Electrical data of rat liver nuclear pellets

	Normality (mM)	P(ml/1)	WB (ml/1)	F(MH$_z$)	WF(Ml/1)	WB/Pg
Control	96.8 ± 0.4	48±4	33±4	491±93	919±5	0.503
HEPATECTOMY	81.±0.6	74±5	37±5	776±125	889±7	0.366
DMNA I	110.4±0.6	49±5	36±5	542±118	915±7	0.538
DMNA II	107.2±0.6	55±5	36±5	573±125	909±7	0.479

These quantities are derived from a model described in details in page

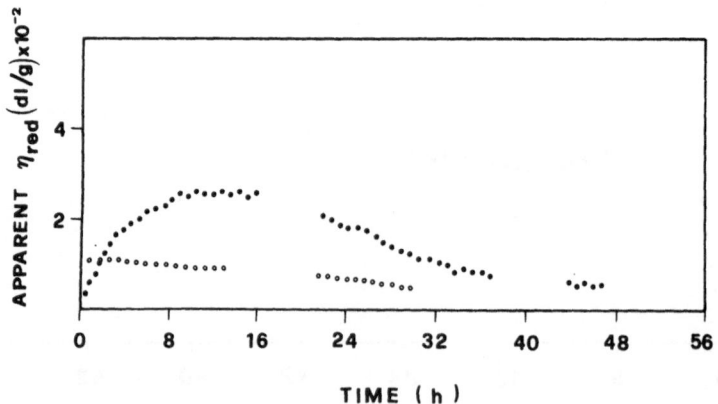

Figure 16 Apparent value of reduced viscosity, η_{red}, as function of incubation time in lysing alkali solution (pH 12.5) of high ionic strength, for liver nuclei obtained from a control rat (....) and from a rat treated i.p. with 5.4 mg/kg DMNA (oo).

the slope of its time-dependent increase were similar in alkaline (Fig. 16) and in neutral (Fig. 17) conditions.

Indeed, it has been proven (17) that the same event, namely the progressive unfolding of superhelical DNA, is responsible for the increase with time of reduced viscosity in both neutral and alkaline conditions, with the plateau value being reached at pH 12.5 in hrs., when the rate of superhelix unfolding (occurring in certain regions of the genome) is compensated by the rate of subsequent strand separation with a decrease in viscosity, which becomes predominant at later times when all DNA is progressively unwinded. The dose-dependent increase in at t = O observed in neutral conditions suggests a significant alteration in chromatin-DNA structure, which indeed occurs (Figs. 13 & 18) as earlier shown by spectropolarimetric assays on rats treated with 5 mg/kg of DMNA (11). At pH 12.5 (Fig. 16) the plateau viscosity value obtained with the carcinogen-treated DNA was significantly smaller than that observed for the control DNA, paralleling the DMNA-induced decrease of DNA molecular weight (17). This plateau value, rather than as previously suggested (15) the slope of viscosity increase, seems therefore to be the quantity apparently related to the average DNA length, while the slope seems to be mostly related to the original DNA superpacking and its unfolding both in alkaline (Fig. 16) and in neutral (Fig. 17) conditions. The size of DNA fragments after the carcinogeninduced damage was so small to make apparent, even in neutral conditions, a dose-dependent decrease of the viscosity plateau levels, which were respectively 6.8 and 7.5 for 48.6 mg/kg and 5.4 mg/kg of DMNA, and were reached in progressively shorter times (48 and 64 hours respectively). On the contrary, the intact giant DNA from liver of control rats continued to increase in viscosity up to 120 hours (12).

It is conforting to notice that in neutral condition the initial reduced viscosity displayed a dramatic increase (from 1 to 2, and 4.5) with increasing DMNA dosage (from 0 to 5.4, and to 48.6 mg/kg), thus showing that not only DNA length was reduced but also chromatin-DNA supercoil was affected by DMNA and accelerates the rate of its unfolding when its higher order superpacking was relaxed by this agent.

Both the high dose of DMNA and the hepatectomy induce a clear increase in the nuclear area for a constant IOD (DNA amount) as compared with the control, suggesting in the chemically treated cells the existence of a chromatin - DNA relaxation and nuclear dispersion similar to the GO -G1 transition already described for human diploid fibroblasts stimulated to proliferate (33).

This pattern seems to be a general phenomenon, affecting the whole population. In fact it is present in the nuclei with a 2C o 4C DNA content (Fig. 13) and also in the population of binucleated cells.

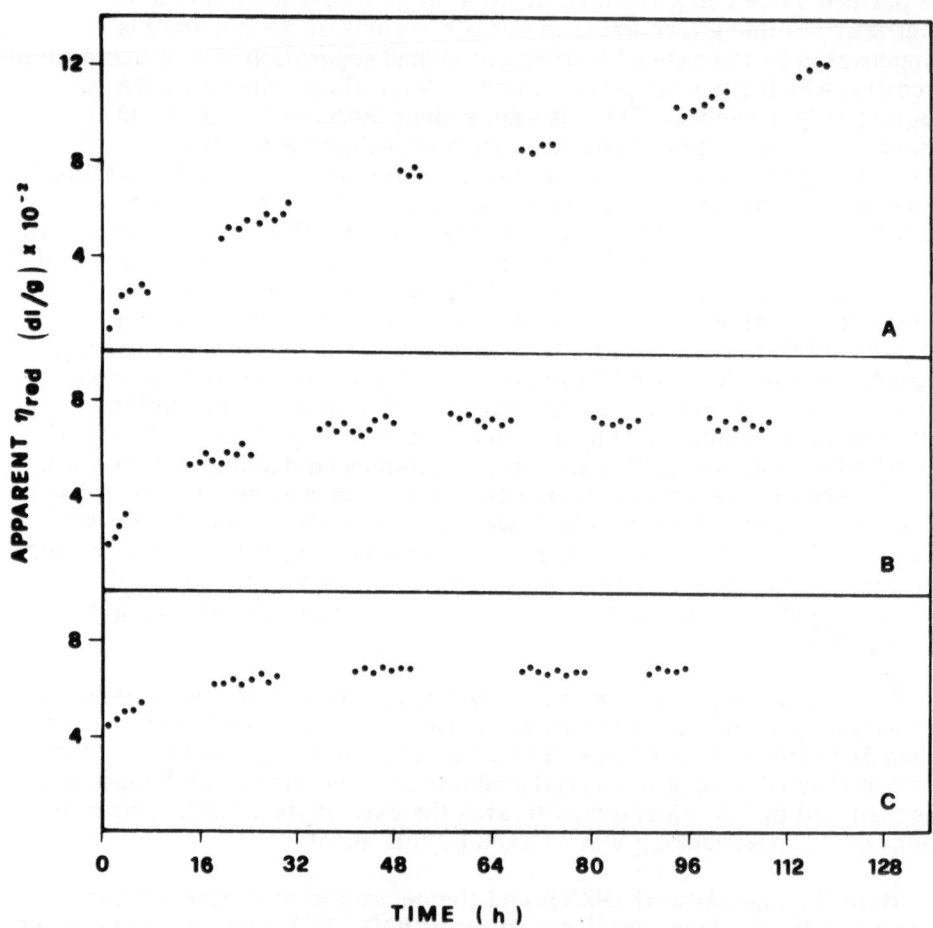

Figure 17 Apparent values of reduced viscosity, red, as function of
incubation time in lysing neutral solution (pH 8) of high ionic strength for
liver nuclei obtained from: A) control rat, B) rat treated i.p. with 5.4
mg/kg DMNA, C) rat treated i.p. with 48.6 mg/kg DMNA.

On the other hand, the area distributions of the low dose treated cells show a little increase (if any), implying only a minor dispersion of the nuclear volume.

The viscosometric data obtained in numerous separate experiments on different nuclei preparations from untreated and carcinogen-treated (either single or double breaking agent) rat liver further clearify the nature of chromatin alteration. Resting G_O liver cells appear to have four transitions occuring, with an exponential decay, respectively between 0 and 9 hrs. (I), 10 and 32 hrs. (II), 33 and 54 hrs. (III), 54 and more than 90 hrs. (IV and last transition). Carcinogen-treated nuclear-DNA displays only the first two transitions and then reaches a plateau value inversely related to its molecular weight (17).

Then, short exposure in vivo (hours) of chromatin-DNA to a damaging agent (such as DMNA or AAF) results in a dose-dependent increase (Figs. 8 and 17) in the initial η_{red} and in $d\eta/dt$, and in a reduced number of step-like η_{red} changes prior to the plateau value, both of which could account for a chemically induced transition from a higher to a lower order of chromatin structure with lower DNA packing ratio. This assumption agrees with the previously reported conformational changes in isolated chromatin and with the obseved increase of chromatin-DNA primary AD-binding sites (Fig. 18) and nuclear dispersion "in situ" (Fig. 13) for rat liver cells exposed to the same carcinogens; interestingly, a parallel increase in putative tightly bound ions and tightly bound water to nuclear DNA, was also observed by measuring for the same liver cell preparation the complex dielectric constant (Table IV).

Table III summarizes the electric data obtained from the model previously described by searching for the four optimized physical parameters P, N, WB and F. The relaxation frequency F of the vicinal bound water dramatically increases for nuclei undergoing the transition from a non-cycling (GO control liver) to cycling (G1 & S phases, 18 hours after partial hepactectomy), increasing also by a dose-dependent significant amount in nuclei exposed to low (o.6 mg/Kg) and high (5.4 mg/Kg) dosage of the carcinogen; these changes may indicate an increased diffusion and decreased microviscosity of the nuclear environment surrounding the suspended macromolecules. Of course other explanations of the data are possible. Curiously, while changes in water content and relaxation frequency go in the same direction for both induced cell proliferation and induced chemical carcinogenesis (where the effect increases with increasing dosage), opposite data are obtained in terms of NaCl equivalent normality (internal ionic strength) and of free ion content N, which decrease during G0-S transition and increase after carcinogen exposure (being actually larger at the lower dosage). Interesting properties can be obtained by defining a quantity I equal to P-T-M: let us suggest for sake of argument that this paramenter is somehow related to the amount of tightly bound ions (see Table IV). It would be then conforting to notice that the amount of

TABLE IV

Derived quantities on liver nuclei

	T_D/v_{DNA}	r	T(ml/1)	T/M	WT(ml/1)		I/M
Control	0.22	0.24	9.6	0.40	961+	1.363	0.62
Hepatectomy	0.49	0.38	14.0	0.36	940+	1.366	0.54
DMNA I	0.	--	7.3	0.23	958	1.363	0.30
DMNA II	0.27	0.28	10.	0.32	955	1.366	0.45

- M is the volumetric fraction of all macromolecules combined, equal to the biochemically assayed amount RNA+DNA+Proteins expressed in mg/ml (25) divided by their average density $\quad$ (g/ml) $\frac{DNA+RNA+Protien}{\frac{DNA}{1.499} + \frac{RNA}{1.66} \quad \frac{+Protein}{1.32}}$

- T is the volumetric fraction of tightly bound water given by $\frac{P-M}{2.5}$ as previously shown (25), where M is biochemically determined and P is electrically determined (Table III);

- WT is the total bound and free water in percentage equal to (T+WB+WF):

- I is the putative volumetric fraction of the ions tightly bound to the marcromolecules, equal to (P-T-M).

- $T_D = (T-T_p)/1.1$ with 1.1 taking into account the effect of RNA ($T_R=T_D x$ 0.1)

- $T_P =(v_p/(v_p+v_r+v_d))x$ WB x R is the amount of the tightly water bound to protein, $v_p+v_R+v_D$ where R is the volumetric ratio of T/WB of total tightly bound water divided by total vicinal bound water, which has been shown to be close to about 0.33+0.02 for both normal and abnormal proteins (26)

- T_D/v_{DNA} is the volumetric ratio of tightly bound water to DNA per unit DNA

- r is the ratio molar (MEB/ MDNA-P) equivalent to the number of intercalating dye (EB) primary binding sites for chromatin DNA, as determined by Scatchard plot analysis (4, 19).

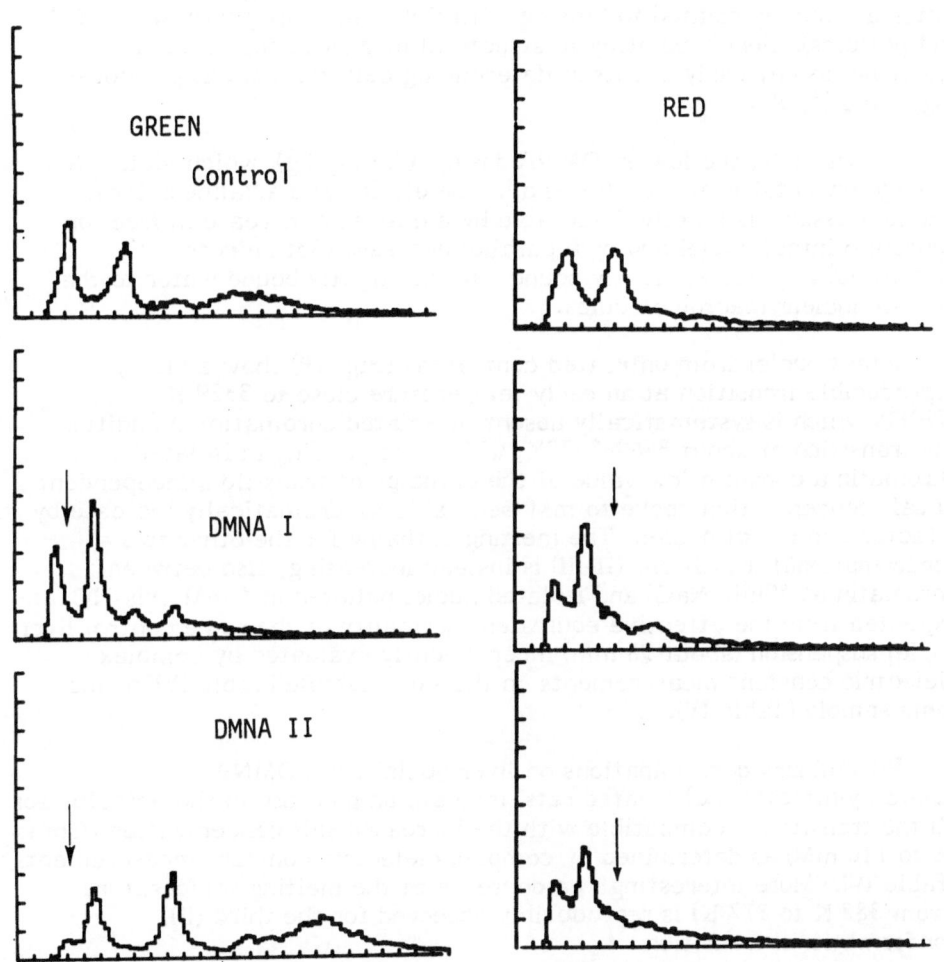

Figure 18 Frequency distribution of green fluorescence per cell as in Figure 14, except for control (A), and from rat treated with 0.6 (DMNA I) and 5.4 (DMNA II) mg/kg DMNA.

tightly bound ions per suspended macromolecule (I/M) would be significantly decreasing with increasing carcinogen dosage, compatible with a redistribution of ions among free and bound compartment, as early event of chemical carcinogenesis.

Interestingly our data (Table IV) show that the changes in tightly bound water are mostly related to binding with DNA (and only partly with RNA and proteins), clearly pointing to structural modifications in this large molecule, as key early events in determining cell function, as previously suggested (5, 38).

Surprisingly, the lowest DMNA dosage (0.6 mg/kg), which yield DNA damage undectable by traditional alkaline elution and alkaline sucrose gradient assays, is readily detectable by a dramatic increase in free ion content o intact nuclei and by a parallel decrease (both electrically monitored) in putative tightly bound ions and tightly bound water to the overall nuclear macromolecules.

Intact nuclei from untreated control rat (Fig. 19) show a highly reproducible transition at an early temperature close to 332° K (59°C), which is systematically absent in isolated chromatin; in addition the transition at about 346°-353°K, which was yielding in isolated chromatin a constant low value of the enthalpy of transition, independent of salt concentration above to mM (see Table II), dramatically increase by a factor 5 in intact nuclei. The melting enthalpy for the other two conformational transitions (II-III) is instead increasing, also between chromatin at 50mM NaCl and isolated nuclei pelleted in 1 mM Tris-HCl, as expected from the effective equivalent normality of the same control liver nuclei suspension (about 98 mM) independently evaluated by complex dielectric constant measurements on the same sample (Table IV) on the same sample (Table IV).

Preliminary determinations on liver nuclei from DMNA (Dimethylnitrosamine) treated rats, indicate an increase in the enthalpy for all the transitions, compatible with the increased salt concentration (from 96 to 110 mM) as determined by complex dielectric constant measurements (Table IV). More interestingly, a decrease of the melting temperature (from 382 K to 377 K) is reproducibly observed for the third (III) conformational transition.

All above data, linked with independently acquired paramenters, in terms of free and bound ions, nuclear morphometry, thermal stability and heat capacity and chromatin organization at angstrom resolution, shed new insight on the mechanisms determing chemically-induced cell transfromation and cell proliferation.

The chromatin alterations occuring at the high DMNA dose

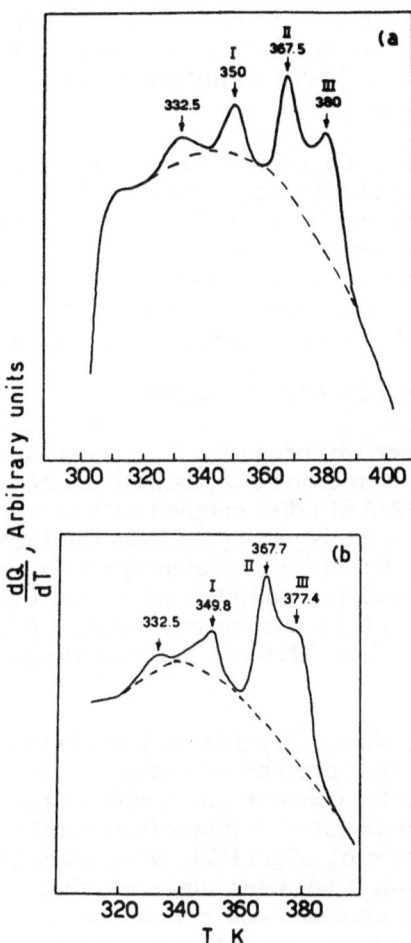

Figure 19 Thermal profiles of intact liver nuclei from untreated (above) and 5.4 mg/kg DMNA treated (below) rats. The dotted lines correspond to the heat capacity profiles of the very same sample after denaturation up to 400°K.

are indeed similar to the one occuring when cells enter G1; it is curious to note that while this single dose not induce cancer in rat liver, repetitive closely spaced administrations of the same dose (without hepatectomy) or of a single dosage after partial hepatectomy does induce cancer of the liver (39). We could then be tempted to speculate that chromatin conformational changes toward a more relaxed uncoiled superstructure could well be a prerequisite for cancer iduction, which is moreover characterized at the level of single cell by an apparent uncoupling between chromatin-DNA structural alteration (increased binding sites) and total RNA synthesis (decreased).

The known fact that even a single large dose of the same chemical on a resting hepatocytes population may induce liver carcinoma at much later times (as compared to cancer induced after partial hepatectomy) can be reconciled with the "relaxed chromatin" prerequisite, noticing hat even in the so-called "resting" control liver a slow turnover is present, i.e. very few cells at the G1/S boundary with relaxed/uncoiled chromatin structure are present and could well be the target priming the carcinogenic process.

PRENEOPLASTIC NODULES AND CANCER

When in the same rat liver we induce the formation of preneoplastic nodules by the Solt-Farber method (40), namely 0.02% 2-acetylaminofluorene (2-AAF) diet coupled with partial hepatectomy, the selected carcinogen-initiated hepatocytes from the focal islands appear to have compeltely different properties (Table V) respect to cycling and early carcinogen-altered hepatocytes, namely a decreased diffusion and increased microviscosity of the nuclear environment (F), combined with a decrease bound water per unit DNA compatible with an increase in chromatin condensation.

It has been recently shown (41) that certain physical properties (NMR relaxation times of hydrogen protons) of water are altered in tumor cells, even independently of water concentration, which since early in this century was known to be elevated in tumor (apparently in the cytoplasm) above that of normal tissue of origin (42). More importantly and consistently with our data, it has been suggested that change in the physical state of water (decreased bound water or increase in the relaxation times of water protons) preceds the increase in water concentration and change in cell function (41).

Preliminary three-dimensional reconstruction of nuclear DNA from thin sections of the intact liver tissue confirms an increase in "average" chromatin condensation, as apparent (Fig. 20) by the shift toward lower transmittance (i.e., higher absorbance) in the frequency distribution of pixel gray levels from nuclear DNA in the preneoplastic nodule regions as compared to nuclear DNA from normal hepatocyte regions, both stained

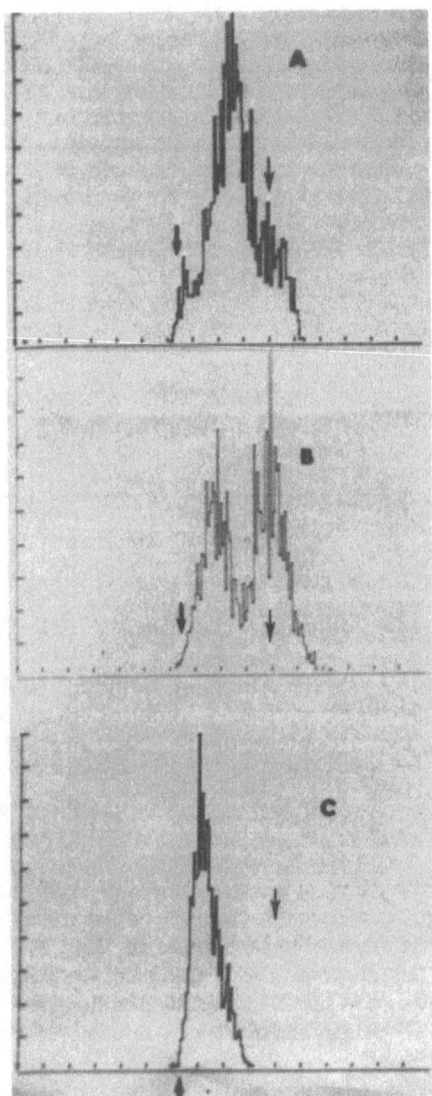

Figure 20 Frequency distributions of pixel transmittance intensity obtained from nuclear image of rat liver tissue sections 3 microns thick in the preneoplastic (A and C) and normal (B) regions. These preliminary data are presently being verified on a larger number of nuclei, Felgen-stained.

TABLE V

Electrical properties of nuclei from rat liver preneoplastic
nodules, being developed using the Solt-Farber method (40). Data
have been acquired between 50 and 1000 MH_z, with 50 MH_z
interval, rather than between 100 and 2000 MHz with 100 MHz
interval (Tables III-IV).

Sample	N	P	WB	WB/P	F	T_D/v_{DNA}
Control	99±1	104±4	300±7	2.1±0.3	71	0.24*
Preneoplastic Lesions	91±1	122±3	540±6	3.3±0.2	69	0.12*
Partial Hepatectomy	104±4	130±3	207±3	1.2	86	0.38*

Nuclei electric properties from control resting and proliferating
liver cells are given as reference.

Units and symbols are identical to Tables III-IV.

In these experiments, nuclei were suspended in high ionic
strength solution (0.1 N) which is known to cause a decrease in
the nuclear volume (with consequent increase in macromolecular
concentration P), as compared to measurements conducted on nuclei
suspended in low ionic strength (0.04 N) and reported in Tables
III-IV.

Nuclei sediment very fast and the electric field goes only across
the bottom of the cylindrical sample holder (a region 5mm high by
7mm wide) containing thereby a constant 0.2 ml nuclear pellet:
progressive dilution with suspending medium or a larger nuclear
pellet do not affect the results and parameters are indeed
uniquely function of a given nuclear environment.

*The values are estimated normalizing to a constant control value
(as reported in Tables III-IV).

Despite the quite different experimental conditions, induced cell
proliferation with partial hepatectomy causes with respect to
control resting liver nuclei a similar increase in tightly bound
water per unit DNA, a similar decrease in vicinal bound water per
unit of macromolecules (WB/P) and a similar increase in
relaxation frequency (F).

within the same liver tissue. Interestingly this apparent increase in
chromatin condensation, usually associated with a change in chromatin
tertiary-quaternary structure toward an higher DNA packing ratio, is a
common denominator in all transformed cells (either genetically,
sponateously or virally induced) when compared to their normal
counterparts (9, 4, 43), suggesting that even in the chemically-induced
neoplastic transformation a decrease in DNA template activity and site
availability is an early prerequisite for the expression of the transformed
phenotype. Studies are presently under way to verify if these preneoplastic
hepatocytes and the hepatoma (later on occasionally developing) display
this and other characteristics of transformed cells, which unequivocally
discriminate them from the normal counterparts at single cell level rather
than as "average" property (as chromatin structure which indeed modulates
significantly during the cycle of both normal and abnormal cells) namely:

a)   the uncoupling between changes in nuclear morphometry and
     changes in cell morphometry (5, 10);

b)   the disruption and/or disorganization of microtubles/ mircofilaments
     (45);

c)   membrane alterations, as monitored with the fluorescamine uptake by
     primary amine in intact cells (20);

d)   the anchorage-independent growth (45) and the uncoupling between
     cell geometry end cell growth (45).

MOLECULAR MECHANISMS

What are the molecular modifications that may eventually lead to cell
proliferation and to cell transformation?

     In recent years a wide number of candidates have been proposed but
only few appear conclusively linked with cell function in general and
particularly with the onset of DNA replication, namely:

-    level of H1 phosprorilation (7)
-    nuclear matrix (46)
-    ions, as Mg^{++}, Ca^{++}, Na^+ and K^+. both in absolute
     concentration (47) and their redistribution among free and bound
     compartment (27);
-    cell geometry in normal cell, but not in transformed cells (45, 48);
     likely related to the presence of oriented-organized
     microtubules-microfilaments (removal of the cytoskeleton causes
     instananeous dispersion/enlargement of nuclear DNA (12)).

     All above changes and others, apparently correlated but not causally
with DNA replication (such as non-histones (51) the level of phosphorilation

(7, 6), c-AMP (7) acetylation (51) and methylation of histones proteins) have as common denominator a dramatic effect on chromatin structure which abruptly relaxes/uncoils immediately before a cell increases its metabolic activity, both in terms of RNA and DNA synthesis (5, 6, 7, and Figs. 13-14) or when a cell is 'initiated' by a chemical carcinogen (Figs. 13-15). Actually it has been shown rather conclusively (7) the existence of a cause-effect relationship between abrupt changes in chromatin structure and cell function (as DNA replication or mitotic condensation); furthermore it is now clear and predictable quantitaively from polyelectrolyte theory (8) how changes in neutralization of phosphate negative charges induced either by modification in bound positive ions or by enzymatic protein modifications cause abrupt changes in the spontaneous bending of supercoiled DNA at quaternary level (being a rope-like or solenoid-like structure).

Very recently (44), chromatin and nuclei were discovered to undergo rapid and reversible structural-volumetric transitions in presence of slight difference in ion concentration, both divalent (Fig. 21) or monovalent, for constant pH and temperature, or in presence of minor variations in pH for constant temperature and ionic strength (44); as shown here (Fig. 22) for intact nuclei volume, the structure of isolated chromatin displays instantaneous phase transitions us function of temperature, ions and pH quite similar to the phase-transitions early reported for polyacrilamide gels (50) and explained from first principles in terms of mean field theory (13). This further corroborates the critical role of chromatin structure and the abrupt nature of its transitions interesting the overall genome. For all fairness, however, a parallel line of thought have produced evidences that the nuclear protein matrix (46) may rather be the determinant of the structural and functional modification of nuclei and chromatin, whose fibers are constrained and modulated by the network of the nuclear protein matrix.

We have then designed a very simple experiment to test which component, chromatin or protein matrix, controls the shrinking and swelling of the overall nuclear volume. If changes in chromatin structure are just a consequence of changes in nuclear volume, being controlled by modifications in the nuclear matrix (whose protein aggregation and network contraction is also dependent on ions concentrations), selective removal of DNA by DNAse enzyme would not affect the shape and volume of liver nuclei, that should still decrease their volume with increasing Ca^{++} concentration and therefore display a phase transition quite similar to the undigested control liver nuclei. This is instead not occuring and digested nuclei display the same constant volume at any Ca^{++} cocentration (Fig. 21), while the undigested control nuclei reduce of several folds their volumes when exposed to identical procedure, temperature and buffer.

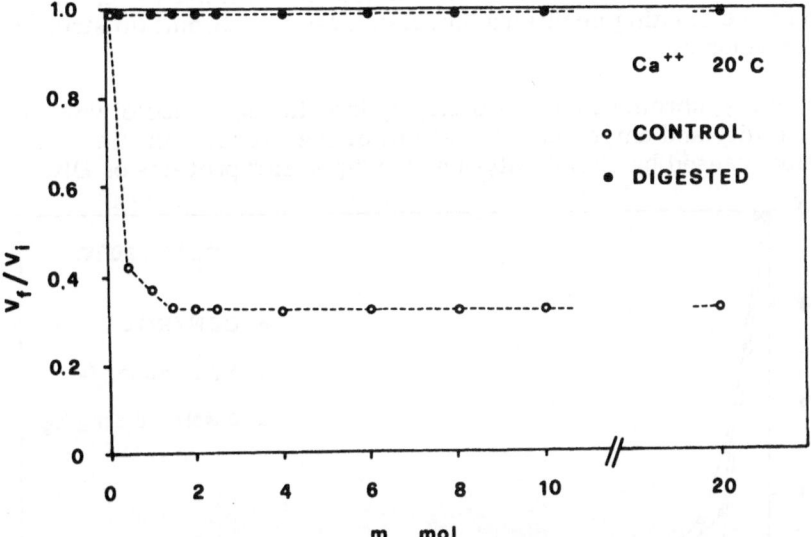

<u>Figure 21</u> Ratio between final and initial volume versus increasing Ca^{++} concentration for isolated liver nuclei before (o---o---o) and after DNAse digestion (— ---). Nuclease digestion has been conducted at 37°C for 30 minutes with 700 Units of DNAse I, while the 5 minutes exposure to various ion concentrations have been carried out at 20°C.

Single (DMNA) and double (AAF) DNA strand breaks, induced by large
dose of chemical carcinogens (4 hours after their administration), cause
immediate increase in nuclear volume (53 and Fig. 13) and substantial
decrease in the degree of nuclei shrinkage associated with the increased
ion concentration (Fig. 22).

It then appears that the chromosome-sized DNA structure altered at
quaternary level, probably in terms of a decreased pitch in the rope-like
fiber (Fig. 5), by the ion neutralization of phosphate charges, controls the
shrinkage of overall nuclear volume through the mediation of drapery-like
chromatin fiber attachment to the nuclear membrane at the pores (Fig. 9
and ref. 5). Removal (DNAse) or simple disruption (chemical carcinogens)
of this long chromatin - DNA fiber would cause the elimination or the
reduction of the existing geometric coupling between chromatin structure
and nuclear volume.

In summary, chromatin appears closely interlinked to nuclei volume
and permeability and any global alterations of the overall genome
organization, caused by chemically-induced "specific" proteins or DNA

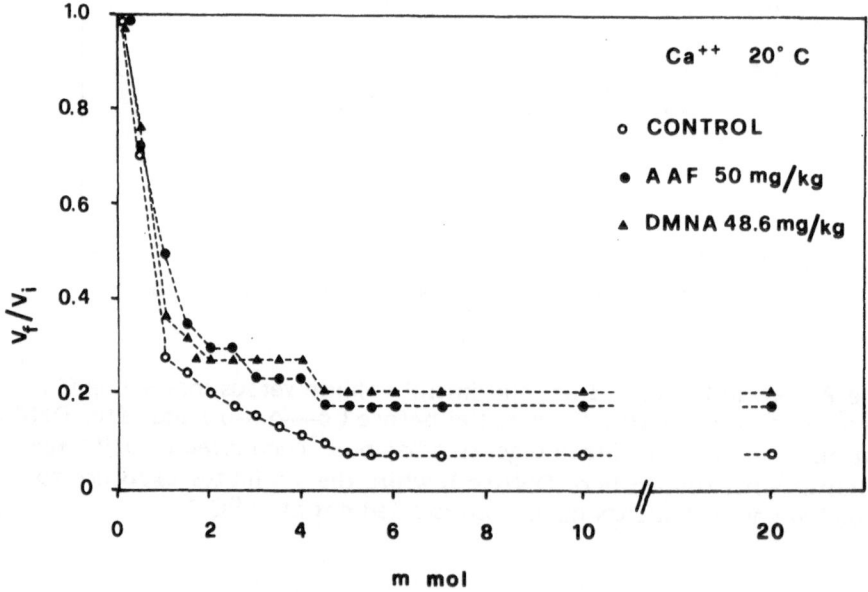

Figure 22 As Figure 21, but for liver nuclei isolated from untreated (o), 50
mg/kg AAF (o) and 48.6 mg/kg DMNA ( ) treated rats.

enzymatic modifications or by "generalized" redistribution of free versus bound water and ions, could then sequentially trigger the random expression of specific genes (yielding the transformed phenotype) and the disruption of microtubules-microfilaments (leading to the uncoupling between cell and nuclear geometry and eventually to the uncontrolled abnormal cell growth).

CONCLUSIONS

In recent years studies of the molecular alterations occuring in cells exposed to chemical carcinogens have received increasing attention (See other chapters in this volume). Among the numerous and possible candidates, DNA strand breaks have been consistently shown to be early events correlated to cell mutation and cancer induction. In few instances, also alterations of isolated chromatin were reported after exposure to a carcinogen (11), but without a clear understanding of the detailed nature of the reported structural alterations and mainly with poor evidence on their causal correlation with the induction of a carcinogenic process. This chapter intended to fill this gap summarizing recent knowledge in the field and in producing new exciting findings, some yet unreported, which shed new light on the organization of the single largest (and most important) molecule within mammalian cells and on its initial role in determining chemically induced neoplastic process, through also the mediation of other dominant cellular component as water and mechanisms such the (cytoskeleton mediated) uncoupling between cell and nuclei geometry.

ACKNOWLEDGEMENTS

The Group of Biostructure consists of the Institute of Pharmacology, Faculty of Medicine; C.N.R. Center for the Physico-chemical studies of Macromolecules, Institute of Industrial Chemistry, Faculty of Science; The section of Biophysical and Electronic Engineering, Institute of Electrotecnics, Faculty of Engineering; Institute of Electronic Circuits, C.N.R.

A. Manzoli and N. Maraldi are from the Institute of Anatomy, University of Bologna
Claudio Nicolini was supported by a Research and Study Leave Award from Temple University and by C.N.R., finalized project "Control of Neoplastic Growth."

REFERENCES

1. Felsenfeld, G., 1978. Nature, 271, 115-121.

2. Finch, J., and Klug, A., 1976. Proc. Nat. Acad. Sci. U.S.A., 73, 1897-1901.

3. Nicolini, C., and Kendall, F., 1977. Physiol. Chem. Phys. 9, 265-283.

4. Nicolini C., 1979. In: 'Chromatin structure and function'. C. Nicolini ed., Plenum Publishing Co., NATO-ASI Series, pp. 613-666,

5. Nicolini, C., 1980. Journal of Submicroscopic Cytology 12 475-505.

6. Ruttle, H., Baldwin, J., Mathews, A., Carpenter B., Suau, P., and Bradbury, E., 1979. In: "Chromatin structure and function'. C. Nicolini ed., Plenum Publishing Co.

7. Dolby, T., Belmont, A., Borun, T., and Nicolini, C., 1981. J. Cell Biolgoy 89, 78-85.

8. Belmont, A., and Nicolini, C., 1981. J. Theoretical Biology 90, 169-179.

9. Kendall, F., Beltrame, and Nicolini, C., 1979. IEEE Transactions Biomed. Eng. 26, 173-175

10. Nicolini, C., and Beltrame, F., 1980. Cell Biology. Intl. Reports (1982) January.

11. Nicolini, ., Ramanhatthan, R., Kendall, F., Murphy, J., Parodi, S., and Sarma, D., 1976, Cancer Research, 36, 1725-1730.

12. Nicolini, C., Grattarola, M., Viviani, R, Martelli, A., Basic and Allied Histoch (1982).

13. Sun, T., Nishio, I., and Tanaka, T., J. Chem. Phys., 1980, 73, 5971-5.

14. Cavazza, B., Conio, G., Patrone, E., Pioli, F., and Trefiletti, V. 1979. Makaromol. Chem., 180, 1607-1609

15. Parodi, S., Carlo, P. Martelli, A., Taningher, M., Finollo, R., Giaretti, 1981 J. Mol. Biol. 147, 501-521

16. Gallina, V., Malvano, R., and Omini, M., 1971, Review Sci. Instrum. 42, 1607-1613.

17. Nicolini, C., Carlo, P., Martelli, A., Finollo, R., Bignone, F., and Brambilla, G., Journal Molecular Biology in Press.

18. Trefiletti, V., Martelli, A., Cavazza, B., Cuniberiti, C., Nicolini, C., and Patrone, E., Internal Report Group Biostructure, 9/81 University of Genova (1981).

19. Nicolini, C., Belmont, A., Parodi, A., Abraham, S., and Lessin, S., 1979. J. Histochem. Cytochem., 21, 102-113.

20. Nicolini, C., 1980. In: 'Advances in neuroblastoma research'. A. Evans ed., Raven Press, New York, pp. 271-285.

21. Nicolini, C., Kendall, F., and Giaretti, W., 1977a. Biophys. J. 19., 163-176.

22. Nicolini, C., Linden, W., Zietz, S., and Wu, S., 1977. Nature 270, 607-609.

23. Kendall, F., Beltrame, F., and Nicolini, C., 1979. In: 'Chromatin structure and function'. Part A., C. Nicolini ed., Plenum Publishing Co., New York-London, pp. 265-292.

24. Beltrame, F., Chiabrera, A., Grattarola, M., Guerrim, P., Parodi, G., Ponta, D., Vernazza, G. and Viviani, R. 2nd Annual Conference of the IEEE Engineering in Medicine and Biology Society, 1980, Washington, D.C.

25. Bianco, B., Drago, G., Marchesi, M., Martini, C., Mela, G., and Ridella, S. 1979. IEEE Transactions Instr. & Measur., 28, 290-294

26. Ridella, S., Intra, E., Mela, G., and Spiga, VI Int. Conference on Electrical Bio-impedence, 1981, Tokyo.

27. Nicolini, C., Carlo, P. and Ridella, S., IEEE Transactions on Biomedical Engineering, 1982, submitted.

28. Widnell, C., and Tata, J., Biochem. J., 1964, 92, 313,317.

29. Nicolini, C., Patrone, E., Cavazza, B., Trefiletti, V., Parodi, G., and Beltrame, F., Internal Report 8/81 Group of Biostructure, University of GenovA (1981) and submitted to P.N.A.S.-U.S.A.

30. Miller, P. Linden, W., and Nicolini, C., Z., 1979. Naturforsch. 34, 442-448.

31. Dolby, T., Borun, T., Gilmour, S., Cohen, A., Zweidler, A., Miller, P., and Nicolini, C., 1979. Biochemistry. 18, 1333-1345.

32. Kendall, F., Beltrame, F., Belmont, A., Zietz, S., Nicolini, C., 1980. Cell Biophysics 2, 373-404.

33. Nicolini, C., Kendall, F., Desaive, C., and Giarretti, W., 1977c. Exp, Cell Res., 106, 199-127.

34. Nicolini, C., 1980. Cell Biophysics, 2, 271-290

35. Beal, P., Hazlewood, P., and Rao, P., Science, 1976. 192, 904-906.

36. Nicolini, C., Kozu, A., Borun, T., and Baserga, R., 1975. J. Biol Chem. 250, 3381-3385.

37. Nicolini, C., Parodi, S., Beltrame, F., and Lessin, S., In Short term Tests for Chemical Carcinogenesis, eds. S. Parodi and Santi, L., Istituto Tumori, Genova (1979)

38. E. Farber, in this volume.

39. Columbano, A., Ledda, G., Rao, P., Rajalashmi, S., and Sarma, D., in this volume.

40. Solt, D., and Farber, E., 1976. Nature 263, 1506-1507.

41. Rao, P., Hazlewood, C., and Beall, P., In Cell Growth, ed., C. Nicolini, Plenum Publishing Co. 1982. New York-London, 535-548.

42. Mellors, R., Kupfer, A., and Hollender, A., 1953. Cancer, 6, 376-384.

43. Nicolini, C., Beltrame, F., and Grattarola, H., In Cell Growth, ed. C. Nicolini, Plenum Publishing Co. New York-London (1982) 587-608.

44. Nicolini, C., Finollo, R., and Carlo, P., submitted to Science.

45. Folkman, J. and Moscona, A., 1978. Nature, 273, 345-348.

46. Pardell, D., Vogelstein, B., and Coffey, D., 1980. Cell, 19, 527-536.

47. Dulbecco, R., and Elkington, J. (1975) P.N.A.S.-USA, 72, 1584-88.

48. Belmont, A., Kendall, F., and Nicolini, C., 1980. Cell Biophys. (1980) 2, 165-175.

49. Puck, T., Waldren, C., Hsie, A., 1972. Proc. Nat. Acad. Sci. U.S.A., 68, 358.

50. Tanaka, T., Scientific American (1980).

51. Bradbury, E., and Matthews, H., in Cell Growth, ed. C. Nicolini, Plenum Publishing Co. NATO-Life Science Series (1982) 411-454.

THE CYTOSKELETON: AN INTERMEDIATE IN THE EXPRESSION OF THE TRANSFORMED PHENOTYPE IN MALIGNANT CELLS

B. R. Brinkley

Department of Cell Biology
Baylor College of Medicine
Houston, Texas   77030

INTRODUCTION

Transformation of cells in vitro by viral or chemical agents is accompanied by a variety of physiological, morphological, and growth-related changes, including altered lectin-binding characteristics and changes in surface proteins (Burger 1973; Pollack and Burger, 1969). In many forms of neoplasia, striking changes occur in cell morphology, including the transition from flattened anisotropic forms that grow as monolayers to rounded pleomorphic forms that pile up as multilayered foci in culture (Temin and Rubin, 1958; Stoker and Abel, 1962). Changes in growth properties include loss of density-dependent control of growth (Todaro et al., 1964), loss of contact-inhibited mobility (Gail and Boone, 1971), and acquisition of anchorage-independent growth (Stoker and Mac-Pherson, 1961; Freedman and Shin, 1974; Benedict et al., 1975; Evans and DiPaolo, 1975; Risser and Pollack 1974). Transformed cells grow well in media containing reduced serum content and are often characterized by reduced cyclic AMP levels (Smith et. al., 1971; Holly and Kiernan, 1968; Anderson et al., 1973; Sheppard, 1972; Mohanhan et al., 1973). Although it is known that various properties in this list are dissociable and are not linked as a group to malignant transformation, taken collectively these findings attest to the molecular complexity of cell transformation. Since most carcinogenic agents are also thought to be mutagens which interact with nuclear DNA producing point mutations and chromosome rearrangements how are these mutations manifested in the broad spectrum of phenotypic changes which accompany transformation?

This article will review evidence indicating that the cytoskeleton is a direct intermediate in the expression of the transformed phenotype. A brief review of the components of the cytoskeleton will be given along with a documentation of the changes in cytoskeletal organization which accompany cell transformation in vitro. Recent evidence which suggests that some cytoskeletal proteins are substrates for viral transforming proteins will also be reviewed.

Components of the Cytoskeleton

Through advances in electron microscopy and immunoctyochemistry as well as through biochemical studies much has been learned about the fibrous components of cytoplasm. The cytoskeleton is a term given to a complex system of anastomosing intertwining filaments and tubules which extend throughout the cytoplasm of eukaryotic cells. There have been many excellent reviews on the cytoskeleton (Goldman et al., 1976; Watson and Albrecht-Buehler,1982; Wilson, 1982) and I will only present an overview of the components in the space that follows. The cytoskeleton can be divided into two functional entities: Structural components which include microtubules, microfilaments and intermediate filaments, and regulatory components consisting of various enzymes, binding proteins and cofactors which modulate cytoskeletal activity. The cytoplasmic ground substance or microtrabeculae (Wolosewick and Porter, 1979) also forms a highly structured lattice in the cytoplasm and contributes to the skeletal material of cytoplasm. In this review however, we will confine our comments to microtubules, microfilaments and intermediate filaments.

The cytoskeleton is involved in many diverse functions including force production, force transduction, cell movement, cell shape, phagocytosis, secretion, axonal transport, and cell surface receptor modulation. More subtle functions including hormone action, gene transcription, DNA synthesis and growth control have been implicated in recent studies. The cytoskeleton's central function in this wide range of cellular activities would suggest its involvement in neoplastic transformation.

Microtubules

Like other developments in the field of cell biology, advances in knowledge of the cytoskeleton was largely made possible by a series of technical achievements dating back over two decades. Although a fibrous network was detected in silver-stained neurons by Cajal in the 19th Century, we generally credit early electron microscopists with the discovery of microtubules and microfilaments. The vast improvements in fixation afforded by glutaraldehyde (Sabatini et al., 1963) led to the widespread recognition of microtubules in most eukaryotic cells. Prior to the glutaraldehyde era, discrete "filaments" were recognized in the mitotic spindles of amoebae (Roth and Daniels, 1962) and even earlier fibrous elements were faintly seen to form a 9+2 pattern in dismembered and sectioned cilia (Manton and Clark, 1952; Fawcett and Porter, 1954).

A significant contribution to our knowledge of microtubule substructures came from electron microscopic (EM) studies in meristematic cells of juniper. As a result of the natural electron opacity afforded by the cell wall material of this plant, Ledbetter and Porter (1964) identified 13 globular subunits in the walls of microtubules a finding which in recent years has been widely confirmed in many diverse species using tannic acid as a stain (Tilney et al., 1973). Much of our current understanding of how subunits are arranged in the microtubule surface lattice has come from optical diffraction studies of negatively stained flagellar microtubules using optical filtering techniques and computer methods of image analysis (Amos and Klug, 1974; Erickson, 1974: Chasey, 1972). In addition, X-ray diffraction studies of unfixed, hydrated material has largely confirmed early EM studies (Mandelkow et al., 1977).

Evidence for oriented polymers in the cytoplasm of living cells came a full decade before the era of electron microscopy. By observing dividing marine oocytes through a polarizing microscope equipped with rectified, stain-free optics, Inoué detected weak form birefringence in the mitotic apparatus which was later shown to be due to highly oriented microtubules. From a series of experimental studies, Inoué and his coworkers (1967, 1975) concluded that soluble subunits were in a dynamic equilibrium with their polymeric forms contained in spindle fibers. Moreover, these investigators proposed that the assembly was entropy-driven and that the subunits were maintained in the polymer by weak hydrophobic bonds. This important study has now been confirmed by three decades of research including in vitro assembly experiments using purified microtubule protein.

Through the use of ^{3}H-colchicine as a probe and the specificity of binding of this drug to microtubule protein, E. W. Taylor and his students (Shelanski and Taylor, 1967; Weisenberg et al., 1968; Borisy and Taylor, 1967a and 1967b) and Wilson and Friedkin (1967) were the first to isolate and characterize a single protein with a sedimentation coefficient of 6S and a M_r of 110-120 Kd. Later it was shown that denaturation of the protein with guanidine hydrochloride produced two similar 55 Kd α and β subunits. It was concluded that in aqueous solutions the larger colchicine binding molecules existed as a dimer which came to be known as tubulin (Mohri, 1968). It was also discovered that α and β tubulin subunits existed in a constant 1:1 molar ratio in microtubules forming an heterodimer (Bryan and Wilson, 1971). A major contribution was made by Weisenberg (1972) who demonstrated that microtubules would form spontaneously from supernatants of brain homogenates when the solution was warmed to 37°C in the presence of GTP and magnesium. The key to his success in achieving in vitro assembly was the addition of the calcium chelating agent EGTA to the reassembly mixture. He concluded that free calcium concentrations as low as 6 uM could inhibit the in vitro assembly of microtubules, an observation which may have physiological relevance concerning cellular

control of microtubule assembly. For assembly to occur, a critical
concentration (Cc) of tubulin (0.2 mg/ml) was essential. The Cc
for in vitro assembly is the lowest level at which cooperative
association of subunits occurs forming structures that nucleate
the assembly of microtubules. Thus, assembly appears to be a two-
step condensation-polymerization process in which nuclei (seeds)
form and then elongate. At steady state polymerized tubulin is
in equilibrium with a critical concentration of soluble tubulin.

Microtubule Associated Proteins

Microtubule-associated protein (MAPs) are a class of proteins
that copurify with tubulin and maintain a constant stoichiometry
with tubulin dimer during purification by the assembly-disassembly
procedure (Shelanski et al., 1973; Borisy et al., 1975). In vertebrate brain approximately 15% of the protein of microtubules is
composed of MAP 1 and MAP 2 which copurify with tubulin (Sloboda
et al., 1976). MAPs have now been identified in a variety of
cultured cells where they differ biochemically and antigentically
from brain MAPs (Bulinski and Borisy, 1980b). The biological
function of MAPs is not completely known but they may play a role
in stabilizing or cross linking microtubules as well as binding
other cytoplasmic components to microtubules. Maps also have been
implicated in the regulation of microtubule assembly (Lockwood,
1975; Murphy and Borisy, 1975; Weingarten et al., 1975). Recently
a new MAP was discovered which appears to bind microtubules to
membrane. Ankyrin, a 210K dalton protein, was originally isolated
from red blood cells where it binds with high affinity to spectrin
and is associated with band 3. Antibodies to ankyrin have been
found to localize on cytoplasmic and spindle microtubules (Bennett
and Davis, 1982) near their interface with membranes.

The Cytoplasmic Microtubule Complex

When many types of cultured cells are stained with antitubulin
antibody and examined by indirect immunofluorescence, they display
an elaborate complex of fine fluorescent filaments throughout the
cytoplasm. In most instances, these filaments associate with one
or two specific foci in the cytoplasm near the nucleus and radiate
out toward the cell periphery, where they either terminate at the
plasma membrane or bend and extend along the cell surface (Figs.
1 and 2). We have termed this array of fluorescent filaments the
cytoplasmic microtubule complex (CMTC) and have identified it in
a wide variety of cells in vitro (Brinkley et al., 1975, Fuller
and Brinkley, 1976). In independent studies, Weber and coworkers
(1975) have described essentially the same complex using antitubulin
immunofluorescence on 3T3 cells in vitro.

The CMTC is present throughout interphase but is disassembled
as the cells enter mitosis. As shown in Fig. 3A, the CMTC begins

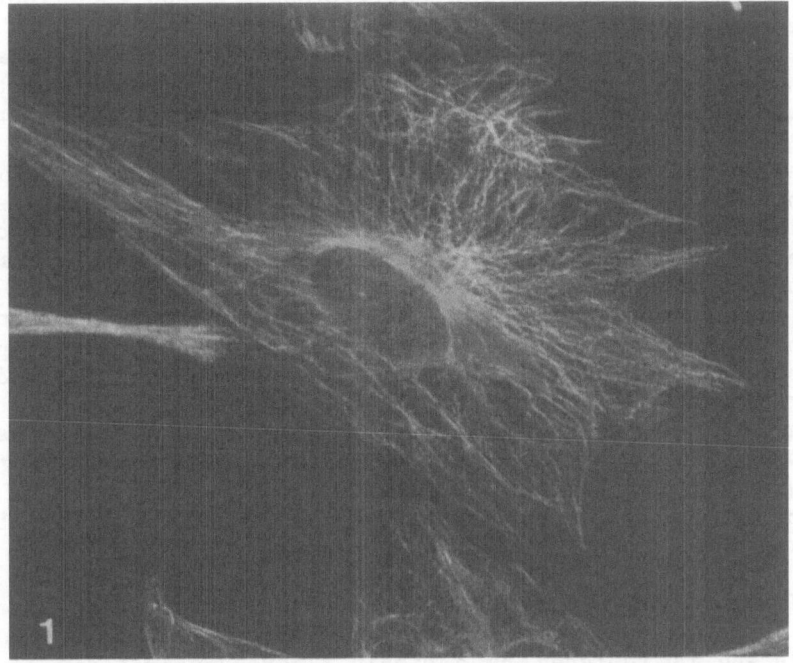

Fig. 1. The cytoplasmic microtubule complex (CMTC)
         in 3T3 cell.

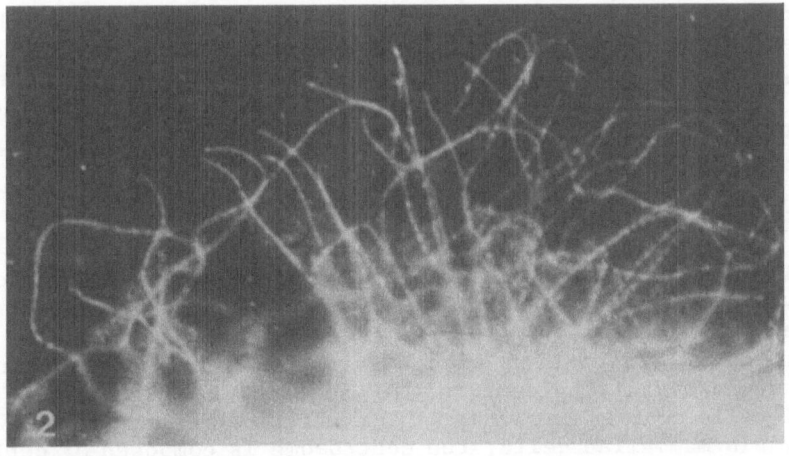

Fig. 2. Higher magnification showing individual
         microtubules terminating near the cell
         surface.

to disassemble in late G_2 or early prophase, and the fluorescent filaments disappear except for those that are associated with the two poles of the spindle. As the cells progress into prometaphase, they become more rounded in appearance, and fluorescence becomes entirely localized within the forming mitotic spindle and the astral fibers (Fig. 3B). At metaphase, the chromosomes become aligned on the equatorial plate, and a clearly defined spindle is present near the center of the cell (Fig. 3C). The cytoplasm surrounding the spindle is totally free of any filamentous components. As the cell progresses through anaphase and into telophase, the chromosomes move to the poles, and cytokinesis occurs (Fig. 3D and 3E). During cytokinesis, the fluorescence becomes concentrated within the midbody, which bridges the two daughter cells (Fig. 3F). This structure is known to contain numerous microtubules and probably represents the rudiments of the interpolar spindle fibers. During late telophase or early G_1, a large aster forms in association with the centriole region of each daughter cell (Fig. 3F). Subsequently, the complete CMTC is generated from each of these regions as the cells become flattened and assume a more fibroblastic appearance (Fig. 3G).

Thus, in all proliferating cells examined, the extensive cytoplasmic microtubule complex is disassembled at the beginning of mitosis and is replaced by a highly fluorescent mitotic apparatus that functions to segregate the chromosomes during mitosis. The entrance of cells into mitosis and the disassembly of the cytoplasmic microtubule apparatus is accompanied by the major alterations in cell shapes from a flattened state to a more rounded appearance. When mitosis is completed, the mitotic apparatus disappears and is replaced by cytoplasmic microtubules that originate at the asters in each daughter cell. The formation of the CMTC in G_1 phase of the cell cycle is accompanied by the return of the cell to a flattened, more fibroblastic appearance. Since both systems are composed of microtubules of similar structure and properties, it appears likely that tubulin is recycled from one apparatus to the other during the mitotic cycle (Brinkley et al., 1975).

Microtubule Organizing Centers

The assembly of microtubules in vitro occurs at random, and involves a two step condensation-polymerization process as described earlier. Microtubule assembly in cells, however, occurs not at random but in association with discrete nucleation sites known as microtubule organizing centers (MTOCs) (Pickett-Heaps, 1969). Most animal cells contain one or two MTOCs which correspond to the centrosomes. In mammalian cells, the centrosome is composed of centrioles and pericentriolar material (Brinkley et al., 1981: Pepper and Brinkley, 1979; Gould and Borisy, 1977; Kuriyama and Borisy, 1981 a,b). Other MTOCs include kinetochores on mammalian chromosomes (Pepper and Brinkley, 1979) and basal bodies.

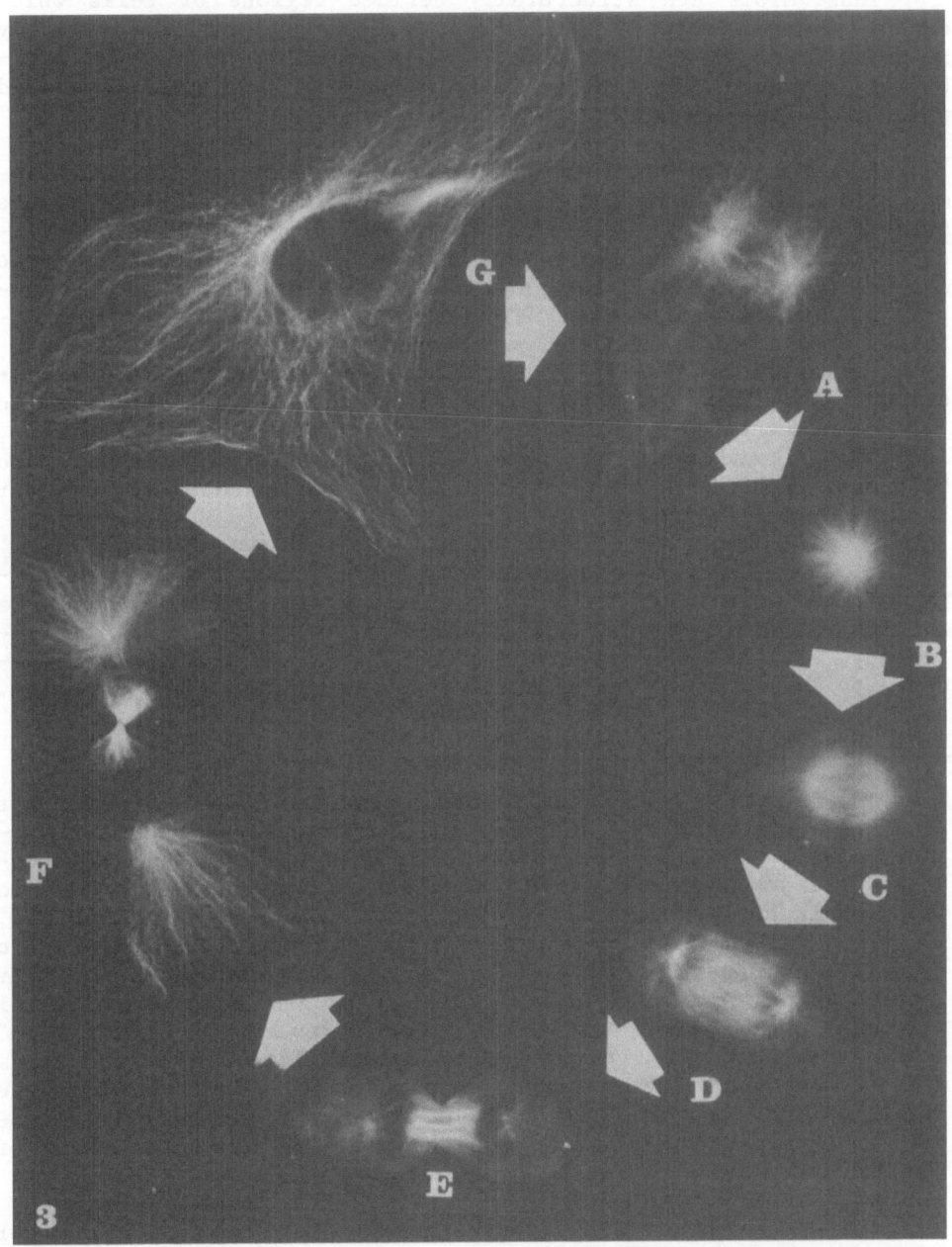

Fig. 3. Microtubule arrays during the cell cycle of 3T3 cell.
A. Late G_2-prophase; B. Prometaphase; C. Metaphase;
D. Anaphase; E. Telophase; F. Late telophase;
G. Interphase.

Thus, MTOCs are structurally defined regions of cells which can be readily detected by electron microscopy and more recently by immunofluorescence (Figs. 4A,B). In addition various autoantibodies from mammalian sources including humans have been identified which react specifically with MTOCs.

In addition to their role as nucleation sites for tubulin polymerization, MTOCs function in part as structural templates for the asssembly of specific microtubule arrays. Since MTOCs are duplicated during the cell cycle, and are systematically segregated to daughter cells, they are thought to be heritable units which are capable of imparting structural "information" as templates for microtubule organization from one cell generation to the next (Soloman, 1981; Brinkley et al.,1981). Regulation of MTOCs is poorly understood at this time but recent success in assaying MTOC activity in lysed cell models or in isolated cell fractions (Brinkley et al., 1981 McGill and Brinkley, 1975; Telzer et al., 1975; Snyder and McIntosh, 1976; Kuriyama and Borisy, 1981 a,b) should improve our knowledge in this area.

Since MTOCs contain nucleic acid and may control, in part, expression of microtubule arrays (Brinkley et al., 1981), they may be targets for carcinogens or transforming factors associated with malignancy. At this time however, there is little experimental evidence to suggest they are directly involved in cell transformation.

Microtubules in Transformed Cells

The fate of microtubules in transformed cells as well as their possible involvement in the transformation process has been the subject of much debate and controversy. Experiments from Puck's laboratory were among the first to suggest that microtubules may be involved in cell transformation (Hsie and Puck, 1971; Puck et al., 1972). These investigators found that after brief exposure to dibutyryl cyclic AMP (cAMP) CHO cells were transformed from their rounded shapes to elongated, flattened forms and underwent parallel alignment with neighboring cells. Such "reverse transformation" could be inhibited by colchicine or cytochalasin B which inhibits microtubules and microfilments respectively. This finding led Puck and his coworkers to conclude that the microtubule-microfilament system in cells might be involved in the expression of the transformed phenotype.

Support for Puck's hypothesis soon came from several other laboratories. When Fonte and Porter (1974) compared rat kidney cells transformed by Kirsten sarcoma virus with normal rat kidney cells they found fewer microtubule profiles in the transformed cells by electron microscopy. Edelman (1976) and Edelman and Yahara (1976) proposed that a network of microtubules and microfilaments which they called surface modulating assemblies (SMA)

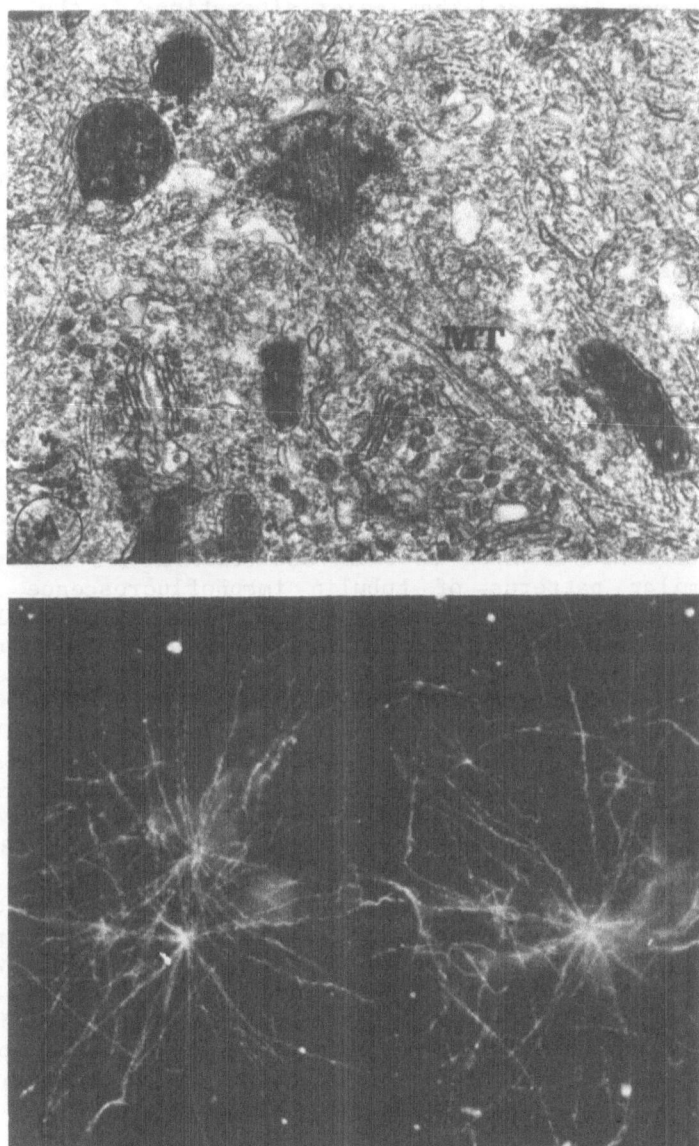

Fig. 4. MTOCs in 3T3 cells.
A. Electron micrograph showing centriole (C) and microtubules (MT);
B. Tubulin immunofluorescence in lysed
3T3 cells incubated with exogenous 6S
tubulin (from Brinkley et al., 1981).

might regulate cell surface receptors and thereby influence growth control. It was concluded that major alterations in the structure and expression of SMA might accompany malignant transformation.

When monospecific antibodies to tubulin became available in the mid 1970s (Fuller et al., 1975; Weber et al., 1975) it was possible to detect microtubules in large populations of cells by indirect immunofluorescence. When Brinkley and coworkers (Brinkley et al., 1976; Fuller and Brinkley, 1976) compared the tubulin immunofluorescence pattern of several matched pairs of normal and transformed cell lines they reported differences in immunofluorscent patterns enabling them to successfully detect transformants in mixed cell populations. Nontransformed cells displayed extensive networks of long sinuous tubules which radiated out from one or two central foci. Transformed cells were smaller and more rounded and displayed mostly short lengths of microtubules and diffuse immunofluorescence throughout. The normal cell was described as having a full CMTC whereas the transformed counterparts displayed a "diminished" network.

In subsequent studies Edelman and Yahara (1976) described somewhat similar patterns of tubulin immunofluorescence in Rous sarcoma virus transformed chicken cells and mouse SV3T3 cells. Of particular interest were microtubule and actin filament networks in chicken cells infected with a temperature sensitive Rous virus. At the restrictive temperature (41°C) the cells displayed extensive actin cables and a "full" radial pattern of microtubules. At the permissive temperature (37°C), these patterns were disordered and staining was more diffuse. Similar staining patterns were noted in normal rat kidney infected with a temperature-sensitive transformation mutant of Moloney murine sarcoma virus (Brown et al., 1981) (Fig. 5). In the latter study. morphological changes in the expression of microtubules and microfilaments accompanied the appearance of a transformation specific 85.000 M_r polyprotein. Evidence for the nuclear origin of the transforming factor was suggested by the study of cytochalasin-enucleated cytoplasts. Enucleation of cells at the nonpermissive temperature and shifting of the cytoplast to the permissive temperature resulted in no change in cytoskeletal morphology or the appearance of the 85,000 M_r protein by gel electrophoresis.

A different interpretation of microtubule patterns in transformed cells has been offered by several other investigators. Using a more rigorous extraction procedure to permeabilize cells, Osborn and Weber (1977) concluded that microtubule networks were abundant in transformed cells. They further concluded that the diffuse or "diminished" staining pattern seen in transformed cells was due to their rounded morphology. Similar conclusions were reached by several other investigators (Tucker et al., 1978; DeMey et al., 1978; Watt et al., 1978). Thus, observations of microtub-

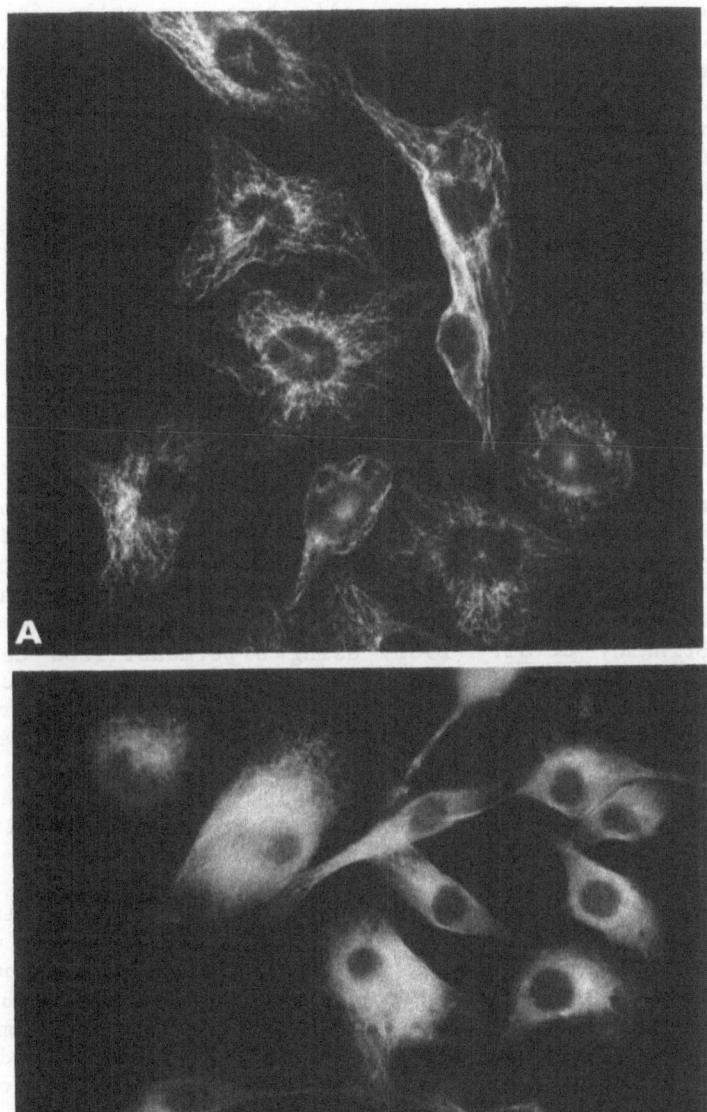

Fig. 5. NRK cell stained by tubulin immunofluorescence.
A. Grown at restrictive temperature
(41°).
B. Grown at permissive temperature
(37°) (from Brown et al., 1981).

ules in normal and transformed cells have generally fallen into
two camps; those who conclude that microtubule patterns have become
altered and those that believe that microtubules are unchanged.
The solution to this dilemma is not clearcut. Obviously for cells
to undergo striking morphological changes as they do in many types
of malignant transformation, microtubule patterns must be altered
or re-arranged. The morphology of some carcinoma cells changes
very little upon transformation. As shown by Asch et al. (1979)
such cells show essentially no change in microtubule and microfilament expression.

Rubin and Warren (1979) utilized morphometric techniques involving electron microscopy to show that normal rat kidney cells
(NRK) had twice the number of microtubules as their Kirsten
sarcoma virus transformed counterparts. In a similar EM morphometric study of mouse BALBc 3T3 and SV 3T3, Zimmer et al. (1981)
concluded that SV 3T3 cells displayed fewer microtubule profiles
in the cortical region of their cytoplasm. The numbers of microtubules associated with the centriole region of 3T3 and SV 3T3
cells were not significantly different. These coworkers concluded
that fewer microtubules extented to the plasma membrane in SV 3T3
cells. The findings of Zimmer et al. (1981) agree in part with a
study by Brinkley et al. (1981) using a permeabilized cell model
of the same 3T3 and SV 3T3 cells. When exogenous 6S tubulin from
bovine brain was added to tubulin-depleted lysed cells, microtubules
reformed from the MTOCs of both cell types. Under identical conditions of tubulin concentration and incubation however, microtubules
which reassembled re-assembled in 3T3 cell models were two to
three fold longer and more numerous than those reconstituted in
lysed SV 3T3 cells.

If microtubule networks are significantly altered in transformed cells, a study by Chafouleas et al. (1981) may offer an
explanation of their diminution. These investigators found that
tubulin levels were unchanged in Swiss mouse 3T3 and SV 3T3 cells
but a 2-fold increase was noted in the level of the calcium binding
protein calmodulin in the transformed cells. Since calmodulin has
been shown to modulate the calcium sensitivity of brain microtubule
assembly-disassembly in vitro, (Marcum et al. 1978) it is possible
that excess calmodulin in transformed cells may in some ways sup-
press the formation of a full CMTC in these cells. Obviously, a
considerable amount of additional work is necessary before the
issue of microtubule changes in cell transformation can be resolved.

Intermediate Filaments

Intermediate filaments (IFs) are characterized by their ubiquitous distribution and uniform size (10 nm) in the cytoplasm of
eukaryotic cells. Biochemically, IFs are defined by their insolubility in low and high salt buffers and non-denaturing detergents.

They have been identified by a variety of synonyms including tono-
filaments, 100A (10 nm) filaments, and cytokeratin filaments.

When viewed by imunofluorescence, IFs display a complex network
throughout the cytoplasm which resembles somewhat the cytoplasmic
microtubule complex (Fig. 6A). In fact, disruption of the CMTC
with colchicine often leads to a collapse of the IF network forming
thick skeins which frequently organize into "caps" near the nucleus
(Fig. 6B). Few if any drugs are known, however, which bind directly
to IFs or their subunits.

The protein content of IFs is highly heterogeneous as shown in
Table 1. The recently adopted classification system for IFs is
based partly upon protein composition and partly upon cellular
distribution (Table 2). Thus, IFs are divided into five major
subclasses based upon biochemical and immunocytochemical criteria,
neurofilaments (neurons), desmin filaments (muscle), α Keratin
filaments (epithelium), vimentin (mesenchyme) and glial filaments
(glial cells). Several studies have shown that IF proteins are
differently expressed during embryonic development (Holtzer et al.,
1982; Lazarides et al., 1982).

Cultured cells, where most of the immunofluorescent studies of
IFs have been carried out, often display more than one class of IF.
Most cultured epithelial cells as well as carcinoma cell lines
appear to contain both α keratin and vimentin (Franke et al., 1981;
Franke et al., 1978a; Fusenig et al., 1978; Summerhayes et al., 1981;
Virtanen et al., 1981). The expression of vimentin in cultured
epithelial cells in vitro may result from adaptation to culture
conditions or from clonal selection of a small population of cells
initially expressing vimentin in vivo (Franke et al., 1978a; Fusenig
et al., 1978; Summerhayes et al., 1981; Virtanen et al., 1981).

Unlike microtubules and actin microfilaments, very little is
known about the polymer-monomer relationships of IF subunits either
in vitro or in situ. Recently investigators have been successful in
achieving in vitro assembly of IFs in several systems including
spinal cord, glial cells, and BHK fibroblasts (Zackeroff and
Goldman 1979).

The morphological proximity of IFs with the centrosome and
centriole lead Goldman and his coworkers (Goldman et al., 1980)
to suggest that MTOCs may also serve as assembly sites for IFs.
Recently, Eckert et al. (1982) have identified an intermediate
filament organizing center (IFOC) in lysed cells near the nucleus
but not coincident with the MTOC in lysed cell models.

The function of IFs is not completely understood but they appear to be closely integrated with other cytoskeletal structures
such as microtubules, stress fibers and microfilaments. They may

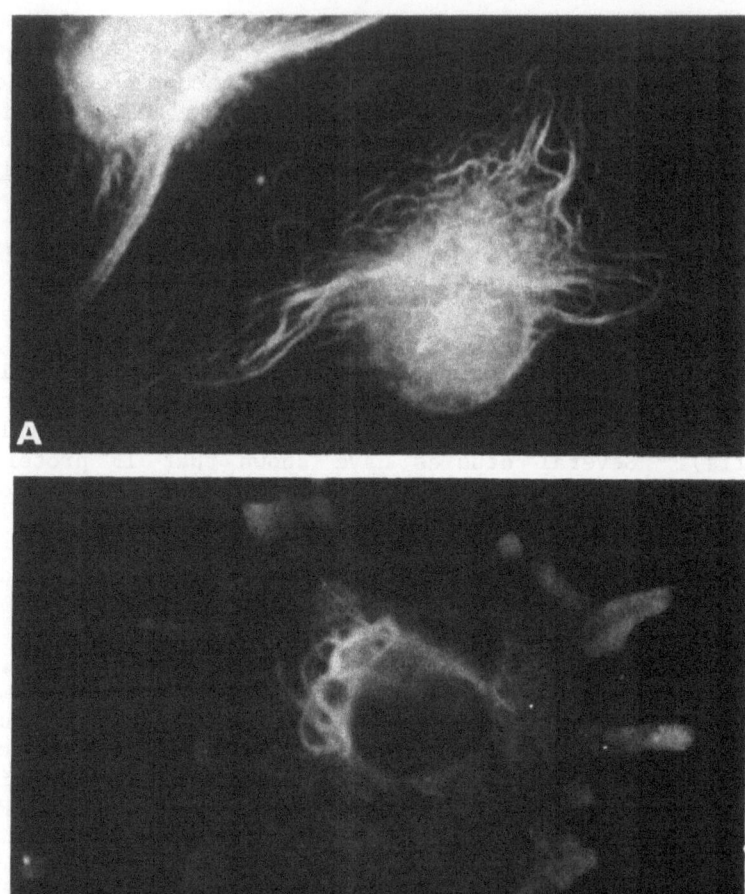

Fig. 6.   Intermediate filaments in PTK$_1$ cells
           shown by indirect immunofluorescence
           using anti-keratin antibodies.
           A.   Interphase pattern;
           B.   Nuclear "cap" after treatment with
           vincristine.

Table 1. Intermediate Filament Nomenclature (From Brinkley, 1982)

Filament type	Major synonym	Tissue (cell)	Molecular weight (x10^{-3})	Reference
α-keratins	cytokeratins prekeratins epidermins	epithelium	68,63,60, 58,54,52	Matoltsy 1965 Franke et al. 1978a
Vimentin	fibroblastic intermediate filament protein (F-IFP) decamin lentin 58-kD protein of fibroblast	mesenchyme	52,57,54,58	Franke et al. 1978b
Desmin	mesosin skeletin 100-Å filament subunit protein	muscle	50,55 85	Lazarides and Hubbard 1976 Small and Sobieszek 1977
Neurofilament protein	filarin 58-kD core protein	neurons	68,160,210	Schmitt 1968
Glial filament protein	glial fibrillary protein (GFP) glial fibriliary acidic protein	glial	51	Huneus and Davison 1970 Eng et al. 1971 Liem et al. 1978 Goldman et al. 1978

function largely as a true cytoskeletal component maintaining cytoplasmic order and organization.

Intermediate Filaments in Transformed Cells

Neoplastic cells express intermediate filaments, and antiserum to various intermediate filament proteins may be useful in defining the tissues from which tumor cells are derived. For example the presence of α-keratin filaments could be useful in confirming the epithelial character of a tumor while vimentin-type filaments would suggest a mesenchymal origin. Whether or not transformation of cells in vitro involves a specific alteration in the expression and organization of intermediate filaments remains uncertain. A non-transformed hamster cell line NIL8 and a sarcoma virus trans-formed counterpart have been studied (Hynes and Destree, 1978) using immunofluorescence. The NIL8 cells contained long extended arrays of filaments while their transformed counterparts contained shorter filaments largely confined to the peri-nuclear region.

In a somewhat similar study involving NRK cells infected with a temperature-sensitive Rous sarcoma virus, Ball and Singer (1981) reported dramatic reorganization of intermediate filaments when cells were grown at permissive (33°) temperature. These investiga-tors utilized double immunfluoresence to observe both microtubules and intermediate filaments in the same cell. At restrictive temper-atures (39°) the two cytoskeletal components were aligned parallel throughout the cell. At permissive temperatures the intermediate filaments were withdrawn to the peri-nuclear area while microtubules appeared to be undisturbed. They concluded that microtubules and microfilaments were closely integrated by cross-linking proteins and such proteins may be substrates for the pp60^{src} kinase. The more we learn about the cytoskeleton, the more it becomes evident that all fibrous components of the cytoplasm are highly crosslinked and closely integrated throughout. Thus, alteration of one cytoskeletal component often leads to changes in expression of other components.

Multiple changes in expression of intermediate filament pro-teins have been observed in other cultured tumor cells. Summerhayes et al. (1981) found a distinct decrease in α-keratin expression and an increase in vimentin expression in rabbit bladder epithelum transformed by benzo(a)pyrene in vitro.

In a carefully controlled study Manger and Heckman (1982) com-pared keratin cytoskeletons in three highly malignant transplantable carcinomas of the rat respiratory tract with three lines of negli-gible malignancy. Their findings suggested that changes in the expression of keratin intermediate filaments along with other archi-tectural changes could be clearly correlated with loss of growth control and tumor progression in carcinomas.

Microfilaments

The consistency of cytoplasm in non-muscle cells is that of a jelly-like fluid capable of being rapidly transformed from a sol to a gel and back again as originally described by Frey-Wessling (1957).

The full range of viscosities displayed by cytoplasm is due largely to actin containing microfilaments and the capacity of actin molecules to exist in several states of polymerization and organization. Actin molecules can exist in three distinct states in the cytoplasm; monomeric G actin, polymerized F-actin (6 nm microfilaments) and higher order microfilament bundles and networks. In monolayer cells in culture actin forms large parallel bundles or stress fibers. Rigid bundles of actin form the core of microvilli and filopodia. Motile cells such as amoebae macrophages or neutrophils may display complex cross-linked actin networks during movement and shape changes. Studies of the morphology and biochemistry of nonmuscle cell actin have progressed greatly in the past decade and many actin binding proteins and gelation factors have been identified as discussed later.

Actin usually comprises approximately 1 to 5% of total cell protein (Hitchcock, 1977; Korn, 1978; Pollard and Weihing, 1974) yet can account for 20 to 30% of total protein in higher motile cells. The differences between muscle actin (α-actin) and the non-muscle form of actin are subtle. Sequence data suggest that all actin have been highly conserved with as little as 6% of the amino acid residues different from cells as evolutionarily distant as Acanthamoeba and rabbit skeletal muscle.

Using isoelectric focusing it can be shown that non-muscle actins exist in two forms called β - and γ actin (Whalen et al., 1976; Rubenstein and Spudich, 1977).

The microheterogeneity of actins may be accountable by the fact that actin genes constitute a large multigene family which is differentially expressed during development (McKeown and Firtel, 1982).

All G-actins (M_r = 42 000) directionally polymerize to form a double stranded helix of F-actin which appears microscopically as a 6 nm microfilament. The process converts 1 mole of bound ATP per mole of G-actin to ADP which remains bound. G-actin monomers exist in a dynamic equilibrium with F-actin as expressed by the equation n(actin) = actin(n). Assembly of actin in vivo proceeds by three reversible steps: (1) nucleation, (2) biased bidirectional elongation and (3) end to end assembly (Oasawa and Asakura, 1975; Pollard et al., 1982). It is possible to determine the polarity of actin filaments and the direction of elongation by decorating F-actin filaments with heavy meromyosin subfragment-1 ($HMMS_1$) as

originally shown by Ishikawa and coworkers (1969). A number of
recent studies suggest that G-actin adds much more readily to one
end of the filament than to the other (Woodrum et al., 1975; Hayashi
and Ip. 1976 Kondo and Ishiwata. 1976; Wegner, 1976; Tilney and
Kellenbach, 1979; Pollard et al., 1982). Decoration with HMMS[1]
produces arrowhead like projections on both sides of the filament.
The "barbed" end of the filament is the preferred or fast growing
end during polymerization. The association and disassociation
rate constants have been calculated for both ends (see Pollard et
al., 1982) and the net rate of polymerization depends upon the
number of free ends available for association. At the steady
state concentration of actin, filament length remains constant with
subunit disassociation balanced by subunit addition. According to
one model, the subunits are proposed to assembly at one end (the
barbed end) flow or "treadmill" through the filament and come off
at the pointed end of the filament (Wegner, 1976; see also Kirschner.
1980). The issue of treadmilling which was also proposed for the
assembly of microtubules (Margolis and Wilson. 1978) is still very
controversial and other investigators support the notion that actin
filaments grow by the addition of G-actin at the fast growing end
(Spudich et al., 1982).

Higher Order of Actin Assemblies in Cells

     Much has been learned about the organization of microfilaments
in cells by observing the association of HMMS[1] decorated filaments
by electron microscopy. Most, if not all, F-actin filaments are
polarized such that their barbed ends are adjacent to membranes
and their pointed ends are extending away from the membranes (Condeelis, 1981; Mooseker et al., 1982). Polymerization occurs by
the addition of G-actin monomers at the membrane associated end as
elegantly shown in Limulus sperm (Tilney et al. 1981). At this
time very little is known about how G-actin is bound to membranes
during the polymerization process. Numerous actin binding proteins
have been identified (Table II) and some calcium sensitive actin
binding proteins such as villin from brush border (Glenney et al.,
1980) and gelsolin from macrophages (Yin and Stossel, 1979) or 90K
protein from platelets (Wang and Bryan. 1980), fragmin from Physarum
(Hasegawa et al., 1980) and a 40K protein from Dictyostelium
(Brown and Spudich , 1980) may function to anchor the growing end
of F-actin to membranes. The growing list of actin binding proteins (Table II: also see Schliwa, 1981) attest to the complexity
of actin organization in cells. Many binding proteins interact
with F-actin at substoichiometric concentrations and appear to regulate the attachment, initiation, polymerization and cross-linking
(bundling) of actin. Some may be metabolic enzymes which bind to
higher ordered actin assemblies to achieve proper spatial order and
sequence for substrate interaction. The glycolytic enzymes aldo-
lase and glyceraldehyde-phosphate dehydrogenase bind to muscle and

Table 2. Actin-binding Proteins (From Brinkley, 1982)

Protein	Subunit Molecular Weight (x10^-3)	Calcium Dependence	Reference
Actin-binding protein	220	−	Hartwig and Stossel 1979
BHK high M_r actin-binding protein	250	−	Schloss and Goldman 1979
Filamin	250	+	Wang 1977
90K protein	90	−	Wang and Bryan 1980
120K protein	120	−	Condeelis 1981
220K protein	220		Bryan and Kane 1978
Fascin	58		Otto et al. 1979
Actinogelin	115	+	Mimura and Asano 1979
Villin	95	+	Bretscher and Weber 1980
Gelsolin	90	+	Yin and Stossel 1979
Cytochalasin B-like protein	65	−	Grumet and Lin 1980
Profilin	16	−	Carlsson et al. 1977
Vinculin	130	−	Geiger 1979
Fimbrin	68	−	Bretscher and Weber 1980a
Acanthamoeba capping protein	31,28	+	Isenberg et al. 1980
Fragmin	50	−	Hasegawa et al. 1980
α-actinin	200	−	Suzuki et al. 1976
β-actinin	42	−	Maruyama et al. 1977
DNase 1	31	−	Hitchcock et al. 1977

nonmuscle actin (Arnold and Pette, 1968; Schwartz, personal communication) and, indeed, other enzymes in the glycolytic system may
use actin bundles and networks for spatial organization. As more
is learned about the various proteins which bind to actin, intermediate filaments, microtubules and the cytomatrix, we may come
to appreciate a new role for the cytoskeleton; that of a spatial
organizer and integrator of complex metabolic pathways involving
multi-enzyme complexes. This view is supported by the growing
evidence for structural complexity of cytoplasm and the notion
that few if any molecules are "free in solution" in the cytoplasm
of intact cells (see Brinkley, 1982). Even water molecules appear
to be highly structured and largely bound to the matrix in the
cytoplasm (Clegg, 1982).

With the development of suitable fluorescent probes for actin,
it became possible to observe various levels of organization in the
cytoplasm by indirect immunofluorescence (Lazarides and Weber,
1974). Through the use of actin antibodies it is possible to
observe long parellel bundles of actin cables or stress fibers in
the cytoplasm of cultured cells (Fig. 7A). The patterns of stress
fibers may vary from many to a few in any cell population and
indeed as cells round up to enter mitosis, the stress fibers disappear and the fluorescence becomes diffuse. Actin can also be
detected in blebs, microvilli and ruffled membranes at the cell
surface.

Microfilaments in Transformed Cells

Cell transformation in vitro is usually, but not always
associated with the general disappearance of actin cables in the
cytoplasm (Pollack et al., 1975a). In general transformed cells
derived from fibroblasts or other mensenchymal cells show a major
diminution of actin cables. Malignant cells of epithelial origin
however, may not show an alteration in stress fiber pattern (Asch
et al. 1979). Figure 7A,B shows a matched pair of SV3T3 and 3T3
cells which illustrate typical patterns of actin stress fibers in
transformed and normal cells. Not all transformed cells, however,
show significant alterations in stress fiber pattern (see Asch et
al., 1979).

In a study of thirteen lines of human breast cancer cells in
vitro Brinkley et al. (1980) found a wide range of stable actin
phenotypes. In general the absence of actin cables was associated
with the rounded morphology of cells. Tumor cells which maintain a
flattened epithelial appearance generally maintained stress fibers.
In studies of chick embryo cells (CEC) infected with transformation-
defective temperature-sensitive (td-ts) mutants of avian sarcoma
virus (ASV) Boschek et al., (1981) observed the time course of change
in actin organization during transformation in vitro. Temperature

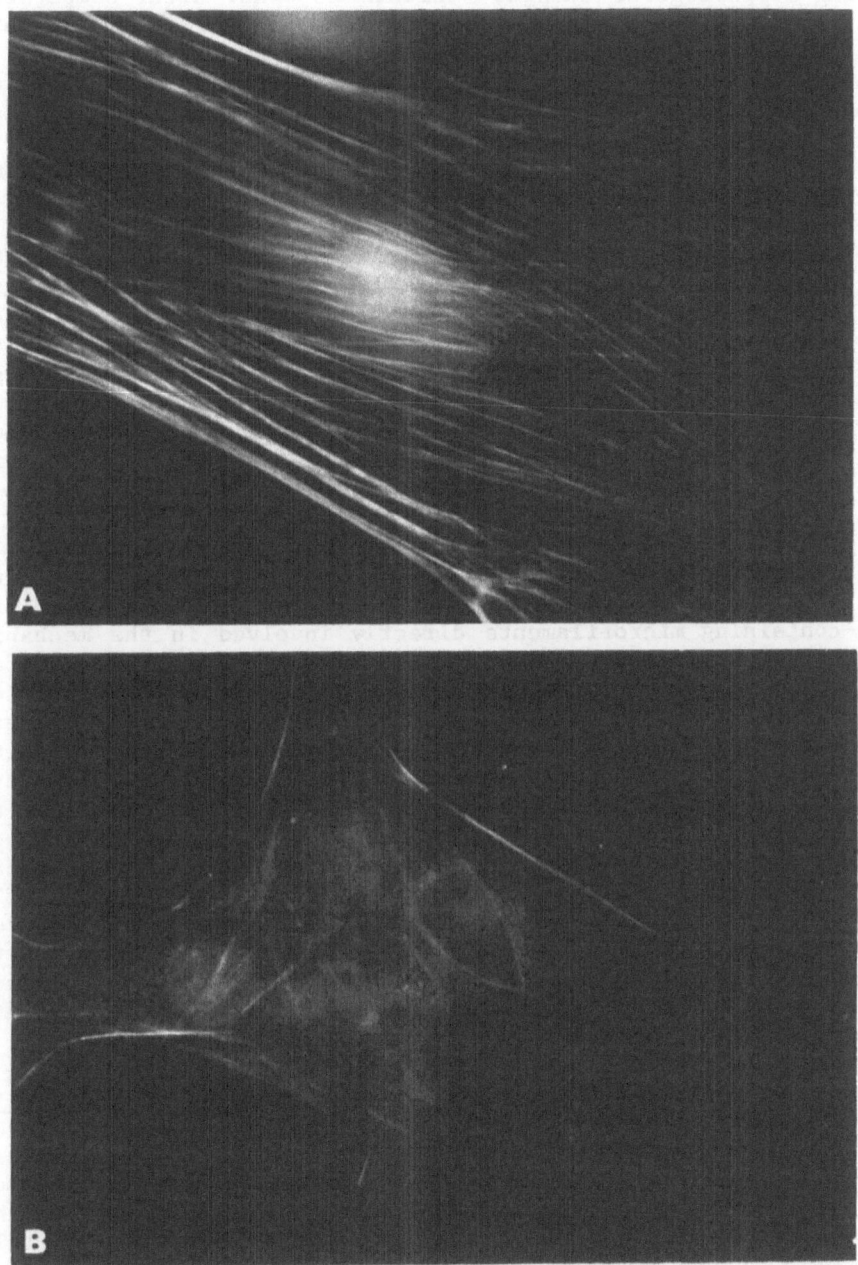

Fig. 7.   Actin stress fibers shown by anti-actin staining.
          A.   3T3 cell;   B.   SV40 3T3 cells.

down-shifts from restrictive to permissive conditions showed two
striking morphological changes. Within 15 mins. after temperature
shift, ruffle-like "flowers" appeared on the cell surface which
contained actin, α-actinin, myosin and tropomyosin. After 6 to
12 hours the stress fibers disappeared and the cells rounded up.
Boschek and coworkers concluded that early changes in actin organization may involve a two step process in which localized actin-
membrane interactions are altered producing the flowers followed
later by a massive shift in F- to G-actin equilibrium.

Somewhat similar findings were reported by Brown et al. (1981)
who followed changes in actin organization in NRK cells infected
with a temperature sensitive Moloney murine sarcoma virus. In their
study new viral proteins, presumed to be transformation-specific
appeared following a down-shift in temperature. Although no changes
in surface morphology were detected immediately, actin stress fibers
fibers were not significantly altered until 24 hours after down-
shift. As discussed in an earlir section, microtubule staining
patterns appeared to be altered after 5 hours.

Pollack and coworkers (1975a, 1975b) have proposed that loss of
anchorage-dependent growth control is related to changes in cytoskeletal organization in viral transformed cells in culture. Are
actin-containing microfilaments directly involved in the mechanism
of cell transformation? In at least one study the altered expression of microfilament patterns in transformed cells is explained
in part by a carcinogen-induced mutation in monomeric actin. Treatment of a human KD cell line with 4-nitroquinolin-1-oxide resulted
in the expression of a mutant α-actin (Hamada et al., 1981; Leavitt
and Kakunada, 1980). A neoplastic cell line HUT-14 expressed the
mutation along with diminished actin cables. A subline HUT-14T was
produced which displayed an even more variant distribution of actin
stress fibers and greater tumorgenicity (Leavitt et al., 1982).
Few studies report on mutations in cytoskeletal proteins however,
and indeed most of the evidence to date suggests that cytoskeletal
changes are brought about by transformation-specific gene products
such as pp60[src] of RSV infected cells which modify cytoskeletal
proteins as discussed later in this review.

Does microfilament organization change in tumor cells in vivo?
Few studies have been seriously concerned with the localization and
organization of cytoskeletal proteins in normal and tumor cells
in vivo. Schenk (1974) reported on microfilaments in squamous
cell carcinomas of the oral cavity in humans and concluded that
invasive cells contained abundant microfilaments. Noninvasive cells
in the same study appeared to lack microfilaments. Similar conclusions were reached by McNutt (1976) who studied basal cell
carcinomas and other human tumor cells. Several investigators
have reported on cytoskeletal alterations in carcinoma cells in

vivo especially on the apparent increase in the appearance of microfilaments in cells near the invasive edge of malignant tumors
(Gabbiani and Chaponnier, 1978; Gabbiani, 1979; Malech and Lentz,
1974; McNutt, 1976).

In a study of adenopolyposis of the colon and rectum (ACR)
Kopelovich et al. (1977) found evidence for altered cytoskeletal
organization in non-tumor tissues (skin fibroblasts) of patients.
Skin fibroblasts from ACR patients were generally deficient in
actin cables when examined by indirect immunofluorescence using
actin antibodies. Since ACR is inherited as an autosomal dominant
trait, 50% of the children are at risk for colon cancer. Their
study showed that approximately 50% displayed normal actin stres
fibers while 50% were identical to their clinically afflicted
parents. These investigators concluded that ARC was systemic and
could produce alterations in the cytoskeleton of non-tumor tissues.
They also concluded that studies of actin organization in fibroblasts might be useful in early detection of some malignancies
such as ACR.

In summary, one of the most consistent cytoskeletal markers
for cell transformation in vitro appears to be the disappearance
or diminution of actin-containing stress fibers. Obviously caution
should be used in using actin stress fibers as markers since considerable variation in stress fiber expression is also seen in non-
transformed cells. At this time, there is good evidence to suggest
that higher ordered assemblies of actin are altered in transformed
cells. If so, this could explain many properties of transformed
cells including altered cell shape, loss of adhesion, altered
motility and surface properties and possibly loss of growth control.
Obviously, the cytoskeletal components are all structurally and
functionally integrated and the organization of the cytoplasm is
maintained by the regulation and control of its structural components. Thus transformation to malignancy must involve general loss
of cell order. In the next section, I will discuss the progress
which has been made in defining the molecular basis of cell transformation and the cytoskeletal components, which may serve as
targets for transforming agents.

IV. Cytoskeletal Proteins - Targets for Transforming Agents

Perhaps the most direct and compelling evidence for a link between the cytoskeleton and a transforming protein comes from the
investigation of Rous sarcoma virus (RSV) transformed chicken cells.
As discussed previously, transformation by RSV leads to the disruption of actin stress fibers and altered staining patterns as determined by immunofluorescence with antibodies to other cytoskeletal
proteins including tubulin, α-actinin, myosin and tropomyosin (Edelman and Yahara, 1976; Ash et al., 1976; Wang and Goldberg, 1976;

Collett and Erickson, 1978; Boschek et al., 1981). Concomitantly,
the cells undergo striking changes in morphology from flattened
fibroblastic forms to more rounded pleomorphic forms. A single
gene product, a 60.000 M_r phosphoprotein called pp60^{src} (Brugge
and Erickson, 1977) is responsibile for transformation in RSV
infected cells (Hanafusa, 1977). It is now known that the pp60^{src}
is a cyclic AMP-independent protein kinase that phosphorylates
tyrosine residues selectively. The phosphorylation of tyrosine
represents a very rare protein modification in normal cells (Sefton
et al., 1980). Phosphotyrosine represents only a 0.05% of the
acid stable phosphate linked to protein with the remainder being
phosphoserine and phosphothreonine (Sefton et al., 1982). Since
RSV transformed cells are characterized by a 5-10 fold increase
in phosphotyrosine levels (Hunter and Sefton, 1980; Sefton et al.,
1980) it is reasonable to conclude that the multiple changes observed in transformation are due to the phoyphorylation of tyrosine
on selected cytoplasmic targets; perhaps the cytoskeleton.

To complicate matters more, normal vertebrate cells contain a
gene which is closely related to RSV src termed the proto-src gene
or pp60 Proto-src (Wang et al., 1978, Vigne et al., 1979). Thus
normal cells produce a gene product which displays a tyrosine-spe-
cific kinase activity (Collett et al., 1978; Hunter and Sefton,
1980) and for all practical purposes is identical to the transforming protein. However pp60 proto-src is present in the cytoplasm
of normal cells at only 1/50th-1/100th the concentration of pp 60
src in RSV transformed cell (Collett et al., 1978; Oppermann et al.,
1979). These observations have led to an explanation of the function of the src gene and especially the preferred substrate and
substrate specifications for pp60^{src}. It also should be pointed
out that RSV is not the only tumor virus which encodes for tyrosine
specific kinase activity. For a current list of tumor viruses
which display src-like kinase activity readers are referred to a
paper by Sefton et al. (1982).

Several lines of evidence suggest pp60^{src} is associated with
the cytoskeleton. Immunofluorescent localization of antibodies to
the src gene product have been reported to occur in the centrosome
and at the inner surface of the plasma membrane under ruffles and
in association with gap junctions between cells (Rohrschneider,
1979; Willingham et al., 1979). After sonication or homogenization
a substantial amount of pp60^{src} activity remains associated with
the membrane fraction although much is lost in the soluble fraction
(Krueger et al., 1980). When cells are extracted with detergents
such as NP-40 or Triton X-100 under conditions which preserve the
cytoskeleton, 75% of the cytoplasmic protein is released. Under
these conditions Burr et al. (1980) found that virtually all of
the pp60^{src} activity remained with the cytoskeleton. When such
cytoskeleton preparations are incubated with ^{32}P-ATP in situ pp60^{src}

is phosphorylated along with other cytoskeletal proteins (Burr et al., 1980).

More recently, Rohrschneider (1980, 1982) reported pp60^{src} was localized within the adhesion plaques of RSV transformed ckicken and mammalian cells. This important discovery suggests a likely target for transforming protein in the cytoplasm which involves the cytoskelton. Adhesion plaques are the termini of stress fibers in normal cells and serve to anchor cells to the substratum (Heaysman and Pegrum, 1973; Heath and Dunn, 1978; Wehland et al., 1979; Geiger, 1979). Stress fibers are important in cell movement, cell contact and in the maintenance of shape and form via their association with the cell surface protein fibronectin (Hynes and Destree, 1978; Burridge and Feramisco, 1980; Singer and Paradiso, 1981).

Biochemical studies support the findings that adhesion plaques are involved in cell transformation. One of the major proteins associated with adhesion plaques is the 130,000 M_r protein vinculin (Geiger, 1979; Burridge and Feramisco, 1979). Immunofluorescent studies indicate that both vinculin and pp60^{src} co-localize in adhesion plaques (Shriver and Rohrschneider, 1980; 1981). In addition vinculin is specifically phosphorylated by pp60^{src} in RSV transformed cells. Sefton and Hunter (1981) and Sefton et al. (1982) found that vinculin from RSV transformed cells contained an 8 fold excess of phosphotyrosine over that found in non-infected cells. Much smaller levels of phosphotyrosine (1% of total phosphate) were detected in normal cells. In addition to vinculin, smaller amounts of phosphotyrosine were found in filamin and vimentin in infected cells. No significant phosphotyrosine activity was noted in tubulin, actin or α-actinin. However, all cytoskeletal proteins need not be phosphorylated to undergo reorganization upon transformation.

When viewed in its most simplistic form, the discovery of a single cytoplasmic target such as vinculin for viral transforming proteins offers for the first time, a logical scheme in cell transformation. The initial transforming event must be the infection of cells with oncogenic viruses and the integration of a portion of the viral genome into the host genome. In the case of the src gene, its product is essentially identical to an endogenous analog (pp60 Proto-^{src}) produced at a much lower level in uninfected cells. Presumably pp60 Proto-^{src} is an important kinase which performs some essential function in cells. Therefore, the viral src gene product (pp60 V -^{src}) must interfere or override the endogenous counterpart due to its elevated activity. The next event in transformation must take place in the cytoplasm. The pp60^{src} phosphorylates tyrosine residues on perferred substrates such as vinculin. Such post-translated modification of vinculin could lead to the loss of critical function such as the assembly of a normal adhesion plaque. Without adhesion plaques, the normal organization and anchorage of stress fibers is lost. Although we still do not yet understand the structure of stress fibers, it is clear that numerous structural proteins are involved including F-actin, myosin, myosin light chain kinase, α-actinin, calmodulin and numerous cross-linking (bundling) proteins. At this time over 20 actin-binding proteins are known (Table 2. also see Brinkley, 1982; Schliwa ,1981) and many of these may be involved in the transcient changes in stress fiber formation. Several lines of evidence suggest that cytoskeletal components are intimately cross-linked and structurally integrated. Thus changes in actin assembles could lead to major reorganization of the entire cytoskeleton. a feature suggested by numerous immunofluorescence studies in transformed cells. The reorganization of the entire cytoplast brought on by cytoskeletal changes along with loss of cell attachment and cell surface changes result in major cell shape changes. Altered cytoskeletal-cell surface properties may account for the loss of surface fibronectin and changes in cell surface receptors.

The cytoskeleton also appears to be directly or indirectly involved in nuclear events including the regulation of gene activity and DNA synthesis. Thus reorganization of the cytoskeleton or loss of regulation of cytoskeletal functions in transformed cells could account for loss of growth control and mobility.

Obviously the pathway suggested by recent discoveries in RSV infected cells may be a gross oversimplification of the events of malignant cell transformation. Certainly in the case of chemical transformation no such logical sequence has been found. Yet chemical-induced cell transformation appears to involve similar morphological and growth related parameters as viral transformation. The possible involvement of the cytoskeleton in cell transformation suggests many fertile avenues for future research. Through recently acquired knowledge of the structural and regulatory components of the cytoskeleton, we have acquired a much improved understanding of cytoplasmic organization and function in normal cells. Since malignancy is a disease involving the basic organization of cells, it is likely that further studies of the cytoskeleton will provide many essential clues in the understanding of neoplastic diseases.

SUMMARY AND CONCLUSIONS

The cytoplasm of eukaryotic cells, once thought to be an amorphous broth bathing the organelles and nucleus, is now known to be highly structured and precisely organized. The elegant structural organization of cytoplasm is maintained largely by an integrated system of tubules and filaments collectively called the cytoskeleton. The dynamic capacity for cytoskeletal proteins such as tubulin, intermediate filament protein and actin to form polymers, to depolymerize, to intertwine and cross-link with neighboring polymers gives cytoplasm its sol-gel characteristics. The central importance of the cytoskeleton in many vital functions including motility and cell division suggests that it well may be a target for carcinogens and viral transforming agents. This view is supported by numerous studies of cytoskeleton expression in normal and transformed cells. Although the molecular basis for cytoskeletal involvement in cell transformation is not well understood, recent progress in defining transformation-specific gene products of oncogenic viruses such as protein kinases which phosphorylate tyrosine-containing residues bring us one step closer to understanding the role of the cytoskeleton in cell transformation.

ACKNOWLEDGEMENT

I am grateful to Linda Wible for technical assistance and to Pat Williams for typing the manuscript. Special thanks are extended to Sari Brenner and Shirley Brinkley for editorial assistance.

REFERENCES

1. Amos, L. A. and Klug, A., 1974, J. Cell. Biol., 14:523.
2. Anderson, W. G., Johnson, G. S. and Paston, I., 1973, Proc. Natl. Acad. Sci. USA, 70:1055.
3. Arnold, H. and Pette, D., 1968, European J. Biochem., 6:163.
4. Asch, B., Medina, D. and Brinkley, B. R., 1979, Cancer Res., 39: 893.
5. Ash, J. F., Vogt, P. K. and Singer, S. J., 1976, Proc. Natl. Acad. Sci. USA, 73:3603.
6. Ball, E. H. and Singer, S. J., 1981, Proc. Natl. Acad. Sci. USA, 78:6986.
7. Benedict, W., Jones, P. and Long, W., 1975, Nature, 256:322.
8. Bennett, V. and Davis, J., 1981, Proc. Natl. Acad. Sci. USA, 78: 7550.
9. Borisy, G. G., Marcum, J. M., Olmsted, J. B., Murphy, D. B. and Johnson, K. A., 1975, Ann. N.Y. Acad. Sci., 253:107.
10. Borisy, G. G. and Taylor, E. W., 1967a, J. Cell Biol., 34:525.
11. Borisy, G. G. and Taylor, E. W., 1967b, J. Cell Biol., 34:535.
12. Boschek, C. B., Jockusch, B. M., Friis, R. R., Back, R., Grundmann, E. and Bauer, H., 1981, Cell, 24:175.
13. Bretscher, A. and Weber, K., 1980, J. Cell. Biol., 86:335.
14. Brinkley, B. R., 1982 in: "Organization of the Cytoplasm" J. D. Watson and G. Albrecht-Buehler, ed., Cold Spring Harbor Symposia on Quantitative Biology, Vol. XLVI (in press).
15. Brinkley, B. R., Beall, P., Wible, L., Mace, M., Turner, D. and and Cailleau, R., 1980, Cancer Res., 40:3118.
16. Brinkley, B. R., Cox, S. M., Pepper, D. A., Wible, L., Brenner, S. L. and Pardue, R. L., 1981, J. Cell Biol., 90:554.

17. Brinkley, B. R., Fuller, G. M., and Highfield, D. P., 1975, Proc. Natl. Acad. Sci. USA, 72:4981.
18. Brown, R. L., Horn, J. P., Wible, L., Arlinghaus, R. B. and Brinkley, B. R., 1981, Proc. Natl. Acad. Sci. USA, 78:5593.
19. Brown, S. S. and Spudich, J. A., 1980, J. Cell. Biol., 87:224a
20. Brugge, J. S. and Erickson, R. L., 1977, Nature, 269:346.
21. Bryan, J. and Kane, R. E., 1978, J. Molec. Biol., 125:207
22. Bryan, J. and Wilson, L., 1971, Proc. Natl. Acad. Sci. USA, 68:1762.
23. Bulinski, J. C. and Borisy, G. G., 1980a, J. Cell Biol., 87:792.
24. Bulinski, J. C. and Borisy, G. G., 1980b, J. Cell Biol., 87:802.
25. Burger, M. M., 1973, Fed. Proc., 32:91.
26. Burr, J. G., Dreyfuss, G., Penman, S. and Buchanan, J. M, 1980, Proc. Natl. Acad. Sci. USA, 77:3484.
27. Burridge, K. and Feramisco, J. R., 1980, Cell, 19:587.
28. Chafouleas, J. C., Pardue, R. L., Brinkley, B. R., Dedman, J. R, and Means, A.R., 1981, Proc. Natl. Acad. Sci. USA 78:996.
29. Chasey, D., 1972, Exp. Cell Res., 74:140.
30. Clegg, J. S., 1982, in "Organization of the Cytoplasm" J. D. Watson and G. Albrecht-Buehler, eds., Cold Spring Harbor Symposia on Quantitative Biology, Vol. XLVI (in press).
31. Collett, M. S., Brugge, J. S., and Erikson, R. L., 1978, Cell, 15:1363.
32. Collett, M. S. and Erickson, R. L., 1978, Proc. Natl. Acad. Sci. USA, 75:2021.
33. Condeelis, J., 1981 in: "International Cell Biology 1980-1981", H. G. Schweiger, ed., Springer-Verlag, Berlin, p. 306.
34. DeMey, J., Janiau, M., DeBrabander, M., Moens, M., and Geuens, J., 1978, Proc. Natl. Acad. Sci. USA, 75:1339.
35. Eckert, B. S., Daley, R. A., and Parysek, L. M., 1982, J. Cell Biol., 92:575.
36. Edelman, G. M., 1976, Science, 192:218.
37. Edelman, G. M. and Yahara, I., 1976, Proc. Natl. Acad. Sci. USA, 73:2047.
38. Eng, L. F., Vanderhaegen, J. J., Bignami, A. and Gersti, B., 1971, Brain Res., 28:351.
39. Erickson, H. P., 1974, J. Cell. Biol., 60:153.
40. Evans, C. H. and DiPaolo, J. A., 1975, Cancer Res., 35:1035.
41. Fawcett, D. W. and Porter, K. R., 1954, J. Morphol., 94:221.
42. Fonte, V. and Porter, K. R., 1974, Int. Congr. Electron Microsc., 8th Aust. Acad. Sci., Canberra, pp. 334.
43. Franke, W. W., Schmid, E., Osborn, M. and Weber, K., 1978a, Proc. Natl. Acad. Sci. USA, 75:5034.
44. Franke, W. W., Schmid, E., Freudenstein, C., Osborn, M. and Weber, K., 1981, Biol., 9:112.
45. Franke, W. W., Weber, K., Osborn, M., Schmid, E. and Freuden-

stein, C., 1978b, Exp. Cell. Res., 116:429.

46. Freedman, V.H. and Shin, S., 1974, Cell, 3:355.

47. Frey-Wessling, A., 1957, "Macromolecules in Cell Structure" Harvard Univ. Press., Cambridge, Mass.

48. Fuller, G. M. and Brinkley, B. R., 1976, J. Supramol. Struct. 5:497.

49. Fuller, G. M., Brinkley, B. R. and Boughter, J. M., 1975, Science, 187:948.

50. Fusenig, N. E., Breiterkreutz, D., Boukamp, P., Lueder, M., Irmscher, G., and Worst, P. K. M., 1978, in: Neoplastic Transformation in Differentiated Epithelial Cell Systems In Vitro", L. M. Franks and C. B. Wigley, ed., Academic Press, London, New York, pp. 37.

51. Gabbiani, G., 1979, in: "Methods and Achievements in Experimental Pathology", G. Jasmin and M. Cantin, eds., S. Karger, New York, Vol. 9, pp. 231.

52. Gabbiani, G. and C. Chaponnier, 1978, in: "Proceedings of the Twenty-Sixth Colloquium, H. Peeters, ed., Pergamon Press, New York, pp. 573.

53. Gail, M. H. and Boone, C. W., 1971, Exp. Cell. Res., 68:226.

54. Geiger, B., 1979, Cell, 18:193.

55. Glenny, J. R., Bretscher, A., and Weber, K., 1980, Proc. Natl. Acad. Sci. USA, 77:6458.

56. Goldman, R. D., Hill, B. F., Steinert, P., Whitman, M. A., and Zackroff, R. V., 1980, in "Microtubules and Microtubule Inhibitors, M. DeBrabander and J. DeMey, eds., Elsevier/North Holland, Amsterdam, p. 91.

57. Goldman, R., Pollard, T. and Rosenbaum, J., 1976, "Cell Motility. Book A, B and C", Cold Spring Harbor Laboratory.

58. Goldman, J. E., Schumberg, H. H. and Norton, W. T., 1978, J. Cell Biol., 78:426.

59. Gould, R. R. and Borisy, G. G., 1978, Exp. Cell Res., 113:369.

60. Hamada, H., Leavitt, J. and Kakunaga, T., 1981, Proc. Natl. Acad. Sci. USA, 78:3634.

61. Hanafusa, H., 1977, in "Comprehensive Virology", H. Fraenkel-Conrat and R. R. Wagner, eds., Vol. 10, Plenum Press, New York, pp. 401.

62. Hartwig, J. H. and Stossel, T. P., 1979, J. Mol. Biol., 134:539.

63. Hasegawa, T., Takahashi, S., Hayashi, H. and Hatano, S., 1980, Biochemistry, 19:2677.

64. Hayashi, T. and Ip, W., 1976, J. Mechanochem. Cell Motil., 3:163.

65. Heath, J. P. and Dunn, G. A., 1978, J. Cell. Biol., 29:197.

66. Heaysman, J. E. and Pegrum, S. M., 1973, Exp. Cell. Res., 78:71.

67. Heneeus, F. C. and Davison, P. F., 1970, J. Mol. Biol., 52:415.

68. Hitchcock, S. E., 1977, J. Cell. Biol., 74:1.

69. Hitchcock, S. E., Carlsson, L. and Lindberg, U., 1977, Cell, 7:531.

70. Holly, R. W. and Kielnan, J. A., 1968, Proc. Natl. Acad. Sci. USA 60:300.
71. Holtzer, H., Bennett, G., Tapscott, S., and Croop, J., 1982, in: "Organization of the Cytoplasm" J. D. Watson and G. Albrecht Buehler, ed., Cold Spring Harbor Symposia on Quantitative Biology, Vol. XLVl, (in press).
72. Hsie, A., Puck, T., 1971, Proc. Natl. Acad. Sci. USA, 68:1648.
73. Hunter, T. and Sefton, B. M., 1980, Proc. Natl. Acad. Sci. USA, 77:1311.
74. Hyashi, T. and Ip, W., 1976, Cell Motil., 3:163.
75. Hynes, R. O. and Destree, A. T., 1978, Cell, 13:151.
76. Inoue, S. and Ritter, H., 1975, in "Molecules and Cell Movements" S. Inoue and R. Stephens, eds., Raven Press, New York, pp. 3.
77. Inoue, S. and Sato, H., 1967, J. Gen. Physiol., 50:259.
78. Isenberg, G. H., Aebi, U. and Pollard, T. D., 1980, Nature, 288: 455.
79. Ishikawa, H., Bischoff, R., and Holtzer, H., 1969, J. Cell. Biol., 43:312.
80. Kirschner, M. W., 1980, J. Cell. Biol., 86:330.
81. Kondo, H. and Ishiwata, S., 1976, J. Biochem., (Tokyo) 79:159.
82. Kopelovich, L., Conlon, S. and Pollack, R., 1977, Proc. Natl. Acad. Sci. USA, 74:3019.
83. Korn, E. D., 1978, Proc. Natl. Acad. Sci. USA, 75:588.
84. Krueger, J. G., Wang, E. and Goldberg, A. R., 1980, Virology, 101:25.
85. Kuriyama, R. and Borisy, G. G., 1981a, J. Cell. Biol., 91:814.
86. Kuriyama, R. and Borisy, G. G., 1981b, J. Cell Biol., 91:822.
87. Lazarides, E., Granger, B. L., Gard, D. L., Gomer, R. H. and Breckler, J., 1982, in "Organization of the Cytoplasm" J. D. Watson and G. Albrecht-Buehler, eds., Cold Spring Harbor Symposia on Quantitative Biology Vol. XLVl (in press).
88. Lazarides, E. and Hubbard, B. D., 1976, Proc. Natl. Acad. Sci. USA, 73:7344.
89. Lazarides, E. and Weber, K., 1974, Proc. Natl. Acad. Sci. USA, 71:2268.
90. Leavitt, J., Bushar, G., Kakunaga, T., Hamada, H., Hirakawa, T., Goldman, D., and Merril, C., 1982, Cell, 28:259.
91. Leavitt, J. and Kakunaga, T., 1980, J. Biol. Chem., 255:1650.
92. Ledbetter, M. C. and Porter, K. R., 1964, Science, 144:872.
93. Leim, R. K. H., Yen, S. H., Salomon, G. D. and Shelanski, M.L., 1978, J. Cell. Biol., 78:426.
94. Lockwood, A. H., 1975, J. Cell Biol., 67:247a.
95. Malech, H. L. and Lentz, T. L., 1974, J. Cell Biol., 60:473.
96. Mandelkow, E., Thomas, E., Bensch, K. G., 1977, Proc. Natl. Acad. Sci. USA, 74:3370.
97. Manger, R. L. and Heckman, C. A., 1982, Cancer Res., (in press).
98. Manton, I. and Clarke, R., 1952, J. Exp. Bot., 3:265.
99. Marcum, J. M., Dedman, J. R., Brinkley, B. R., and Means, A. R., 1978, Proc. Natl. Acad. Sci. USA, 75:3771.

100. Margolis, R. L. and Wilson, L., 1978, Cell, 13:1.
101. Matoltsy, A. G., 1965, Nature, 201:1130.
102. McGill, M. and Brinkley, B. R., 1975, J. Cell Biol., 67:189.
103. McKeown, M. and Firtel, R. A., 1982, in: "Organization of Cyto-
        plasm", J. D. Watson and G. Albrecht-Buehler, eds., Cold
        Spring Harbor Symposia on Quantitaive Biology, Vol. XLVl
        (in press).
104. McNutt, N. S., 1976, Lab Invest., 35:132.
105. Mimura, N. and Asand, A., 1977, Nature, 282:44.
106. Mohri, H., 1968, Nature, 217:1053.
107. Monahan, T. M., Fritz, R. R. and Abell, C. R., 1973, Biochem.
        Biophys. Res. Commun., 55:642.
108. Mooseker, M., Keller, T., Howe, C., Wharton, K., and Grimwade,
        B., 1982, in "Organization of the Cytoplasm", J. D. Watson
        and G. Albrecht-Buehler, ed., Cold Spring Harbor Symposia
        on Quant-
        itative Biology, Vol. XLVl, (in press).
109. Murphy, D. B. and Borisy, G. G., 1975, Proc. Natl. Acad. Sci.
        USA., 72:2696.
110. Oosawa, F. and Asakura, S., 1975, "Theromodynamics of the Poly-
        merization of Protein" Academic Press, N.Y.
111. Opperman, H., Levinson, A. D., Varmus, H. E., Levintow, L. and
        Bishop, J. M., 1979, Proc. Natl. Acad. Sci. USA, 76:1804.
112. Otto, J., Kane, R. and Bryan, J., 1979, Cell, 17:285.
113. Osborn, M., Weber, 1977, Cell, 12:561.
114. Pepper, D. A. and Brinkley, B. R., 1979, J. Cell Biol., 82:585.
115. Pickett-Heaps, J. D., 1969, Cytobiologie, 3:257.
116. Pollack, R. E. and Burger, M. M., 1969, Proc. Natl. Acad. Sci.
        USA, 62:1074.
117. Pollack, R., Osborn, M. and Weber, K., 1975a, Proc. Natl. Acad.
        Sci. USA, 72:994.
118. Pollack, R. and Rifkin, D., 1975b, Cell, 6:495.
119. Pollard, T. D., Aebi, V., Cooper, J. A., Fowler, W. E., and
        Tseng, P., 1982, in "Organization of the Cytoplasm", J. D.
        Watson and G. Albrecht-Buehler, eds., Cold Spring Harbor
        Symposia on Quantitative Biology, Vol. XLVl, (in press).
120. Pollard, T. D. and Weihing, R. R., 1974, CRC Crit. Rev. Bio-
        chem., 10:590.
121. Puck, T. T., Waldren, C. A., Hsie, A. W., 1972, Proc. Natl. Acad.
        Sci. USA, 69:1943.
122. Risser, R. and Pollack, R., 1974, Virology, 59:477.
123. Rohrschneider, L. R., 1979, Cell, 16:11.
124. Rohrschneider, L. R., 1980, Proc. Natl. Acad. Sci. USA, 77:3514.
125. Rohrschneider, L. R., Rosok, L. R. M. and Shriver, K., 1982,
        in "Organization of the Cytoplasm", G. Albrecht-Buehler and
        J. D. Watson, ed., Cold Spring Harbor Symposium on Quant-
        itative Biology, Vol. XLVI, (in press).
126. Roth, L. E. and Daniels, E. W., 1962, J. Cell Biol., 12:57.
127. Rubenstein, P. A. and Spudich, J. A., 1977, Proc. Natl. Acad.
        Sci. USA, 74:120.
128. Rubin, R. W. and Warren, R. H., 1979, J. Cell. Biol., 82:103.

129. Sabatini, D. D., Bensch, K. and Barrnett, R. J., 1963, J. Cell Biol., 17:19.
130. Schenk, P., 1974, Z. Krebs Forsch, 84:241.
131. Schliwa, M., 1981, Cell, 25:587.
132. Schloss, J. A. and Goldman, R. D., 1979, Proc. Natl. Acad. Sci. USA, 76:4484.
133. Schmitt, F. D., 1968, Proc. Natl. Acad. Sci. USA, 60:1092.
134. Sefton, B. W. and Hunter, R., 1981, Cell, 24:165.
135. Sefton, B. M., Hunter, T., Beemon, K. and Eckhart, W., 1980, Cell, 20:807.
136. Sefton, B. M., Hunter, T., Nigg, E.H., Singer, S. J., and Walter, G., 1982, in "Organization of the Cytoplasm", Cold Spring Harbor Symposium on Quantitative Biology, Cold Spring Harbor Press,Vol. XLVI, (in press).
137. Shelanski, M. L., Gaskin, F. and Cantor, C. R., 1973, Proc. Natl. Acad. Sci. USA, 70:765.
138. Shelanski, M. L. and Taylor, E. W., 1967, J. Cell Biol., 38:304.
139. Sheppard, T., 1972, Nature, 236:14.
140. Shriver, M. K. and Rohrschneider, L. R., 1980, Cell Proliferation, 8: in press.
141. Shriver, M. K. and Rohrschneider, L. R., 1981, J. Cell Biol., 89:525.
142. Singer, I. L. and Paradiso, P. R., 1981, Cell, 24:481.
143. Sloboda, R. D., Dentler, W. L., Rosenbaum, J. L., 1976, Biochem., 15:4497.
144. Small, J. V. and Sobieszek, A., 1977, J. Cell Sci., 23:243.
145. Snyder, J. A. and McIntosh, J. R., 1976, Ann. Rev. Biochem., 45:699.
146. Solomon, F., 1981, J. Cell Biol., 90:554.
147. Spudich, J. A., Simpson, P. A., Pardee, J., Stryder, L., Brown, S. S., Yamamoto, K., Weeds, A. and Kugzmarski, E. R., 1982, in "Organization of the Cytoplasm", J. D. Watson and G. Albrecht-Buehler, eds., Cold Spring Harbor Symposia on Quantitative Biology, Vol. XLVl, (in press).
148. Stoker, M. and Abel, P., 1962, in "Cold Spring Harbor Symp. Quant. Biol. 27:375.
149. Stoker, M. and MacPherson, I., 1961, Virology, 14:359.
150. Summerhayes, I. C., Cheng, J.-S. E., Sun, T.-T. and Chen, L. B., 1981, J. Cell Biol., 90:63.
151. Suzuki, A., Goll, D. E., Singh, I., Allen, R. E., Robson, R. M. and Stromer, M. H., 1976, J. Biological Chemistry, 251:6860.
152. Telzer, B. R., Moses, M. J., and Rosenbaum, J. L., 1975, Proc. Natl. Acad. Sci. USA, 72:4023.
153. Temin, H. M., and Rubin, H., 1958, Virology, 6:669.
154. Tilney, L. G., Bonder, E. M. and DeRosier, D. J., 1981, J. Cell Biol., 90:485.
155. Tilney, L. G., Bryan, J., Bush, D. J., Fujiwara, K. and Mooseker, M., 1973, J. Cell Biol., 59:109.

156. Tilney, L. G. and Kullenbach, N., 1979, J. Cell Biol., 81:608.
     Todaro, G. J., Green, H. and Goldberg, B. D., 1964, Proc. Natl.
          Acad. Sci. USA, 51:66.
157. Tucker, R. W., Sanford, K. K. and Frankel, F. k., 1978, Cell,
          13:629.
158. Vigne, R., Breitman, M. L., Moscovici, C. and Vogt, P. K., 1979,
          Virology, 93:413.
159. Virtanen, I., Lehto, V.-P., Lehtonen, E., Vartio, T., Stenman,
          S., Kurki, P., Small, J. V., Dahl, D. and Bradley, R. A.,
          1981, J. Cell Sci., 50:45.
160. Wang, E. and Goldberg, A. R., 1976, Proc. Natl. Acad. Sci. USA,
          73:4065.
161. Wang, K., 1977, Biochemistry, 16:1857.
162. Wang, L.-H., Halpern, C. C., Nadel, M., and Hanafusa, H., 1978,
          Proc. Natl. Acad. Sci. USA, 75:5812.
163. Wang, L. L., and Bryan, J., 1980, Eur. J. Cell Biol., 22:329.
164. Watson, J. D. and Albrecht-Buehler, G., 1982, in "Organization
          of the Cytoplasm", Cold Spring Harbor Symposia on Quantit-
          ative Biology, Vol. XLVl, (in press).
165. Watt, F. A., Harris, H., Weber, K. and Osborn, M., 1978, J. Cell
          Sci., 32:419.
166. Weber, K., Bibring, T. and Osborn, M., 1975, Exp. Cell Res., 95:
          111.
167. Wegner, A., 1976, J. Mol. Biol., 108:139.
168. Wehland, J., Osborn, M. and Weber, K., 1979, J. Cell Sci., 37:
          257.
169. Weingarten, M. D., Lockwood, A., Hwo, S.-Y., and Kirschner,
          M. W., 1975, Proc. Natl. Acad. Sci. USA, 72:1858.
170. Weisenberg, R. C., 1972, Science, 177:1104.
171. Weisenberg, R. C., Borisy, G. G. and Taylor, E. W., 1968, Bio-
          chem., 7:4466.
172. Whalen, R. B., Butler-Browne, G. S., and Gros, F., 1976, Proc.
          Natl. Acad. Sci. USA, 73:2012.
173. Willingham, M. C., Jay, G., Pastan, I., 1979, Cell, 18:125.
174. Wilson, L., 1982, "Methods in Cell Biology" Vol. 24 A,B,
          Academic Press, Inc., New York.
175. Wilson, L. and Friedkin, M., 1967, Biochem., 6:3126.
176. Wolosewick, J. J. and Porter, K. R., 1979, J. Cell Biol., 82:
          114.
177. Woodrum, D. I., Rich, S. A., and Pollard, T. D., 1975, J. Cell
          Biol., 67:231.
178. Yin, H. L. and Stossel, T. P., 1979, Nature, 281:583.
179. Zackroff, R. V. and Goldman, R. D., 1979, Proc. Natl. Acad. Sci.
          USA, 76:6226.
180. Zimmer, D. B., Turner, D. S., Goldstein, M. A., and Brinkley,
          B. R., 1981, Cell Biol. Interna. Repts., 5:1115.

DISCUSSION

Dr.Rajewsky : *The elegant techniques and the strategy chosen will*
not be able to pinpoint subtle alterations in gene products,
e.g.,conformational consequences of simple amino acid changes
in cell surface proteins.How are you planning to approach this
analytical problem?

Dr.Ts'O : Using 2D gel electrophoresis,you can measure the 2nd level
of gene expression,that is,changes in proteins,using the methodology described above.

Dr.Farber : The problem with the system described is that it does
not take into account a) the heterogenicity of the tumor or
b) the fact that the cells will be at different stages in the
cell cycle and therefore,there will be differences in the protein content of the various cells in the population.The problem
will be to screen out other cells from the tumor cells.

Dr.Nicolini : *Are your cell populations that is tumors versus*
normal kinetically matched?Those differences in 2D gels could
indeed be related merely to differences in cell proliferation
rather than cell transformation as shown previously for several
comparable studies.Indeed it would appear to me that this is
what will determine the above differences with such an experimen-
tal design,without going to single cell level.Cell heterogeneity
will furthermore complicate the picture for tumors.

Dr.Ts'O : Your point is well taken.However,I would like to clarify
that we were not trying to characterize a tumor but the genetic
expression of a cell.

Dr.Rueff : *I would use a different approach to the problem you*
raised.I would do a shot-gun experiment of tumor DNA and once
I have the library of cloned tumor genes,I would use them
for transformation by DNA-transfection and if I am lucky I would
obtain a homogeneous population of transformed cells expressing,
with luck,just one protein or a very few which could be easily
identified by electrophoretic techniques.What do you think about

such proposal?

Dr.*Ts'O* : There are problems associated with experimental techniques and interpretation of results with DNA transfection experiments. However,we are carrying out similar experiments using Herpes Simplex Virus II isolated from human cervical cancer and with a genome of 100×10^6.This is cut with restriction enzymes to a genome of 15×10^6 and each individual fragment is used for transforming hamster cells;the expression of viral gene products and internal gene products is locked when using the techniques described earlier.At present,no data is available about the results.

Dr.*Hall* : *First, how do you demostrate that your selected foci are actually the ones that give rise to tumors in the liver?Secondly, is your correlation of the presence of selected foci and the tumor incidence just a step removed from a correlation between the presence of DNA adducts and the presence of a tumor in that particular organ?*

Dr.*Farber* : We see   very little bile duct proliferation very early in the process and this disappears.At almost any stage after the selection,you see a normal looking liver with foci that you can follow daily.They became progressively larger and generate nodules.Most of these remodel with a few persisting and,if you go further, you can see inside a few further steps and inside a few cancer.So,at the moment,there is what we call a linear continuity in which one can follow progressively the different cell populations.It is not simply the matter of having a few changes early and then a way down the pipe,something else happens.As far as the second question,yes,we are a long way.However, unlike adducts,one do not have a long gap between the first visible foci and cancer.As I indicated in answer to your first question,we can trace a next sequence,admittedly with some gap but nevertheless a clear-cut sequence from fair,resistant hepatocytes to hepatocellular carcinoma.One cannot do this with adducts or with their immediant possible consequences,such as mutation,transpositions,rearrangements etc.

Dr.*Weinstein* :*In the stage when you added the AAF to perform the selection,how do you know it is differential inhibition of the surrounding versus preferential stimulation of the cells?*

Dr.*Farber* : Well,if you leave out the partial hepatectomy nothing does happen.Thus the AAF by itself does not do anything.If you do a partial hepatectomy without AAF,nothing happens.You have to use the two toghether.

Dr.*Weinstein* : You might need the proliferative stimulus,partial hepatectomy plus AAF,and it preferentialy stimulates the ini-

tiated cells.They may still require growth stimuli and AAF makes
it.You do not really know if the drug resistace of the liver is
really the mechanism.What you score is the product of the AAF
treated cells,not the target of AAF-treated cells.You have to
take out the markers and then you score for these markers.You
really do not know what the target of AAF is.

Dr.Farber : No.All we know is the phenotype after a few cell cycles.
We can begin to see this around the fourth and fifth cell cycles.
We would assume that cancer begins as a doublet.If you need cell
proliferation you begin with two initiated cells.We do not
know what the phenotypes of those two cells are.All we know
is the phenotype after third and fourth cell cycles.

*Dr.Weinstein : I would like to raise an alternative mechanism to
that of yours.Your initiated cell which occurs in response to
AAF and partial hepatectomy,undergoes a preferential growth
in response to those two agents.But,it is not because AAF kills
the surrounding normal cells.The initiated cells just grow out
because they are resistant.*

Dr.Farber :Against this is the following: if you vary the AAF to
allow the normal cell regeneration,you inhibit the foci.You
need a certain level of AAF.If you drop to 1%,that will not
inhibit the surrounding efficiently to inhibit regeneration.
You do not see foci.There seems to be a clear inverse relationship between the degree to which the liver will respond to
partial hepatectomy by growing and the number of foci.The simplest
hypothesis for us,is that the resistance is handled,but until
we can isolate the initiated cells,we won't be absolutely certain.

*Dr.Diamond :What about transplantation experiments.Do you select
only for a certain cell type?For instance,it is known in the
case of the Novikoff hepatoma,that from primary tumor only a
very few of the cells are transplantable while from the transplanted tumor,all cells are.Thus you initially select for a very
rare cell the one that can be transplanted.*

Dr.Farber : That is true,and probably this is also true in the case
in which people try to make tissue culture from many human
tumors and see their response to chemotherapeutic agents.
They probably get only a very few cells to grow and thus are
selecting out a population.It might be that these are the most
malignant,but that is not known.In our case,we also do not know,
but recently we confirmed experiments in which normal liver cells
were put into the spleen and they grew.If you take the nodule
cells they grow much better.

*Dr.Weinstein : The model you presented at the end of your lecture
suggests that when B(a)P is used as a complete carcinogen (in the*

*absence of TPA),carcinomas might be produced without going
through the papilloma stage,since the stage of clonal expansion
does not occur.Do your data indicate that this is the case?*

Dr.*Burns* : In fact,we have a deficiency in papillomas in the combined
exposure from what we expect from the initiation/promotion expe-
riment.The theoretical analysis suggested that the amount of
clonal expansion to produce this amount of displacement need not
be very great,not anywhere near a detectable mass of cells.

Dr.*Weinstein* : An alternative to your model is that when B(a)P is
used as a complete carcinogen,it acts as both an initiator and
promoter,and that although the dose response curve for its initiating action is linear,the dose response curve for its role
as promoter is curvilinear.The latter might be particularly true
if B(a)P is a poor promoter in comparison to TPA.

Dr.*Burns* : It is certainly possible that you need to include the
dose response for the promoter activity in   this.My only comment
on this is that we have selected a dose of TPA that produces the
maximal possible effect.

Dr.*Hubert-Habart* : *Did you try TPA alone,for a long time,and if
you did,did you observe the formation of papillomas?*

Dr.*Burns* : We have approximately 0.2 papilloma per animal at 300
days with just TPA treatment.We have observed one carcinoma or
two in these animals but not enough to make a statistical value.
I believe that so called spontaneous initiation is about 0.2
tumor per mouse.

Dr.*Farber* : I cannot think of carcinogenesis exclusively in terms
of irreversible changes in DNA,some alterations in differentiation,and so on.It is all of these things at the appropriate time.
At one stage you may get altered differentiation,or normal differentiation,at other steps some reversible or irreversible things.
For instance in the liver a large part of the population of
nodules disappear.The same happens of course in the skin,so
called regression.We also thought it was regression we saw in
the liver,but in fact this is not a regression.The liver cells do
not disappear,they stay there although they may be changed in
some of their patterns.So,clearly,it is not regression,it is
changing into somthing else.Do you want to say somthing about
regression,Burns?

Dr.*Burns* :The idea in the epidermis is that the basal cells prolife-
rate.The labelling index is 3%,this means that 3% of the cells
are synthesizing DNA at a given moment.If we apply TPA to this
tissue we get an increase in labelling index,within 24 hours,
to 15%.In addition,you get hyperplasia.Ultimately you have 3
or 4 layers of cells that still differentiate and keratinise.

If one of these cells became initiated and proliferates more rapidly,then the rest is pushed out to a papule.The keratinising process still continues within this papilloma.The labelling index in the basal cells of the papilloma is about 30%.Three weeks after stopping the TPA treatment,in the normal epidermis there is a decrease to the normal number of cells that are synthesizing DNA,that is 3%.However,three weeks after stopping the TPA treatment,half of the papillomas have regressed,but the surviving papillomas have a labelling index that is not detectably below that of the papillomas during promotion.So there is reversibility of the same type as is seen in the normal epidermis.The existence of these cells within this population means that a great deal of the cells that are produced within the papilloma do not contribute to the growth of the papilloma. The rest of it is keratinization or some other form of cell loss. So,a very small decrease in the rate of proliferation could tip the balance and lead to regression.At the moment we do not know what is actually responsible for this and we really should study this more.

Dr.Sarma : Concerning the remodelling of nodules in the liver,I consider three possibilities:one is necrosis or cell death of those remodelling nodules,another may be that normal liver cells are growing into the remodelling nodules,third may be that the programming of the remodelling nodules is such that it gets accommodated into normal architecture of the liver.So one will not see it as a nodule but those cells would be still there.

Dr.Schulte-Hermann : I would like to comment on the question of regression-remodelling of liver cells.Dr.Farber takes the view that foci cells do not regress,do not die.But,do remodel.I think that one should not exclude these two possibilities.I think both are correct and I believe that you still have some proliferation in your remodelling foci.So,if you take this proliferation index in the range of 1-2% you should still have an increase in size of the remodelling nodules and a doubling time of about 1-2 months.I do not see why only the normal liver cell should die and not the foci cell.This may be a physiological process and is not so unique for hyperplastic nodules in the liver.A similar process may occur as physiological program in various organs after the removal of a functional stimulus or load.As an example, the adrenal cortex looses most of its functional capabilities such as P450 catalysed reactions,and many of its cells after surgical removal of the pituitary gland which eliminates ACTH. The loss of phenotypic markers in the liver foci may indicate likewise the removal of a certain "Differentiating or Adapting" pressure.You remove something that keeps the cell in a certain functional state and end up with both loss of a certain phenotypic appearence of the cell and loss of extra cells.

Dr.Rueff : *What it would be very interesting to see in Dr.Rajewsky elegant system is if there would be any difference in tumor yield,when applying a promoter,between fetal or embryonic cells and more developed ones.Of course ENU is a complete carcinogen and you do not need a promoter.But I wonder if it could be possible to try that experiment in your system?*

Dr.Rajewsky : We should select a suitable carcinogen which is not complete in its action.You could give it in such low dose that by itself it would not produce tumors in the animal's life time. Then you could combine it with a promoter.But the other alternative would be to choose a different carcinogen which by itself would not be complete and then combine it with a promoter.

Dr.Brambilla : *In comparison with the liver,the brain is a relatively well protected area concerning the host immune response. Do you think that this fact may play at least a minor role, besides.the slower repair of alkylated bases,in assuring the formation of high frequency of brain tumors after ENU treatment?*

Dr.Rajewsky : It is very interesting question.The brain for some reason does not excise the 0-6 while the other tissues do.One possibility would be that during evolution the brain has been protected.The organism gives the impression that there is not much damage possible to the brain:this is apparently wrong,since agents such as ENU can get there very well.A possibility is that the brain likes to maintain changes like 0-6;they may.be important for the brain cells and not to other cells.

Dr.Farber : It is worth emphasizing,as you mentioned,that MNU will induce liver cancer if coupled with cell proliferation.Perhaps the kinetics of alkylation and dealkylation are also very important in the larger context of cell aging.

Dr.Rajewsky : In terms of promotion,my personal feelings are that the MNU is working so efficiently in the brain system as if it was a promoter.Maybe we should consider the possibility that the system inherently contains the functions that are created in the other systems by promoter addition.Maybe the system has a built-in promoter which is the developing differentiating cell system itself.

Dr.Sarma : It is possible that in these rats you do have initiated cells in the liver.Maybe you should subject these rats to selection regimens and determine.whether you obtain any preneoplastic or neoplastic cell populations.Also we should re-do the experiments concerning the miscoding of templates containing 0-6-alkylguanine and 0-4-alkylthymine using the full complement of DNA replicating enzymes.Recently,in viral systems the fidelity of replication was shown to increase when using the full complement of replication enzymes.

Dr. King : your development of this system lends itself to the utilization of agents that require metabolic activation. Such an appoach might well aid in identifying specific cells that are involved in the transformation process. By appropriate selection you could introduce the same or different lesions, with or without the participation of a wide range of enzymes (i.e. soluble and microsomal).

Dr. Rajewsky : We can do this with fluorescent antibodies very nicely for the whole tissues and distinguish the different cell types.

Dr. Dragsted : If the early initiated cell has a lower RNA production it would mean that you should be able to have a marker for these cells at an extremely early stage. As Dr. Rajewsky has said, some workers have shown that at early stage of cancer you might have a change in the altered bases of t-RNA that cannot be explained at the moment. Is it not true that if one has less t-RNA one may have more altered bases? Can this be used as marker?

Dr. Nicolini : The acridine orange stained cells after short exposure to a carcinogen display an increase in chromatin-DNA binding sites paralleled by a decrease in the overall cytoplasmic RNA. This uncoupling, never occuring during normal cell proliferation, is a marker of cell-carcinogen interaction. However, even if chromatin relaxation appears a prerequisite of cancer induction, this decrease of RNA does not and appear rather an index of cell "toxicity" generalizable to every cell intaracting with the carcinogen. What is instead linked with the specific development of neoplastic lesions is a later decrease of chromatin template activity coupled with an increase in chromatin-DNA condensation, which appear consistently associated with the expression of a transformed phenotype. In this case, however, we have a complication, since both DNA primary binding sites and RNA synthesis decrease as for non-cycling or slowly cycling normal cells. RNA does indeed significantly change during the cell cycle, being low in early G1, high in G2 and very low for non-cycling cells, G0 or Q . So one has a complication in this respect at the single cell level, without an indipendent estimate of cell cycle stage. Therefore, even if you have much less RNA in the average initiated cell, alone is not a single cell marker for initiation.

Dr. Rueff : Do you have more precise data about the modifications which occur in microfilaments and microtubules?

Dr. Nicolini : You may find them in numerous publications by Brinkley, Hsie and Puck. They have shown in quite few systems that in normal cells the microfilaments and microtubules are extremely organized and oriented, while are highly disorganized and /or disrupted

in transformed cells.The cytoskeleton could then be physically
responsible of the observed coupling between cell geometry and
nuclear morphometry,which is indeed present only in normal cells
and absent in transformed cells.Other mechanisms could obviously
cause such coupling and uncoupling,which indeed we stress as a
unique feature of the neoplastic process regardless of the actual
molecular mechanism,being the cytoskeleton,ion fluxes,membrane
alterations or something else.

Dr. *Pinarci : Does the chromatin change from a state of relaxation
to a state of condensation mean also a change from high entropy
level to low entropy level? Also the changes in condensation-
relaxation of the cellular and nuclear architecture are
homogeneous or heterogeneous?*

Dr. Nicolini : Yes and they appear homogeneous . Three-dimensional
reconstruction of nuclear DNA images from resting liver cells,
both at the light microscope and electron microscope resolution,
shows that chromatin fibers exist in more than one state of
condensation/supercoil which modulate synchronously and homoge-
neously with subsequent changes in cell function. It would then
seem that,contrary to traditional view,large part of the genome
and not just few specialized segments undergo abrupt structural
transition in correspondence to specific cell metabolic activity.
For istance immediatly preceeding induced cell proliferation
or upon interaction with chemical carcinogens the overral genome
abruptly relaxes from an high supercoil to a lower order structure,
yielding a similar degree of DNA superpacking in every region
of the nucleus. A change in metabolic activity then does not
involve only few DNA segments(genes),with the largest majority
remaining as spectators,but rather interest the genome as a whole.
An other example is the structural modulation occuring during
cell cycle for the Barr body,which rather than remaining in the
same state of high condensation,as expected from its putative
constantly low transcription capability,parallels the interphase
changes occuring in the overall nuclear DNA.

Dr. *Parodi : When you look at chromatin at the light microscope
level essentially you distinguish condensed and decondensed
chromatin.There are hundred of different types of differentiated
cells both at the physiological and at the pathological level,
as different cell cycle phases,differnt normal and malignant
cells,different preneoplastic cells,all different differentiated states. How can you explain all the great variety of situations we are confronted with only a two stage conditions?*

Dr. Nicolini : Let me first clarify that at the resolution of light
microscopy there appear to be more than two states of condensation ,which are furthemore continously changing during cell
cycle progression.Similarly can be said for the nuclear DNA chan-

ges during differentiation,transformation or expression of
metastaic potential.All our work with nuclear imaging does
indeed question the validity of traditional dicotomy of hetere-
chromatin versus euchromatin.Recently using DNAse I,an enzyme
which specifically attacks active genes,we have shown that both
regions are similarly digested at the same rate and only chromatin-DNA in a third very disperse state(less than 3% of the genome) is preferentially digested at early times. The two stages
condition in rat liver nuclei,which after stimulation becomes
only one stage(from high resolution image analysis of electron
micrographs),appears then related to chromatin-DNA in two distinct structures of different packing ratio not directly reflecting
different degree of actual gene availability for transcription
and replication . A further structural modification(at the level
of the nucleofilament)appears required,which occurs only after
a quantal chromatin transition from an highly condensed state
("rope-like") to a disperse state ('nucleofilaments') containing
similar fraction of active genes. Moreover, in the model proposed
the quinternary chromatin-DNA structure is mantained by fixed
site attachments at the nuclear pores, regularly spaced every
5000 A° (or more in G1 and S phase cells)within the fiber;conse-
quently more than 100,000 DNA regions may be identified undergoing <u>local</u> structural transitions leading to gene activation.
A large number of combinations of transcrible genes are then
possible,since activation or inactivation of each specific gene
depends on which DNA sequences are 'properly' relaxed and which
are more or less supercoiled;and this may vary from time to time
(during cell cycle) and from cell type to cell type. Actual transcription will obviously depend on other conditions,such as
substrate concentration,enzyme activity or association constants.
In general we may then say that global effect,determined by ions,
water and enzymatic protein modifications,are important in that
they may be changing the local availability of the DNA sequences
along the DNA chain.In native chromatin DNA is highly supercoiled;
global or local molecular alterations induce changes in the
higher and lower order structures which then may cause specific
gene availability and transcribility.

*Dr. Durante : I think that your observations on DNA transcription
in order to discriminate normal and tumor cells are not sufficient.
A higher rate of RNA translation or other translational controls
can balance the effect due the lower quantity of transcribed
RNAs,if they are the same in the two systems.In this case there
may be a quantitative change,low as judged from the data presented,but it is more important to know if there also is a qualitative change. I think that this fact can be better elucidated
through biochemical techniques as,for istance, ROT analysis and
may be in vitro translation and subsequent electrophoresis.*

Dr. Nicolini : You may be right,but biochemical analysis are carried

out on bulk preparation and not at single cell level,where
alterations due to cell proliferation can only be discriminated
from those related to cell transformation. Furthemore our data
pointing to the significance of global changes are not at the
exclusion of specific local molecular changes;a more completed
view may lead to a better understanding of the molecular
and cellular events causally related to the control of cell
function and of neoplastic transformation. Toward this end a
constant interplay between in vivo and in vitro biomolecular
characterization is called for.

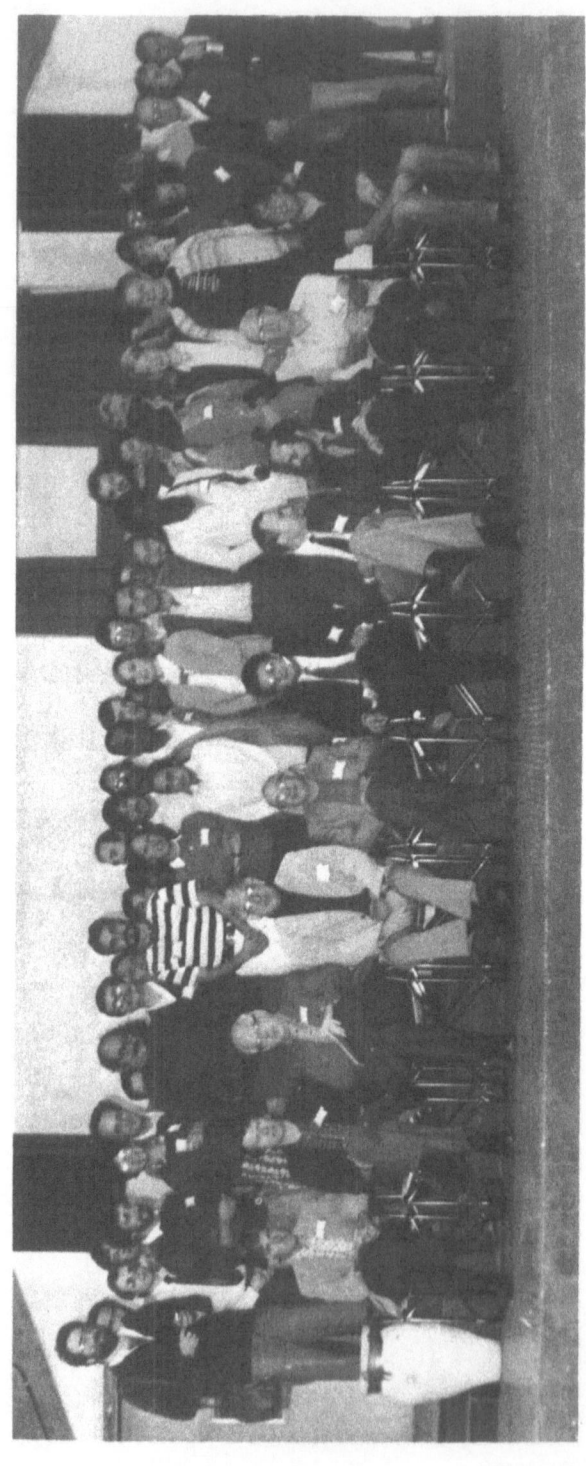

PARTICIPANTS AT ERICE ASI ON CHEMICAL CARCINOGENESIS,1981

(II Course of the International School of Biostructure)

Sitting from left to right,First Row:P.Cerutti,F.J.Burns,C.M.King,G.Wogan,
E.Farber,C.Nicolini,R.Schulte-Hermann,F.Oesch,W.Taylor and E.,Patrone.

ETTORE MAJORANA – CENTER FOR SCIENTIFIC CULTURE

INTERNATIONAL SCHOOL OF PURE AND APPLIED BIOSTRUCTURE:
    Director: C. Nicolini – 2nd course – "Chemical Carcinogenesis"
    Directors: E. FARBER, C. NICOLINI – 18–30 October 1981,
    A NATO ADVANCED STUDY INSTITUTE

LIST OF PARTICIPANTS

Gianni BRAMBILLA   Istituto di Farmacologia
                                 Viale Benedetto XV, 2
                                 16132 Genova, Italy

Fredic BURNS   Institute of Environmental Medicine
                                 New York University
                                 Medical Center
                                 550 First Avenue
                                 New York, N.Y. 10016, USA

Peter CERUTTI   Dept. Carcinogenesis
                                 Swiss Inst. for Explt. Cancer Res.
                                 Ch. de Boveresses
                                 CH-1066 Epalinges sur Lausanne,
                                 Switzerland

Giovanni DELLA PORTA   Istituto Nazionale Tumori
                                 Via Venezian, 1
                                 Milano, Italy

Emanuel FARBER   Dept. of Pathology
                                 School of Medicine
                                 University of Toronto
                                 100 College Street
                                 Toronto, Canada

Charles KING   Dept. of Chemistry and Carcinogenesis
                                 Michigan Cancer Foundation

481

110 E. Warren
Detroit, MI.   48201, USA

Roberto MONTESANO   IARC
                               Lyon, France

Claudio NICOLINI   Istituto di Farmacologia
                               Viale Benedetto XV, 2
                               16132 Genova, Italy

Franz OESCH   Vorsteher der Abt. Moledularpharma-
                               kologia
                               Pharmakologisches Inst. der Univer-
                               sitat
                               Obere Zahlbacher Strasse 67
                               D-6500 Mainz, FRG

Silvio PARODI   Istituto Scientifica Studio e Cura
                               Tumori
                               Viale Benedetto XV, 10
                               16132 Genova, Italy

Manfred RAJEWSKY   Inst. fur Zellbiologie
                               University of Essen
                               Hufelanstrasse 55
                               D-4300 Essen 1, FRG

Ditta Kavi SARMA   Dept. of Pathology
                               Faculty of Medicine
                               University of Toronto
                               100 College Street
                               Toronto, Canada

Ron SCHULTE-HERMANN   Inst. fur Toxikologie und Pharmako-
                               logie
                               der Phillips Universitat
                               Marburg, FRG

Paul TS'O   Division Biophysics
                               School of Public Health
                               John Hopkins University
                               Baltimore, MD   21205, USA

Bernard WEINSTEIN   Dept. of Medicine
                               Columbia University
                               College of Physicians and Surgeons
                               New York, NY 10032, USA

Gerald WOGAN

Dept. of Nutrition and Food Sciences
Massachuettes Inst. of Technology
Room 16-333
Cambridge, MA 02139, USA

Peter ABBOTT

Imperial Cancer Res. Fund Laboratories
P.O. Box n. 123 -
Lincoln's Inn Fields
London WC 2A 3PX, UK

Charles ARUS

Univ. Autonoma de Barcelona
Dept. Bioquimica (Ciencias)
Bellaterra - Barcelona, Spain

Cecilia BALBI

Istituto Scientifico Studio
Tumori
Viale Bebedetto XV, 10
Genova, Italy

Franco BIGNONE

Istituto Giannina Gaslini
Via V Maggio
Genova - Quarto, Italy

Claudio Blonda

Istituto di Genetica
Universita degli Studi
Via Amendola 165
Bari, Italy

Stefania BONATTI

Istituto di Mutagenesi e Differen-
ziamento
CNR - Via Svezia, 10
56100 Pisa, Italy

Franco M. BUONAGURO

Istituto di Patologia Generale
Piazzette Sant' ndrea delle Dame, 2
80138 Napoli, Italy

Marco CAVANNA

Istituto di Farmacologia
Viale Benedetto XV, 2
16132 Genova, Italy

Britta CHRISTENSEN

The Danish Cancer Society
Laboratory of Environmental Carcino-
genesis
Ndr. Frihavnsgade 70
DK 2100 Copenhagen, Denmark

Lorenzo CITTI

Istituto di Mutagenesi e Differenzia-
mento
CNR
Via Svezia, 10
56100 Pisa, Italy

Amedeo COLUMBANO

Istituto di Patologia Generale I
Universita di Cagliari
09100 Cagliari, Italy

Helene COULOMB

Institut de Recherches Scientifiques
sur le Cancer
Boite Postal n. 8
7 rue Guy Mocquet
94800 Villejuif, France

Jacques DE GERLACHE

Unit of Biochemical Toxicology and
Cancerology
Universite' Catholique de Louvain
U.C.L. 73.69
B - 1200 Brussels, Belgium

Alain DELEENER

Universiteit Brussel
Faculteit der Wetenschappen
Algemene Dierkunde
Pleinlaan 2
1050 Bruxelles, Belgium

Silvio DE FLORA

Istituto di Igiene
Via Pastore, 9
16132 Genova, Italy

Leila DIAMOND

The Wistar Institute
Thirty-Sixth Street at Spruce
Philadelphia, PA. 19104, USA

Eugenia DOGLIOTTI

Istituto Superiore di Sanita'
Roma, Italy

Lars DRAGSTEN

Arbejdsmiljø Instituttet
Produktregisteret
Blegdamsves 104 C
2100 Copenhagen Denmark

Cecile DREVON

Centre International de Recherche
sur le Cancer
150 Cours Albert-Thomas
69372 Lyon Cedex 2, France

Mauro DURANTE

Istituto di Genetica
Via Matteotti 1/A
56100 Pisa, Italy

Mine ENGINUN

I.U. Kimya Fakultesi
Analitik Kimya Kirsusu
Istanbul, Turkey

Joseph FRIEDMAN

Institut Suisse de Recherches
Experimentales sur le Cancer
rue des Boveresses
CH-1066 Epalinges s./
Lausanne, Switzerland

Chiara GERI

Istituto di Genetica
Via Matteotti 1/A
56100 Pisa, Italy

Walter GIARETTI

Istituto di Fisica Sperimentale
Politecnico di Torino
Via Duca degli Abruzzi 24
10129 Torino, Italy

Maria Ignacia GOMES

Universidade Nova de Lisboa
Dep. Bioquimica
Campo de Santana 130
1198 Lisboa Codex, Portugal

Vahdet GUL

T.C. Bursa Universitesi
Tip Fakultesi
Patologi Ve Adli Tip Kursusu
Bursa, Turkey

Stephen Thomas HADFIELD

Imperial Cancer Research Fund Labs.
P.O. Box n. 123
Lincoln's Inn Fields
London, WC 2A 3PX, UK

Janet A. HALL

Christie Hospital & Holt Radium Inst.
Manchester Area Health Authority
South District
Manchester M20 9BX, UL

J.B. HANSEN

Kemisk Laboratorium II
H.C. Ørsted Institutet
Universitetsparken 5
2100 Capenhagen, Denmark

Filiz HINCAL

Faculty of Pharmacy
Dept. of Analytical Toxicology
Hacettepe University
Hacettepe, Ankara, Turkey

Michael A. HUBERT-HABART

Istitut Curie - Laboratoire Curie
11 rue Pierre et Marie Curie
75231 Paris Cedex 05, France

Don JENS

Duphar B.V.
P.O. Box 2
1380 AA Weesp, The Netherlands

Marc LANS

Unit of Biochemical Toxicology and
Cancerology
Universite' Catholique de Louvain
U.C.L. 73.69
B-1200 Brussels, Belgium

Giovanna Maria LEDDA

Istituto di Patologia Generale I
Universita' di Cagliari
09100 Cagliari, Italy

S. LIMBOSCH

Universite' Libre de Bruxelles
Dept. de Biologie Moleculaire
Rue de Chevaux 67
1640 Rhode-St-Genese,
Bruxelles, Belgium

Walter LUTZ

Institute fur Toxicologie
Universitat Zurich
Schorenstrasse 16
CH 8603 Schwerzenbach bei Zurich,
Switzerland

Ottar MADSLIEN

Norwegian State Pollution Control
P.O. Box 8100
Oslo, Norway

John Hendrick MEERMAN

Dept. of Pharmacology
State University of Groningen
Bleomsingel 1
9713 BZ Groningen, The Netherlands

Dorcas OKOR

University of Benin
Department of Chemistry
P.M.B. 1154
Benin City, Nigeria

Paolo PANI

Cattedra di Patologia Generale I
Via Porcell 4
09100 Cagliari, Italy

Eligio PATRONE

Centro di Studi Chimico-Fisici
Istituto di Chimica Industriale
Via A. Pastore, 3
Genova, Italy

Veronique PREAT

Unit of Biochemical Toxicology and
Cancerology
Universite' Catholique de Louvain
U.C.L. 73.69
B-1200 Brussles, Belgium

Paola PRINCIPE

Istituto Superiore di Sanita'
Viale Regina Elena 299
00161 Roma, Italy

Srinivasan RAJALAKSHMI

University of Toronto
Dapt. of Pathology
Medical Sciences Building
1 Kings College Circle
Toronto, M5S 1A8, Canada

Edgar RIVEDAL

Lab. for Environmental and
Occupational Cancer
NHIK - The Norwegial Radium Hospital
Montebello, Oslo 3, Norwey

Luigi ROBBIANO

Istituto di Farmacologia
Universita' di Genova
Viale Benedetto XV, 2
16132 Genova, Italy

Jose' RUEFF

Universidade Nova de Lisboa
Facultade de Ciencias Medicas,
Departmento de Bioquimica
Lisboa, Portugal

Andrzey SAWARYN

Freie Universitat Berlin
Institut fur Kristalographie
Takustrasse 6
1000 Berlin 33/ West Germany

Pev-Olov SCHULTZ

Foretagshalsan, Mellangatan
S-57100 Nassjo Sweden

Avishay-Abraham STARK   Tel Aviv University
                               Dept. of Biochemistry
                               Ramat-Aviv, Tel Aviv, Israel

Maurizio TANINGHER   Istituto di Oncologia
                               Universita di Genova
                               Viale Benedetto XV 10
                               16132 Genova, Italy

Willy TAYLOR   Department of Physiology
                               The Medical School the University
                               Newcastle upon Tyne NE1 7RU UK

Sven Arne THOREN   Institute of Hygiene
                               Faculty of Medicine
                               21 Blegdamsves, DK-2100
                               Copenhagen ø Denmark

Jean Jacques TOULME   Museum National d'Histoire Naturelle
                               Laboratoire de Biophysique, INSERM
                               61 rue Buffon, 75005 Paris, France

Gino TURCHI   Istituto di Mutagenesi e Differen-
                               ziamento
                               CNR, Via Svezia 10
                               56100 Pisa, Italy

Luigi VALDATTA   Via Emilia Pavese 117, Castle S.
                               Giovanni
                               29015 Piacenza, Italy

Franz WATJEN   Kemisk Laboratorium II
                               KØ Benhavns Universitet
                               H.C. Ørsted Institutet
                               Universitetsparken 5
                               2100 Copenhagen ø Denmark

William Peter WATSON   Sittinbourne Research Centre
                               Sittinbourne, Kent ME9 8AG, UK

A. Kamil PINARCI   Environmental Engineering Dept.
                               Meddle East Technical University
                               Inonu Bulvari
                               Ankara, Turkey

SUBJECT INDEX